ECHOCARDIOGRAPHY IN HEART FAILURE AND CARDIAC ELECTROPHYSIOLOGY

Edited by **Umashankar Lakshmanadoss**

Echocardiography in Heart Failure and Cardiac Electrophysiology
http://dx.doi.org/10.5772/61427
Edited by Umashankar Lakshmanadoss

Contributors

Zoltan Szabo, Veronika Sebestyen, Iacopo Fabiani, Nicola Riccardo Pugliese, Lorenzo Conte, Vitantonio Di Bello, Santini Veronica, Ming-Chon Hsiung, Dai-Yin Lu, Masanori Kawasaki, Silvia Lupu, Lucia Agoston-Coldea, Dan Dobreanu, Mariana Floria, Tanase Daniela Maria, Tomoko Sugiyama Kato, Takashi Nishimura, Shunei Kyo, Kenji Kuwaki, Hiroyuki Dada, Atsushi Amano, Gunjan Choudhary, Arushi A Malik, Dwight Stapleton, Pratap C Reddy, Manivannan Veerasamy, Umashankar Lakshmanadoss

Published by InTech

Janeza Trdine 9, 51000 Rijeka, Croatia

Publishing Process Manager Iva Lipovic

Technical Editor SPi Global

Cover InTech Design team

First published October, 2016
Printed in Croatia

Additional hard copies can be obtained from orders@intechopen.com

Echocardiography in Heart Failure and Cardiac Electrophysiology, Edited by Umashankar Lakshmanadoss

p. cm.

Print ISBN 978-953-51-2738-3
Online ISBN 978-953-51-2739-0

For EU product safety concerns:
IN TECH d.o.o., Prolaz Marije Krucifikse Kozulić 3, 51000 Rijeka, Croatia,
info@intechopen.com or visit our website at intechopen.com.

Meet the editor

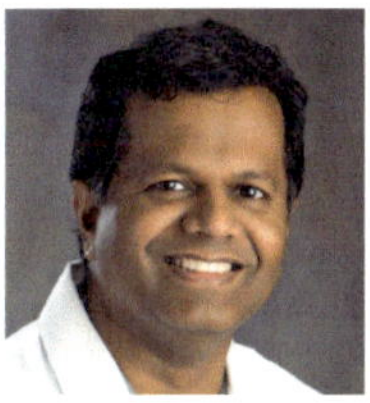

Dr. Umashankar Lakshmanadoss completed his training from Madras Medical College, India, and from University of Rochester, NY, USA. He served as director of inpatient medical consult service at Johns Hopkins University School of Medicine and then joined the Division of Cardiovascular Medicine at Guthrie Clinic, Sayre, PA, USA. Then he pursued training in cardiac electrophysiology at Oakland University William Beaumont School of Medicine and continued his advanced cardiac electrophysiology training at Mayo Clinic, Rochester, MN. Currently, he is an assistant professor of medicine in the Division of Cardiology, Louisiana State University Health Sciences Center, Shreveport, LA. He also serves as the director of complex arrhythmia ablation program. His research interest is in the field of clinical cardiac electrophysiology.

Contents

Preface

The world of echocardiography continues to be full of exciting new technological developments with an ultimate goal of better patient care. In this book, titled "Echocardiography in Heart Failure and Cardiac Electrophysiology", authors from different parts of the world contributed to the advancement of the field. We have authors who describe the basics of speckle tracking echocardiography and its recent applications and estimating strain pattern. Clinically relevant topics such as multimodality imaging in the diagnosis and management of hypertrophic cardiomyopathy have been discussed very nicely. Despite improvements in medical therapy, the mortality rate in congestive heart failure is still unacceptably high. Early diagnosis and management would be the key in reducing the mortality rate. An entire chapter is dedicated to the noninvasive measurement of pulmonary capillary wedge pressure. By early identification of this increased wedge pressure, clinicians may be in a position to diagnose heart failure in the earlier phase. In patients who have advanced heart failure, the obvious options include a bridging therapy such as left ventricular assist device or a destination therapy such as a cardiac transplantation. We have included a chapter that is entirely dedicated to the role of echocardiography in the management of patients with left ventricular assist device and possible cardiac transplantation. When we talk about congestive heart failure, we typically think about left ventricular heart failure. However, the recent data clearly suggest that the right ventricle plays a major role and is often neglected, unfortunately. Hence, we have included an excellent chapter describing the various modalities of processing the right ventricular function by echocardiography. Echocardiography could be very useful in critically ill patients and for early diagnosis, management, and possible differential diagnosis. One dedicated chapter describes the use of echocardiography in this sicker population. In patients with progressive heart failure and electromechanical disturbances, cardiac resynchronization therapy could be very useful to improve their quality of life and reduce the mortality. One of the authors has a dedicated chapter about the various noninvasive imaging technologies involving cardiac resynchronization therapy. We clearly know that atrial fibrillation and congestive heart failure go hand in hand. We have included a basic chapter describing the role of electrocardiographic markers for atrial arrhythmias. The patient with patrons in relation could be a good candidate for atrial fibrillation ablation, which is a highly advanced and complex procedure. One of our authors put together an excellent review about the multimodality echocardiographic assessment of patients undergoing atrial fibrillation. These topics would be of great interest to the clinicians whether they are trainees, physicians, advanced care providers, or anyone involved in patient care.

This work was made possible because of the contributors who have worked assiduously to help us produce an excellent book. I am indebted to Ms. Iva Lipović, publishing process manager at InTech, for the constant support. I dedicate this book to my mother Jana, my source of inspiration and encouragement, wife Gini and son Babboo, for their understanding, support, and unconditional love.

Umashankar Lakshmanadoss, MD, CCDS
Assistant Professor of Medicine,
Director, Complex Arrhythmia Ablation Program,
Louisiana State University Health Sciences Center,
Shreveport, LA, USA

Section 1

Echocardiography in Electrophysiology

Chapter 1

Introductory Chapter: Practical Approach to the Use of Intracardiac Echocardiography in Invasive Electrophysiology Procedures

Umashankar Lakshmanadoss

Additional information is available at the end of the chapter

http://dx.doi.org/10.5772/65243

1. Introduction

Use of intracardiac echocardiography (ICE) has been significantly increased with the advent of invasive electrophysiology and interventional procedures. In this day and age, we as a clinician are focused more on efficient and safe procedures for the patient. Intracardiac echocardiography plays a major role in doing these interventional procedures in a safe and efficient way. In addition to this, the use of ICE significantly reduced the need for fluoroscopy and hence reduced the occupational hazards of radiation and lead aprons for the physicians. It changed the way of doing these interventional procedures and one could easily say that this is one of the paradigm shift for us. In this chapter, I intend to review the basics of intracardiac echocardiography and also describe the various views and applications of intracardiac echocardiography in invasive electrophysiological procedures.

Several types of ice catheters are available in the market currently. They could be broadly divided into two different modalities. One catheter is a mechanical non-steerable catheter, which utilizes a rotating element to create a video 360° imaging claim perpendicular to the long axis of the catheter (UltraICE® Boston Scientific). This is 9 Fr catheter using 9 MHz. The second group of the catheter is a 64 element phased array 4-way steerable catheter. AcuNav® catheter (Biosense – Webster) is one of the commonly available phased out a catheter with the frequency range of 5.5–10 MHz. This is available in 8 and 10 Fr sizes. The system uses gray scale and has the facility for performing color Doppler, tissue Doppler and 3-D localization with Cartosound®. The images from this catheter result in a 90° sector image in the form of pie. ClearICE® catheter (St. Jude Medical) is another form of 64 elements phased array site looking highly steerable catheter with two sets of electrodes for integration of 3-D localization with NavX®. In addition to the gray scale and tissue Doppler, this can also do synchronization mapping which speckles tracking. In our electrophysiology laboratory, we commonly use the phased array 8 or 10 Fr AcuNav® catheter. For the purpose of this chapter, one the images from phased array system is included.

2. What are all the moments possible with the ICE catheter?

There are totally eight movements possible with this steerable catheter. With these eight movements, an experienced operator should be able to navigate through the important structures of the heart.

1. Clockwise: rotation of the catheter away from the operator
2. Counterclockwise: rotation of the catheter towards the operator
3. Anterior flexion: catheter bends forward
4. Posterior flexion: catheter bends backward
5. Right tilt: catheter bends towards the right side
6. Left tilt: catheter bends towards the left side
7. Push: catheter is advanced in further
8. Pull: catheter is withdrawn

3. How to advance the ICE catheter into the heart?

In our laboratory, the imaging catheter is mostly advanced, either from the right or left femoral vein into the right atrium. This could be performed without the use of fluoroscopy. After getting a venous access, the ICE catheter is advanced through the sheath into the femoral vein. Once the catheter is out of the venous access sheath, one should be able to visualize the lumen of the venous system. We typically advance the catheter making sure that there is a sufficient lumen seen at the tip of the catheter. To negotiate the side branches and tortuous veins, we use the knob of the ice catheter to do the various possible movements as described above. While advancing the catheter, one could clearly visualize the structures including liver. Once we reached right atrium, we typically leave the catheter to get the home you as described below. Fluoroscopy guidance should be used by less experienced operators as the catheter tip is not soft.

http://dx.doi.org/10.5772/65243

4. What settings does one need to have to optimize the ice images?

It is also important to understand the basics and physical principles of echocardiography to optimize the images obtained.

1. Frequency: the frequency range of the ice catheter is 5.5–10 MHz. High frequency lengthens the near field and hence has higher resolution. However, the depth of the penetration is reduced and thereby limiting its usefulness. A frequency setting of 7.5 MHz is a good starting point for most of the electrophysiological procedures. If we need to examine one particular area with a higher resolution, then the operator could use higher frequency mode. For example, lower frequencies (5.5 MHz) may be required to visualize distant structures such as the inferior and lateral wall of the left ventricle in the dilated heart. Similarly, higher frequencies (8.5–10.0 MHz) may be required to visualize a near field structure with a high resolution as in the case of outflow tract tachycardia.
2. Depth: depth of the imaging sector could be either increased or decreased to include the area of interest. For the purpose of transseptal access and imaging of the right-sided pulmonary veins from the right atrium, and the setting of 60–80 mm would be sufficient. For imaging, the left-sided pulmonary veins and left atrial appendage from the right atrium at the setting of 80–100 mm would be optimal. If the operator wants to evaluate the pericardium for the purpose of pericardial effusion, a depth setting of 100–120 mm could be sufficient. For the purpose of imaging right ventricle and left ventricle from the right atrium, a wide range of depth setting of 100–120 mm could be used depending on the size of the ventricles.
3. Gain: gain is the amplitude of the received signal. When the gain is increased, we are amplifying the received signal, and hence the image becomes brighter. However, an excessive increase in grain and noise to the image and hence lateral resolution is not great. Hence, to enhance lateral resolution, the minimum amount of system gain should be used.
4. Focus: usually, it is not needed to adjust focus. Most of the imaging sectors have the focal zone set to a region that is 2/3 of the total. If the how to evaluate the near-field structure is with more detailed analysis (visualizing right atrium lead thrombus from the right atrium)], then we have to adjust the focus.
5. Dynamic range: dynamic range refers to the range of ultrasound intensities that can be displayed; it is one of the methods of controlling the contrast of the image. The higher the dynamic range, the better the contrast resolution. During ablation, if there is any doubt of the thickness of the structures, one could reduce the dynamic range and see if the thickness of the structures is increased or not. This could be very helpful to assess the catheter contact with a left atrial appendage, left the atrial ridge and other endocavitary structures.
6. Mechanical index: during an ablation procedure, ablationist would be interested in looking for the bubbles from the tissue which could be an impending sign of steam pop. If the mechanical index is very high, these microbubbles could be destructed with the subsequent admission of high intensive signals. Hence, the mechanical index should be kept as intermediate if one wants to see the microbubbles.

7. Tissue Doppler: tissue Doppler could be used to find the area of scar or fibrosis. This could be of vital importance in ventricular tachycardia ablation.

8. Color Doppler and continuous wave Doppler: this could be used in evaluating pulmonary veins and valves.

5. What are all the structures one could view using ICE catheter?

Right atrium:

Superior vena cava

Eustachian valve

Crista terminalis

Right atrium appendage

Tricuspid valve

Ostium of the coronary sinus

Cavotricuspid isthmus

Right ventricle:

Right ventricular inflow

Tricuspid valve attachments

Papillary muscle

Moderator band

Right ventricular inferior wall, apex, and lateral wall

Para Hisian region

Right ventricular outflow tract

Pulmonic valve

Left atrium:

Inter atrial septum

Left-sided pulmonary veins

Right-sided pulmonary veins

Left atrial appendage

http://dx.doi.org/10.5772/65243

Left atrial posterior wall

Mitral annulus

Coronary sinus

Left ventricle:

Left ventricular inflow

Anterolateral and posteromedial papillary muscle

Left ventricle apex

Left ventricular outflow tract

Aortic valve

Aorta

Miscellaneous:

Pericardial effusion

Thrombus or mass attached to the intracardiac leads

Adequate contact of the catheter with the tissue

Echogenicity of the tissue during ablation

Left atrial appendage closure device

Atrial septal defect closure device

Esophagus

6. How does one use the ICE catheter in atrial fibrillation ablation?

While advancing the ice catheter from the femoral vein, one could visualize the liver. At this time, the catheter is slightly advanced into the mid-right atrium. When the catheter in this position, we could visualize most of the right atrium, tricuspid valve, and right ventricle. This is referred to "home position". The catheter is left over here in an unlocked are a neutral position. This whole meal allows the assessment of the tricuspid valve structure, function and estimation of pulmonary artery systolic pressure using tricuspid regurgitation. This view also gives a better sense about right atrium and the right ventricle leads. Whenever the operator feels that he is lost secondary to the unfamiliar imaging plane, he just needs to put on the catheter to the home view by removing all catheter deflections and gently rotating the ice catheter in the clockwise and counterclockwise rotation until the tricuspid valve is visualized (**Figure 1**).

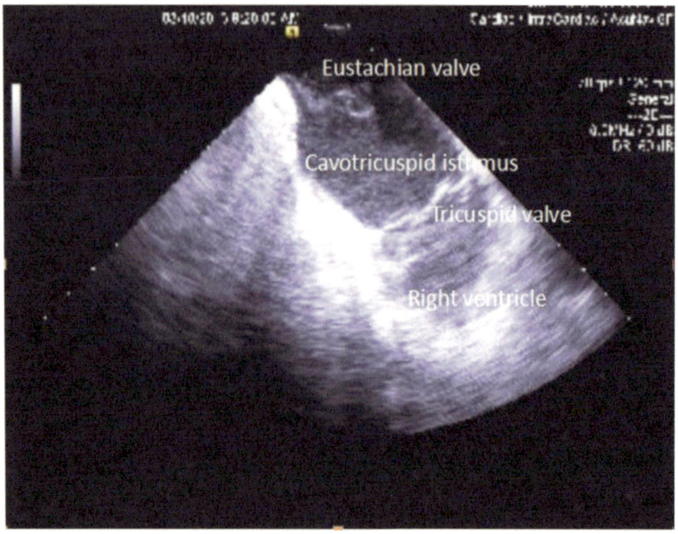

Figure 1. Home position.

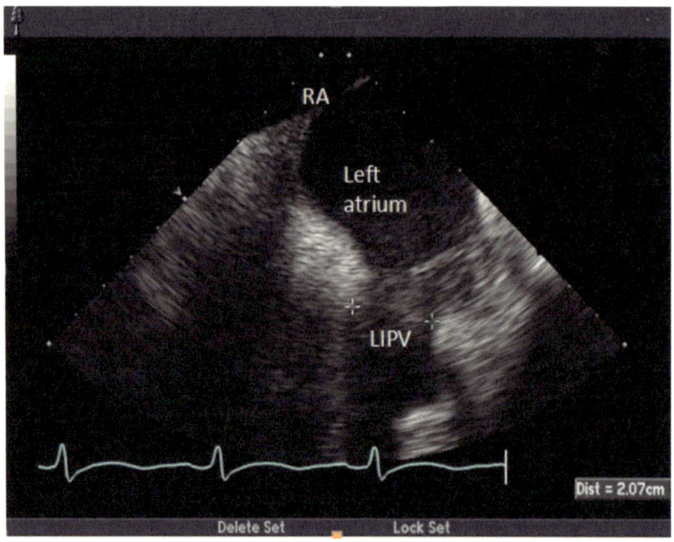

Figure 2. Left atrium and pulmonary veins.

From the home position, with the mild clockwise rotation, we can direct imaging plane posteriorly and left the ward. Initially, we can see the aortic valve, right ventricle inflow and right ventricle outflow just below the aortic valve. From this view, for the clockwise rotation of the catheter with about 45°, we can see the long axis of the aortic root. Here, we can analyze any atheroma of the aorta. This could be of vital importance when the operator is planning for a retrograde aortic approach. The aortic valve is also visualized well in this view. This is a good view to look for any regurgitation through the aortic valve. Just behind the aortic valve, one may be able to see the pulmonary artery and pulmonic valve. A continued clockwise rotation from this view will direct the image plane more posteriorly. This view is a good view to visualize left atrial appendage, mitral annulus and ostium of the coronary sinus. Many operators use this view to interrogating left atrial appendage for any thrombus. This view can also be used to help in cannulation of the coronary sinus in the case of any technical difficulties (**Figures 2** and **3**).

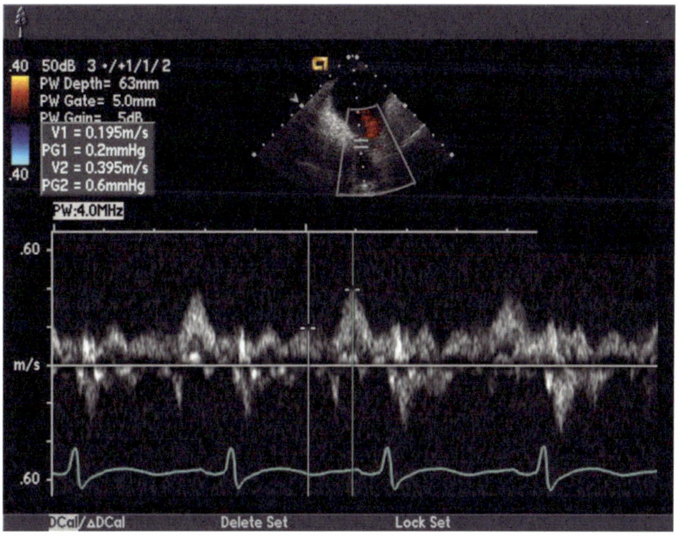

Figure 3. Continuous wave Doppler of the pulmonary veins.

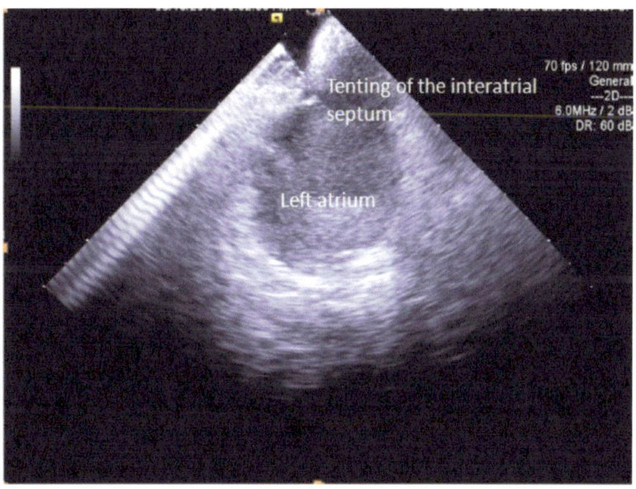

Figure 4. Tenting of the interatrial septum.

From this view, the catheter is slightly rotated clockwise. In this plane, one could visualize both left-sided pulmonary veins. The left superior pulmonary vein is usually visualized earlier and further clockwise rotation from that angle will bring left inferior pulmonary vein into visualization. This is a good view to measure the dimensions of the pulmonary vein, color Doppler of the pulmonary vein and continuous wave Doppler to evaluate the velocity of the pulmonary vein. During atrial fibrillation ablation, this view could be used to avoid ablation deep into the veins (**Figure 4**).

For the clockwise rotation of the ice catheter from this view will typically show the posterior wall of the left atrium. In this view, one could visualize esophagus and descend aorta. Esophageal temperature probe catheter can be visualized in the esophagus from the right atrium using this view. During ablation of the posterior wall of the right atrium, it would be easy to visualize the echogenicity of the lesion and proximity to the esophagus. Continued clockwise rotation of the ice catheter from this view will bring the right-sided pulmonary veins closer to the imaging surface of the ice catheter. The right-sided pulmonary veins will be visualized in a short axis. Using color Doppler, we could identify the pulmonary vein flow. Further advancement of the catheter into the right atrium and continued clockwise rotation from this level will bring up the right superior pulmonary vein in a better imaging plane. We will be able to see both right-sided pulmonary veins and pulmonary artery at this level. Usually, the right superior pulmonary vein is one of the most difficult veins to visualize. Sometimes the addition of a slight posterior tilt and right or left steering can further optimize this image to visualize the right superior pulmonary vein. Further clockwise rotation from this view will bring the catheter to the home view.

From the home position, ice catheter is advanced with a little bit of posterior flexion and rightward tilt. At this view, one could visualize the junction of the superior vena cava with right atrium. This view is commonly used to advance the guidewire into the superior vena cava before transseptal puncture. From here, the ice catheter is pulled down a little bit with continued posterior and right tilt. Now, they can clearly visualize interatrial septum including limbus and fossa ovalis. Typically, the operator advances the transseptal access needle in this view. One will be able to identify the tenting of the interatrial septum and further advancement of the transseptal needle into the left atrium. Slight clockwise rotation over here will help the operator to visualize and estimate the distance between the transseptal access site and posterior left atrial wall, thereby avoiding perforation into the left atrial posterior wall during transseptal access. Similarly, the distance between the transseptal access and left lateral wall can also be assessed in the previous imaging plane and hence avoiding left atrial perforation during transseptal access.

7. How does one use ICE catheter in ventricular tachycardia ablation?

From the home view, the catheter is tilted anteriorly. Now, we can visualize the posterior tricuspid leaflet and inferior wall of the right ventricle. The catheter is further advanced through the tricuspid valve into the right ventricle with continuous monitoring of the ICE

http://dx.doi.org/10.5772/65243

imaging. Once the catheter is just below the aortic valve in this view, further anterior tilt will make the catheter flex towards the inferior part of the right ventricle. This view is a good view to visualize the long axis of the posteromedial papillary muscle. From here, the anterior tilt is gently released in the catheter is further advanced towards the right ventricular apical region. Here, the catheter is brought to a neutral position with no tension on the knob. From here, clockwise rotation of the catheter will help us in visualizing the interventricular septum. This is also a good view of the epicardial axis as the right ventricular apical region is well visualized over here. With continuous clocking from here, we could visualize the posteromedial papillary muscle, and further clocking will bring the popular anterolateral muscle. The left ventricle cavity will be well visualized. Further clocking will also bring aortomitral continuity into the picture. Further advancement of the catheter into the right ventricle outflow tract with continued clockwise rotation will bring left ventricular outflow tract into the picture in a short axis view. We will be able to see all the three cusps of the aortic valve. Here noncoronary cusp will be adjacent to the inter-atrial septum; right coro-

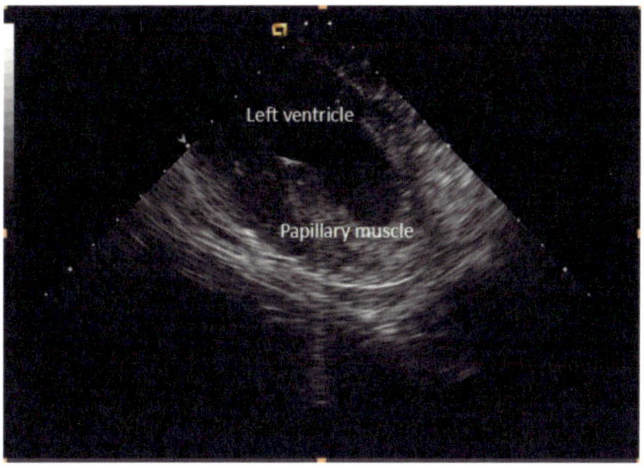

Figure 5. Left ventricle.

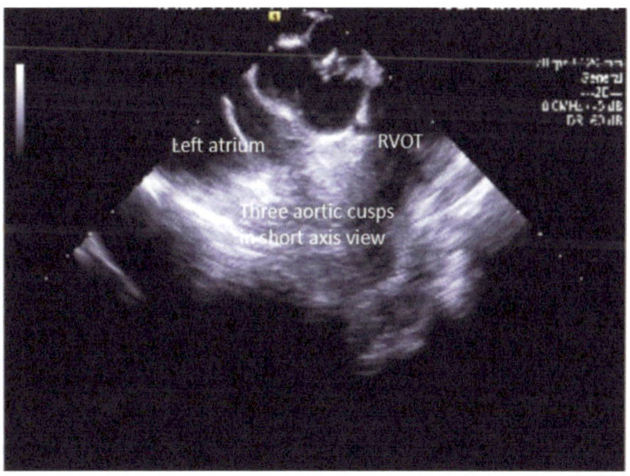

Figure 6. Aortic cusps.

nary cusp will be adjacent to the right ventricular outflow tract and left coronary cusp will be adjacent to the left ventricular outflow tract. In this view, one can also visualize left atrial appendage. In between the left coronary cusp on the left atrial appendage, we may be able to see left main coronary artery or left anterior descending artery. Further clockwise rotation over here will bring the aortic valve and ascending aorta in long axis (**Figures 5** and **6**).

8. How does one use ICE catheter to avoid complications during electrophysiological procedures?

Ice catheter can be used to monitor the catheter contact with the tissue. This helps us to make sure that they are ablating the right structure. It also helps us to maintain a better stability during respiration or with cardiac motion. With the help of the near field lesion visualization, one could avoid over ablating a region. Steam pops can happen during ablation secondary to high temperatures in the tissue. Impending signs of steam pop like increased echogenicity and microbubbles can be seen using ice catheter and hence avoiding imminent complications including perforation. Ice catheters also help us in negotiating through the valves safely without getting entangled in the valve apparatus. During ablation, continuous monitoring of the pericardial space can identify an early pericardial effusion thereby avoiding a less optimal outcome for the patient.

9. Conclusion

Imaging using intracardiac echocardiography has led to significant improvement in the safety and efficacy of the complex local physiological procedures. In addition to this, less dependence on the fluoroscopy also produces the occupational hazards for the physicians and the patients.

Author details

Umashankar Lakshmanadoss

Address all correspondence to: drlumashankar@gmail.com

Louisiana State University Health Science Center, Shreveport, USA

Chapter 2

The Role of Electrocardiographic Markers in the Prevention of Atrial and Ventricular Arrhythmias

Veronika Sebestyén and Zoltán Szabó

Additional information is available at the end of the chapter

http://dx.doi.org/10.5772/64460

Abstract

In our chapter, we overview the main clinical conditions that increase arrhythmogenicity, and we present the surface electrocardiogram (ECG) markers that could be suitable for the prediction of atrial and ventricular arrhythmias. We highlight the clinical value of the prolongation of the P-wave duration and P dispersion (Pd) in the prediction of atrial fibrillation, and we also expound the utility of QT interval, T-wave peak-to-end interval (Tpe), and Tpe/QT ratio (known as arrhythmogenic index (AIX)) in the prediction of ventricular arrhythmias. Furthermore, we present the results of our clinical investigations with regard to surface ECG markers among patients with increased arrhythmia vulnerability. Moreover, we mention other, novel, effectively used ECG markers.

Keywords: atrial fibrillation, P dispersion, P-wave interval, QT interval, T-wave peak-to-end interval, ECG markers, ventricular arrhythmias

1. Introduction

There are several diseases which may affect the pulse generation and the conduction in the heart. Patients suffering from these clinical conditions have increased probability for the occurrence of atrial and ventricular arrhythmias [1–4]. Numerous studies have been dealing with certain surface electrocardiogram (ECG) markers which could be suitable for the prevention of various cardiac rhythm disturbances [5–7]. Previously, it has been shown that the prolongation of the P-wave duration and P dispersion (Pd) can predict atrial arrhythmias [5, 8, 9]. Moreover, it has also been demonstrated that the prolongation of QT interval, T-wave peak-to-end interval (Tpe) and Tpe/QT ratio (known as arrhythmogenic index—AIX) could predict ventricular arrhythmias [6, 7]. In our chapter we would like to present the electrophysiological substrates and pathogenetic factors taking part in arrhythmogenesis and to demonstrate ECG-based diagnostic opportunities that can help in the prediction and prevention of arrhythmias. Furthermore, we present the results of our studies to demonstrate the clinical use of these ECG markers.

2. Non-invasive electrocardiographic markers in the prediction of atrial fibrillation

2.1. Epidemiology and electrophysiological background of atrial fibrillation

The most common form of rhythm disturbances is atrial fibrillation (AF). Its prevalence is 0.12–0.16% among people younger than 49 years, 3.7–4.2% with regard to people aged 60–70 years and 10–17% among people aged 80 years or older [10]. Age, gender, hypertension, diabetes mellitus, heart failure and valvular heart disease are independent risk factors that may play a role in arrhythmogenesis. Moreover, AF may be caused by hyperthyroidism and excessive alcohol consumption [11, 12] (**Table 1**).

Cardiovascular causes of atrial fibrillation (%)	
Ischemic heart disease	17
Hypertensive cardiomyopathy	21
Valvulopathies	15
Dilated cardiomyopathy	9
Hypertrophic cardiomyopathy	5
Other structural heart diseases	9
Non-structural heart diseases	29

Table 1. Cardiovascular causes of atrial fibrillation.

In patients with end-stage renal failure, its prevalence is approximately 13%. Interestingly, 10% of subjects suffering from 'lone' AF have no comorbidity, detectable underlying structural or functional heart disease. Previous studies have also demonstrated that nearly 30% of patients with atrial fibrillation may have a positive family history. The predisposition for arrhythmia events was shown to be inherited in an autosomal dominant pattern. In a small proportion of familial AF, specific mutant genes were identified, and mutations were detected mainly in KCNE2, KCNJ2, and KCNQ1. While encoding the protein products of certain potassium channels, these are suggested to play a role in the maintenance of sinus rhythm [13–16].

Atrial anisotropy is thought to be one of the key points of increased atrial arrhythmia vulnerability, where the inhomogeneous spreading of atrial impulses can be secondary to an altered histological structure of the atrial myocardium (hypertrophy, fibrosis, and fatty degeneration)

[17–19]. Consequently, the dilation of both atria may appear representing an increased susceptibility for atrial arrhythmias [20]. Furthermore, increase in cardiac preload and afterload and electrolyte imbalances may also have an additive role in the increase of atrial arrhythmogenicity and reentry mechanism, where the latter is the electrophysiological substrate for atrial fibrillation.

2.2. Clinical consequences of atrial fibrillation

Irregular and high ventricular response due to AF, atrioventricular dissociation and the lack of atrial systole may contribute to low cardiac output syndrome. Patients usually complain about palpitation, fatigue, dyspnea, vertigo/dizziness, and chest pain. However, 11% of these patients are asymptomatic. Decrease in atrial blood flow velocity gives the chance for atrial thrombus formation. Mortality caused by atrial fibrillation is primarily connected with an increased risk for thromboembolic events and stroke (**Figure 1**) [10, 11, 21].

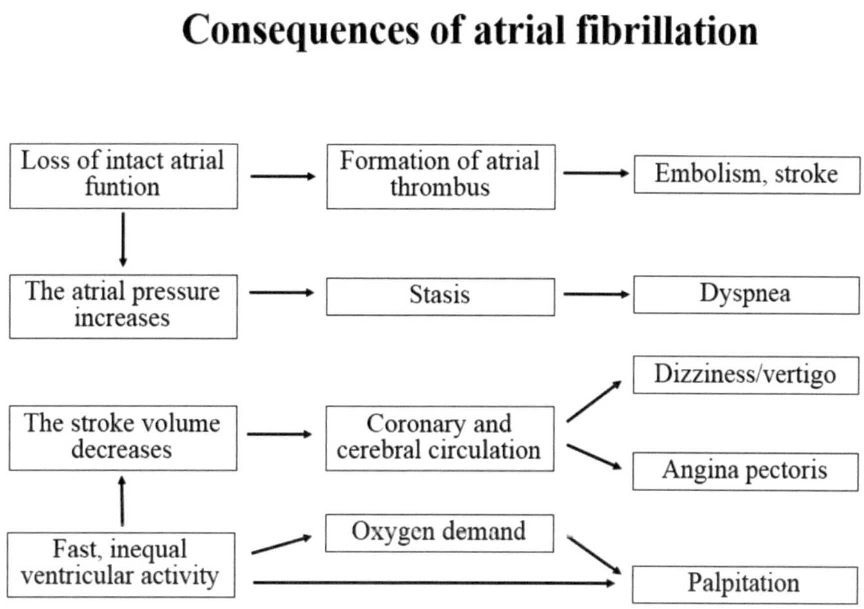

Figure 1. Pathomechanism and consequences of atrial fibrillation.

2.3. Electrocardiographic prediction of AF

2.3.1. P-wave duration and P dispersion

Due to the structural and electrophysiological heterogeneity of the left atrium, unidirectional block can occur, which plays a role in the genesis of atrial microreentry and premature beats. In patients with paroxysmal atrial fibrillation during sinus rhythm, the intra- and interatrial conduction time of the sinus impulse were shown to lengthen, and the duration of the P wave measured on a surface electrocardiogram (ECG) is increased, where the prolongation of atrial conduction time is proportional with the duration of P-wave interval. Previously, it has also been shown that the prolongation of P-wave duration and P dispersion (Pd) can predict atrial arrhythmias. P-wave duration of the surface electrocardiogram is specified as the section from the first electrical activity following the T wave (or the U wave) to the intersection of the P wave's descending branch and the isoelectric line. The investigator should analyze three consecutive P waves each lead and calculate their average duration, where the result is the P wave duration in the given lead (**Figure 2**). P dispersion (Pd) is determined as the difference between the longest and shortest P interval. P interval and Pd can be corrected to the heart rate (Pmaxc, Pdc) according to Bazett's formula (Pmaxc = Pmax/√RR (ms), Pdc = Pd/√RR (ms)) (**Figure 2**) [5, 8, 9].

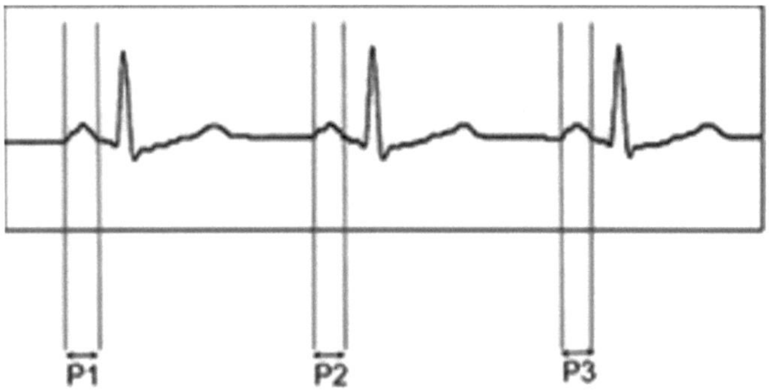

Figure 2. Measurement of P-wave duration on the surface ECG.

2.3.2. Alterations of P-wave duration and P dispersion among patients participating renal replacement therapy

The incidence of atrial fibrillation is increased during hemodialysis (HD), and the prolongation of P-wave duration has been shown to be a valuable indicator of atrial conduction disturbances. Based on the aforementioned, we analyzed the length of P-wave interval and P dispersion on the surface ECG of 28 patients with end-stage renal failure on extracorporeal renal replacement therapies. According to our results, P-wave duration and P dispersion increased significantly at the end of the hemodialysis sessions compared to those measured at the beginning, and they remained lengthened 2 hours after the treatment [22]. Previously, a novel convective-transport-based renal replacement method, the hemodiafiltration (HDF), has been introduced. Lately, convective treatment has been proven to reduce mortality of these particular patients with end-stage kidney disease. This favorable effect of HDF may be partly caused by the decreased occurrence of atrial and ventricular arrhythmias. We intended to examine whether these suggested differences between hemodialysis and hemodiafiltration with regard to arrhythmia vulnerability could be shown as alterations of P interval and P dispersion on the surface ECG. We obtained clinical data from 30 patients receiving HDF over a period of 3 months; and the same group of patients was then evaluated during treatment with conventional HD for at least another 3 months. The duration of the P wave and Pd increased significantly during HD, but no such significant prolongations were observed in the case of HDF (**Figure 3**) [23].

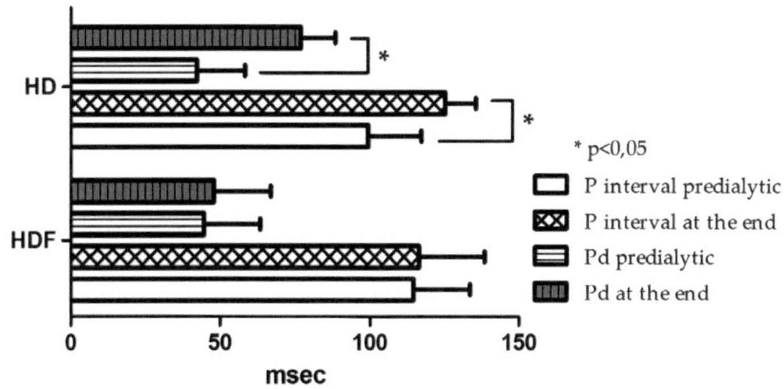

Figure 3. Changes in corrected P-wave duration (P interval) and corrected P dispersion (Pd) during hemodialysis and hemodiafiltration.

2.3.3. Biphasic P wave

Slow and inhomogeneous atrial conduction, thus atrial anisotropy, can appear as biphasic P wave in the inferior electrocardiographic leads (leads II, III, and aVF). In nearly 75% of patients with paroxysmal, AF has an increased duration of the initial portion of P wave in lead III [24]. Various investigations have reported the clinical value of P-wave measurements in the prediction of AF (**Table 2**) [22, 23, 25–30].

Underlying clinical condition	References
Hyperthyroidism	[25, 26]
Postcardiac surgery	[27, 28]
Renal failure and renal replacement therapy	[22, 23]
Pulmonary diseases	[29, 30]

Table 2. Studies which investigated alterations of the atrial phase of surface ECG.

2.3.4. Investigation of Ta wave

Inhomogeneous atrial repolarization may also play an additive role in the genesis of atrial arrhythmias and paroxysmal atrial fibrillation. Therefore, ECG analysis of atrial repolarization may provide further data on atrial arrhythmia vulnerability. Recently, a novel electrocardiographic marker the atrial T wave, also known Ta wave, has been shown to characterize atrial repolarization in patients with sinus rhythm. Due to its small amplitude within the PQ segment, signal averaging is necessary to soften the measurements. Moreover, in patients with physiologic atrioventricular conduction, it is generally localized in the subsequent QRS complex (name for the combination of three of the graphical deflections seen on a surface ECG which corresponds to the ventricular depolarization) holding the measurements to be impossible. Nevertheless, characteristics of the detectable atrial repolarization phase of the ECG have been compared between individuals with sinus rhythm and paroxysmal AF. However, no significant differences with regard to the morphology, amplitude and length of Ta wave have been clearly elucidated yet [31].

3. Ventricular arrhythmias and sudden cardiac death

3.1. The role of electrocardiographic markers in the prevention of ventricular rhythm disturbances and sudden cardiac death

Despite the improvement in statistical data, cardiovascular diseases are responsible for approximately 17 million deaths every year in the world, where approximately 25% is related to sudden cardiac death [32]. Malignant ventricular arrhythmias (e.g. ventricular tachycardia and ventricular fibrillation) are the most important underlying rhythm disturbances responsible for these unfavorable statistics. The incidence of these ventricular arrhythmias correlates with age primarily due to the higher prevalence of coronary artery disease [33]. Sudden cardiac death has an estimated incidence of 1100–9000 in Europe and 800–6200 in the United States every year [32].

3.2. Pathomechanism of ventricular arrhythmias and sudden cardiac death

Various factors have been shown to play a role in the genesis of ventricular arrhythmias. Both congenital factors and acquired pathophysiological mechanisms can provoke these cardiac rhythm disturbances [33]. Previously, it has been demonstrated that *genetic predisposition* can contribute to the genesis of sudden cardiac death. Fifty percent increase has been confirmed in the likelihood of the occurrence of malignant ventricular arrhythmias in the presence of a family history of sudden cardiac death [34]. Furthermore, it has been shown that familial sudden death appears more frequently in patients resuscitated from primary ventricular fibrillation [35]. Previously, single nucleotide polymorphisms located in the 21q21 and 2q24.2 loci have been also shown to increase the risk of sudden cardiac death [36, 37]. However, certain concerns were raised with regard to these results, and further investigations are needed. The risk of sudden cardiac death is higher in males [38, 39]. On the other hand, coronary artery disease, ischemic cardiomyopathy and heart failure, hypertensive heart disease, and lipid abnormalities are the most important *acquired* provoking factors with regard to ventricular arrhythmogenesis and sudden cardiac death [3, 38]. Interestingly, kidney disease and hemodialysis itself have been demonstrated to be significant underlying substrates for the genesis of ventricular arrhythmias. The incidence of sudden cardiac death in patients suffering from kidney diseases was shown to be approximately 1.4–25% [4]. Furthermore, physical inactivity, smoking, alcohol abuse, and inadequate alimentation are significant pathophysiologic factors that may contribute to ventricular arrhythmogenesis [39] (**Table 3**). Most importantly 50% of sudden death appears in patients without a previously known heart disease, but most of these individuals suffer from ischemic heart disease. Therefore, 40% of the reduction in sudden

http://dx.doi.org/10.5772/64460

arrhythmia death is due to the effective management and prevention of coronary artery disease [38, 39]. Left ventricular systolic dysfunction has also been proven to be an important underlying factor for ventricular arrhythmogenesis. Left ventricular ejection fraction, an echocardiographic parameter, has been shown in association with increased probability for sudden cardiac death mainly in patients with myocardial infarction. Related to heart failure, certain biochemical indicators such as the B-type natriuretic peptide and N-terminal pro-B-type natriuretic peptide have also been shown to be useful in the risk stratification of sudden cardiac death [40, 41].

Congenital or acquired causes	**Temporary factors**
• Coronary artery disease	• Electrolyte imbalance
	◦ Hypokalemia, hypomagnesemia
• Hypertensive heart disease	• Endocrinological disorders
	◦ Thyroid
	◦ Suprarenal gland
• Cardiomyopathies	• Myocarditis
◦ Hypertrophic	• Pericarditis
◦ Dilated	
◦ Right ventricular dysplasia	
• Valvular diseases	• Toxic effects
	◦ Alcohol
	◦ Certain antibiotics
	◦ Antifungal agents
	◦ Antidepressants
• Primary electrophysiologic causes (channelopathies)	• PH abnormalities
◦ Brugada syndrome	• Smoking
◦ Long QT syndrome	
◦ Short QT syndrome	
• Congenital heart diseases	• Postoperative period
• Comorbid factors	• Malnutrition
◦ Pulmonary diseases	• Abdominal distension
◦ Kidney disease	

Table 3. Common causes of ventricular arrhythmias are shown. Congenital and acquired diseases may play a role in ventricular arrhythmogenesis; furthermore, temporary factors can additionally increase the susceptibility for rhythm disturbances.

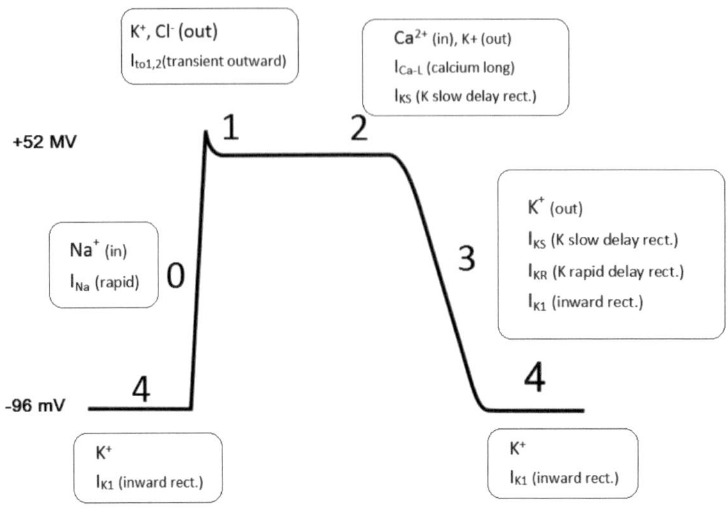

Figure 4. The monophasic action potential of a ventricular myocardial cell is shown. The plateau phase largely depends on the potassium and the calcium ion channel activity. The longer the plateau phase, the more increased the myocardial cell's repolarization. M cells show a prominent prolongation in action potential diameter and develop early after depolarizations in response to rapidly activating delayed rectifier potassium current (IKr) blockers.

3.3. Ventricular repolarization and cardiac arrhythmias

Secondary to the pathophysiologic factors, the electrophysiological properties of the myocardial cells can change, resulting in the modification of the duration and amplitude of the monophasic action potential featuring the myocardial cell's electrical properties (**Figure 4**) [42]. As a result, inhomogeneous ventricular repolarization and anisotropy may appear, which seem to be one of the electrophysiological key points in the genesis of ventricular arrhythmias. Previously, it has been shown that a mid-myocardial population of cardiac myocytes (e.g. M cells) can play an important role in the prolongation of repolarizational dispersion [43, 44]. From an electrophysiologic point of view, these special cells have been shown to be between Purkinje and ventricular myocytes, while they show a significant prolongation in action potential diameter and develop early after depolarizations in response to rapidly activating delayed rectifier potassium current (IKr) blockers [45]. In the meantime epicardial and endocardial myocytes are less likely to do so. Accordingly, due to certain drug therapies (e.g. amiodarone and sotalol) or other provoking factors, an exaggerated dispersion in transmural action potential duration may come alive, resulting in an increased danger of transmural inhomogeneity of ventricular repolarization and an increased susceptibility for ventricular arrhythmias (**Figure 4**) [42, 46].

3.4. QT interval and dispersion

QT interval represents the electrical repolarization of the ventricular myocardium. Patients with increased susceptibility for the development of malignant ventricular dysrhythmias can be identified with the determination of QT interval [47]. Duration of the QT interval is changing in the different leads of the surface electrocardiogram. QT dispersion (QTd) is derived from the interlead alterations of QT intervals. This is a useful parameter to describe the differences in ventricular recovery times representing the prolongation of myocardial repolarization [48]. QT dispersion has also been proven to correlate with the duration of the monophasic action potential of the epicardial myocardial cells. Since these electrocardiographic markers have been introduced to predict ventricular arrhythmias and sudden cardiac death, they are considered to be among one of the non-invasive parameters [49]. The prolongation of QT interval can be congenital (e.g. Romano-Ward or Jervell and Lange-Nielsen syndromes) or acquired. Congenital syndromes are caused by mutations in at least five different ion channel genes resulting in the defects in the sodium channel (SCN5A, LQT3), the rapidly activating delayed rectifier channel (IKr) (HERG, LQT2 or KCNE2, LQT6), and the slowly activating delayed rectifier channel (IKs) (KvLQT1, LQT1 or KCNE1, LQT5), respectively [50]. QT prolongation can be acquired and may occur after acute myocardial infarction, congestive heath failure, dyslipidemia, diabetes mellitus, sudden sympathetic autonomic activation (triggered activity) and renal failure [6, 51–55]. In individuals with liver cirrhosis, the lengthening of QT interval has not been shown to be related to the etiology of the liver disease and seems to appear both in alcoholic and nonalcoholic patients [46]. In addition, QT prolongation may be associated to certain drug interactions (e.g. haloperidol, methadone, amiodarone, sotalol, selective serotonin reuptake inhibitors, macrolide antibiotics, and antifungal agents) [56]. QT dispersion may also be affected by various diseases (amyloidosis, sarcoidosis, carcinoid, hemochromatosis, diabetes mellitus, thyroid dysfunction, or Parkinson's disease) [57–63].

3.5. QT measurements and their clinical use

Since these repolarizational variables are modified by numerous causes, the thorough investigation of patient's history is one of the leading points during the determination of arrhythmia risk. Considering the required standards for precision, the measurement of QT interval still remains subjective as the terminal point of the T wave usually cannot be clearly defined. QT interval can be measured manually or automatically [49, 64]. During manual investigations, improvement in consistency of the results and the minimization of interobserver variability may be achieved by the measurements performed by one examiner. During the threshold method, the point where the T wave reaches the isoelectric line is determined as its end. According to the tangent method, the end of T wave is defined as the point where a given tangent line overtakes the isoelectric line, where the tangent line is the last part of the T wave at its maximum downslope. To get more accurate data, the average of three sequential periods in a given lead is calculated and defined as QT interval [47, 48] (**Figure 5**). QT measurements may also be performed by means of computers with the superimposed median beat method, where an electrocardiographic complex is constructed for each of the 12 leads. These medians are superimposed on each other. Afterwards, QT interval is determined from the earliest onset of the Q wave to the latest offset of the T wave. Moreover, QT interval can be measured from the point of maximum convergence for the Q-wave onset to the T-wave offset [48].

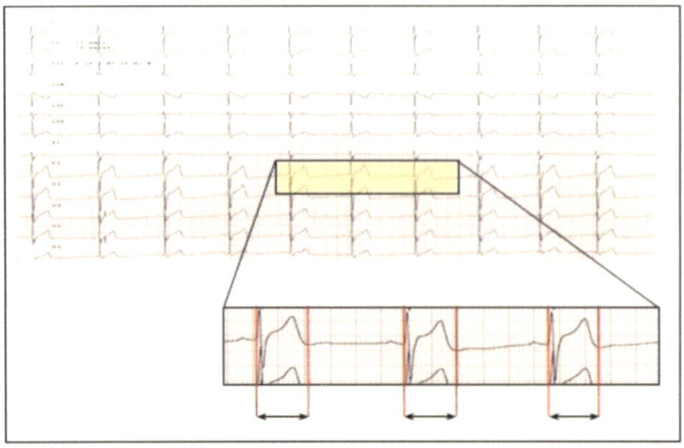

Figure 5. The manual measurement of the QT interval of the 12-lead surface electrocardiogram. The calculation and averaging of three consecutive sections may provide a more accurate result in the given lead.

Ventricular rate has a significant influence on QT interval's duration. When heart rate accelerates, QT interval shortens. Therefore, QT interval has to be corrected to heart rate (QTc) using the Bazett's formula ($QTc = QT/\sqrt{RR}$) (borderline QTc, male 431–450 ms and female 451–470 ms; abnormal QTc, male ≥ 451 ms and female ≥471 ms). Normal values of QT dispersion vary in a very wide range from 10 to 71 ms. The QTc >450 ms value has been reported to have an increased risk for ventricular arrhythmias [49]. With regard to patients suffering from liver cirrhosis, a special relationship between QT interval duration and heart rate exists; thus, a specific 'cirrhosis formula'—similar to the Fridericia's—should be used. Measurement of QT interval and dispersion can help in the monitoring of antiarrhythmic therapy especially with the widely used antiarrhythmic drugs, amiodarone and sotalol [46, 56]. Previously, the prolongation of the QT dispersion has been shown to represent recurrent ischemia after percutaneous transluminal coronary angioplasty. Lately, the eligibility of QT dispersion in the evaluation of long-term outcome of patients waiting for cardiac transplantation has also been discussed. Life-threatening ventricular rhythm disturbances of patients with long QT syndromes often caused by a sudden increase in sympathetic activity, and beta-blockers have been shown to significantly reduce these arrhythmic episodes. In patients who remain symptomatic despite treatment with beta-blockers (mostly patients with LQT2 and LQT3), left cardiac sympathetic denervation may be a therapeutic solution. In the case of cardiac arrest, ICD should be implanted; however, there are controversial data regarding the ICD therapy in subjects with no such previous history [47, 49, 50].

3.5.1. Changes in QT interval and QT dispersion in hyperlipidemia and kidney disease

The susceptibility to malignant ventricular arrhythmias increases proportionally with the lengthening of QT interval. Progressive atherosclerosis is an independent risk factor of the occurrence of sudden cardiac death. In our study clinical data of 96 patients with hyperlipidemia were compared to 103 controls. Serum LDL-C (low density lipoprotein – cholesterol) and Tg levels were positively correlated with corrected QT interval and QT dispersion, so lipid parameters may affect these ECG markers [65]. Furthermore, we investigated the ECG parameters representing ventricular repolarization in the case of 30 patients receiving hemodiafiltration (HDF) over a period of 3 months, and we obtained data from the same patients after treatment with conventional hemodialysis (HD) for at least another 3 months. The duration of the QT interval and QT dispersion was only increased significantly in the case of HD, but no similar significant prolongations in the case of HDF could be observed (**Figure 6**) [66].

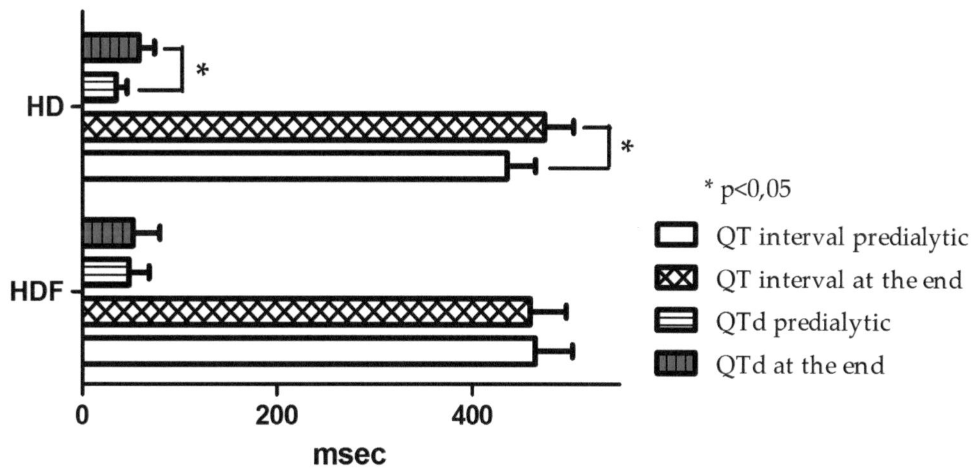

Figure 6. Prolongation of corrected QT interval and corrected QT dispersion (QTd) during different renal replacement therapies.

3.6. QT variability

Previously, numerous studies have been dealing with the beat-to-beat variability in QT interval of the surface electrocardiogram in order to quantify temporal dispersion of ventricular repolarization [67]. Its increase has been associated to long QT syndrome, heart failure, myocardial ischemia, hypertrophic cardiomyopathy, and panic disorder [68–72]. Increased QT variability has also been shown to predict appropriate implantable cardioverter-defibrillator shocks. Moreover, increased variability has been observed with regard to sudden cardiac death in patients with myocardial infarction without ICD therapy [73, 74]. QT variability may also increase in healthy people with postural change from the supine to standing position and after activities that increase beta-adrenergic tone [75]. QT variability is measured by a special computer algorithm that is able to analyze QT-interval signals that are derived from multiple channels [76].

3.7. Short QT syndrome

Short QT syndrome, an inherited disease, is characterized by QT interval <300 ms and an increased risk for paroxysmal atrial fibrillation and ventricular arrhythmias. Short QT syndrome is also related to an increased risk of sudden cardiac death, likely caused by ventricular fibrillation [77]. More genetic mutations of sodium and calcium channels have been reported to be an underlying substrate for this clinical entity (KCNH2, KCNQ1 and KCNJ2). Increased activity of outward potassium currents in phase 2 and phase 3 leads to the decreased duration of cardiac action potential, resulting in the shortening of refractory periods. This mechanism is thought to be responsible for the genesis of reentry mechanism and increased dispersion of ventricular repolarization [77, 78]. Besides ICD, antiarrhythmic drug therapy also has to be taken into consideration. Only quinidine, a sodium channel blocker, has been shown to normalize the QT interval at resting heart rates, while it restored the heart rate dependence of QT interval towards an adaptation range of healthy individuals by prolonging the duration of cardiac action potential [79, 80]. However its further effects remain to be elucidated.

3.8. Early repolarization

Recently, a J-point elevation of ≥0.1 mV in two adjacent leads occurring on the surface electrocardiogram manifested as terminal QRS slurring (the transition from the QRS segment to the ST segment) or notching (a positive deflection inscribed on terminal QRS complex) associated with concave upward ST-segment elevation and prominent T waves has been introduced as an early-repolarization (ER) pattern [81, 82]. A transmural voltage gradient between the ventricular epicardium and endocardium may be responsible for this phenomenon [83, 84]. ER commonly occurs in the general population (approximately 10%) and often exists in athletes and youngsters and at slower heart rates in individuals without known cardiac diseases [85]. However, recently, studies have emphasized a possible link between ER and life-threatening ventricular dysrhythmias [86]. The electrocardiographic signs of ER may be associated with a shorter QT interval and can display high dynamicity affected by ventricular rate and pauses, mediators of autonomic nervous system, androgen hormones and certain drugs (sodium channel blockers, beta-blockers, quinidine and isoproterenol) [87–91]. Importantly, a distinction between ER, short QT and Brugada syndromes sometimes proves to be difficult on the basis of electrocardiography, where genetic tests may be valuable in identifying the underlying ion channel defect [89, 92, 93]. Subjects with ECG signs of classic ER have minimal risk for ventricular arrhythmias, and the recognition of high-risk patients is often a real challenge [93, 94]. The susceptibility for ventricular arrhythmias may increase when ER is associated with heart failure, hypokalemia or acute coronary syndrome [95, 96]. Furthermore, the family history of ERS or sudden death, the extension of electrocardiographic signs of ER into a Brugada syndrome pattern, the presence of horizontal ST segment following the J wave, ER signs localized in inferior or infero-lateral leads, the presence of coupled ventricular premature beats, increase in parasympathetic tone, also the association of ER with short QT intervals, young age and male gender draw the attention to a higher arrhythmia risk [94, 97–99]. In high-risk patients with ER syndrome and a family history of sudden death, quinidine and/or ICD implantation can be a therapeutic solution. Furthermore, cilostazol, a phosphodiesterase III inhibitor, has been shown to normalize the aforementioned ECG changes. In the case of ER syndrome-mediated electrical changes, a beta-adrenergic agent (e.g. isoproterenol) may be a useful therapeutic solution [100].

http://dx.doi.org/10.5772/64460

3.9. T-wave alternans (TWA) and T-wave peak-to-end interval

T-wave alternans is defined as an alteration in the morphology of the T wave in an AB-AB or every-other-beat pattern (**Figure 7**). It has been introduced as a non-invasive ECG marker for evaluating spatiotemporal heterogeneity of ventricular repolarization [101]. By reflecting the intracellular changes in calcium handling and showing beat-to-beat alternations of action potential duration of the ventricular cells, this electrocardiographic parameter seems to be capable for the prediction of ventricular repolarizational heterogeneity and the predisposition for ventricular arrhythmias [102].

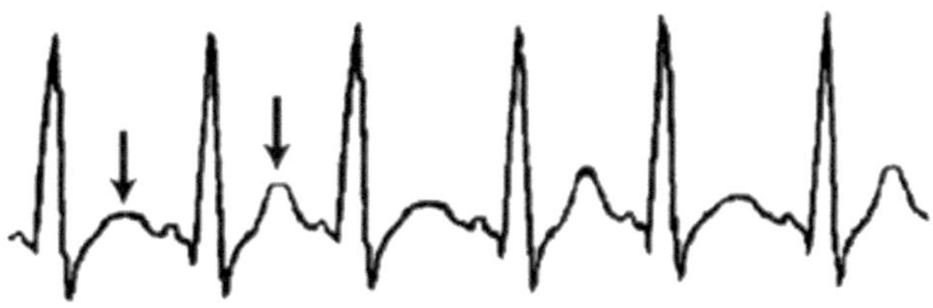

Figure 7. Alternation in the morphology of T waves on the surface electrocardiogram. Based on Narayan [101].

The electronic filtering of the T wave on a 'microvolt level' (i.e. microvolt T-wave alternans (MTWA)) creates even greater applicability of this non-invasive electrocardiographic method [103]. Therefore, MTWA has also been introduced as a valuable tool for the risk stratification of sudden cardiac death. Importantly, MTWA seems to have a particular role in the risk stratification between patients who need implantable cardiac defibrillators and those who do not [103–105]. TWA test is usually conducted during treadmill or bicycle exercise or with the administration of chronotropic agents in order to achieve an optimal ventricular rate, since TWA may occur in normal individuals at heart rates >120 beats/min. Occasionally, pacemaker stimulation required to maintain stable ventricular frequency. A target ventricular rate range of 105–110/min was determined for pathologic alternans in adults. If ectopic or premature beats constitute >10% of beats, the affected portion of the electrocardiogram is not recommended for TWA examination [106–108]. MTWA tests' results can be positive, negative or indeterminate. Patients with indeterminate results have to be investigated again [109]. In the case of a negative test, the probability of malignant ventricular arrhythmias and sudden cardiac death are low (with 98% accuracy for follow-up periods of 12–24 months in clinical studies) [110]. However, these patients have to undergo a repeated investigation every 12–24 months. Subjects with a negative MTWA test are not likely to require a defibrillator. Importantly, TWA testing may be equivalent to an electrophysiology study. Nevertheless, at present there is no definitive evidence available that can prove the real effectiveness of this method in guiding the antiarrhythmic treatment [107]. Previously a novel electrocardiographic marker, T-wave peak-to-end interval (Tpe) has been reported to represent the transmural dispersion of repolarization of the left ventricle and the vulnerability to ventricular arrhythmias [6, 111]. The prolongation of Tpe has been shown to be associated with increased mortality rates in long QT syndrome, acute myocardial infarction, sleep apnea and hypertrophic cardiomyopathy [6, 111, 112].

Reference value of T-wave peak-to-end interval is considered to be 94 ms in the case of male and 92 ms with regard to female subjects [113]. In addition, the Tpe/QT ratio is used as an arrhythmogenic index (AIX) of ventricular arrhythmogenesis [7, 114]. It has been demonstrated that in patients with acquired QT syndrome, the Tpe/QT ratio is superior to QT interval and QT dispersion in the prediction of torsades de pointes ventricular tachycardia [115]. Also, Tpe/QT ratio was shown to be a valuable predictor of sudden cardiac death [116–118].

Author details

Veronika Sebestyén and Zoltán Szabó*

*Address all correspondence to: szaboz.med@gmail.com

Division of Emergency Medicine, Faculty of Medicine, Clinical Centre, Institute of Medicine, University of Debrecen, Debrecen, Hungary

References

[1] Bruere H, Fauchier L, Clementy N. History of thyroid disorders in relation to clinical outcomes in atrial fibrillation. Am J Med. 2015;128(1):30-37.

[2] Goichot B, Caron P, Bouée S. Clinical presentation of hyperthyroidism in a large representative sample of outpatients in France: relationships with age, aetiology and hormonal parameters. Clin Endocrinol (Oxf). 2016;84(3):445-451.

[3] Rosamond WD. Invited commentary: trends in coronary heart disease mortality-location, location, location. Am J Epidemiol. 2003;157:771-773.

[4] Abe S, Yoshizawa M, Sloman G. Electrocardiographic abnormalities in patients receiving hemodialysis. Am Heart J. 1996;131:1137-1144.

[5] Dilaveris PE, Gialafos EJ, Sideris SK. Simple electrocardiographic markers for the prediction of paroxysmal idiopathic atrial fibrillation. Am Heart J. 1998;135(5):733-738.

[6] Puddu PE, Bourassa MG. Prediction of sudden death from QTc interval prolongation in patients with chronic ischemic heart disease. J Electrocardiol. 1986;19:203-211.

[7] Gupta P, Patel C, Patel H. T(p-e)/QT ratio as an index of arrhythmogenesis. J Electrocardiol. 2008;41:567-574.

[8] Andrikopoulos GK, Dilaveris PE, Richter DJ. Increased variance of P wave duration on the electrocardiogram distinguishes patients with idiopathic paroxysmal atrial fibrillation. Pacing Clin Electrophysiol. 2000;23(7):1127-1132.

[9] Aytemir K, Ozer N, Atalar E. P wave dispersion on 12-lead electrocardiography in patients with paroxysmal atrial fibrillation. Pacing Clin Electrophysiol. 2000;23(7): 1109-1112.

[10] Piccini JP, Hammill BG, Sinner MF. Incidence and prevalence of atrial fibrillation and associated mortality among Medicare beneficiaries, 1993–2007. Circ Cardiovascular Qual Outcomes. 2012;5:85-93.

[11] Genovesi S, Vincenti A, Rossi E. Atrial fibrillation and morbidity and mortality in a cohort of long-term hemodialysis patients. Am J Kidney Dis. 2008;51(2):255-262.

[12] McCullough PA, Steigerwalt S, Tolia K. Cardiovascular disease in chronic kidney disease: data from the Kidney Early Evaluation Program (KEEP). Curr Diab Rep. 2011;11(1):47-55.

[13] Chen YH, Xu SJ, Huang W. KCNQ1 gain-of-function mutation in familial atrial fibrillation. Science. 2003;299(5604):251-154.

[14] Ellinor PT,Petrov-Kondratov VI, MacRae CA. Potassium channel gene mutations rarely cause atrial fibrillation. BMC Med Genet. 2006;7:70.

[15] Roberts R. Mechanisms of disease: genetic mechanisms of atrial fibrillation. Nat Clin Pract Cardiovasc Med. 2006;3(5):276-282.

[16] Wiesfeld AC, Hemels ME, Van Gelder IC. Genetic aspects of atrial fibrillation. Cardiovasc Res. 2005;67(3):414-418.

[17] Allessie MA, Bonke FIM, Schopman FJG. Circus movement in rabbit atrial muscle as a mechanism of tachycardia, II: the role of nonuniform recovery of excitability in the occurrence of unidirectional block as studied with multiple microelectrodes. Circ Res. 1976;39:168-177.

[18] Boineau JP, Schuessler RB, Brockus CW. Natural and evoked atrial flutter due to circus movement in dogs. Role of abnormal atrial pathways, slow conduction, nonuniform refractory period distribution and premature beats. Am J Cardiol. 1980;45:1167-1181.

[19] Olgin JE, Kalman JM, Lesh MD. Role of atrial endocardial structures as barriers to conduction during human type I atrial flutter: activation and entrainment mapping guided by intracardiac echocardiography. Circulation. 1995;92:1839-1848.

[20] Dittrich HC, Pearce LA, Hart RG. Left atrial diameter in nonvalvular atrial fibrillation: an echocardiographic study. Am Heart J. 1999;137:494-499.

[21] Marx J, Hockberger R, Walls R, editors. Rosen's Emergency Medicine-Concepts and Clinical Practice. 7th ed. Philadelphia: Mosby by Elsevier; 2010. 2731 p.

[22] Szabo Z, Kakuk G, Lorincz I. Effects of hemodialysis on maximum P wave duration and P wave dispersion. Nephrol Dial Transplant. 2002;17(9):1634-1638.

[23] Pall A, Czifra A, Sebestyen V, Szabo Z. Hemodiafiltration and hemodialysis differently affect P wave duration and dispersion on the surface electrocardiogram. Int Urol Nephrol. 2016;48(2):271-277.

[24] Hayashi H, Horie M. Biphasic P wave in inferior leads and the development of atrial fibrillation. J Arrhythm . 2015;31(6):376-380.

[25] Guntekin U, Gunes Y, Arslan S. P wave duration and dispersion in patients with hyperthyroidism and the short-term effects of antithyroid treatment. Indian Pacing Electrophysiol J. 2009;9(5):251-259.

[26] Aras D, Maden O, Korkmaz S. Simple electrocardiographic markers for the prediction of paroxysmal atrial fibrillation in hyperthyroidism. Int J Cardiol. 2005;99(1):59-64.

[27] Hashemi Jazi M, Amirpour A, Gharipour M. Predictive value of P wave duration and dispersion in post coronary artery bypass surgery atrial fibrillation. ARYA Atheroscler. 2012;8(2):59-62.

[28] Baspinar O, Sucu M, Kilinc M. P wave dispersion between transcatheter and surgical closure of secundum-type atrial septal defect in childhood. Cardiol Young. 2011;21(1): 15-18.

[29] Sievi NA, Clarenbach CF, Kohler M. Chronic obstructive pulmonary disease and cardiac repolarization: data from a randomized controlled trial. Respiration. 2016;91(4): 288-295.

[30] Sap F, Karatas Z, Karaarslan S. Dispersion durations of P wave and QT interval in children with congenital heart disease and pulmonary arterial hypertension. Pediatr Cardiol. 2013;34(3):591-596.

[31] Giacopelli D, Bourke JP, Langley P. Characteristics of the atrial repolarization phase of the ECG in paroxysmal atrial fibrillation patients and controls. Acta Cardiol. 2015;70(6): 672-677.

[32] Mendis SPP, Norrving B. Global Atlas on Cardiovascular Disease Prevention and Control. Section A, Chapter 1. [Internet]. World Health Organization 2011 Available: http://www.world-heart-federation.org/fileadmin/user_upload/documents/Publications/Global_CVD_Atlas.pdf. [Accessed: 2016.03.10].

[33] Jouven X, Desnos M, Ducimetiere P. Predicting sudden death in the population: the Paris Prospective Study I. Circulation. 1999;99:1978-1983.

[34] Friedlander Y, Siscovick DS, Cobb LA. Family history as a risk factor for primary cardiac arrest. Circulation. 1998;97:155-160.

[35] Dekker LR, Bezzina CR, Wilde AA. Familial sudden death is an important risk factor for primary ventricular fibrillation: a case-control study in acute myocardial infarction patients. Circulation. 2006;114:1140-1145.

[36] Bezzina CR, Pazoki R, Wilde AA. Genome-wide association study identifies a susceptibility locus at 21q21 for ventricular fibrillation in acute myocardial infarction. Nat Genet. 2010;42:688-691.

[37] Arking DE, Junttila MJ, Chugh SS. Identification of a sudden cardiac death susceptibility locus at 2q24.2 through genome-wide association in European ancestry individuals. PLoS Genet. 2011;7(6):e1002158. DOI: 10.1371/journal.pgen.1002158.

[38] Perk J, De Backer G, Zannad F. European guidelines on cardiovascular disease prevention in clinical practice (version 2012). The Fifth Joint Task Force of the European Society of Cardiology and Other Societies on Cardiovascular Disease Prevention in Clinical Practice (constituted by representatives of nine societies and by invited experts). Eur Heart J. 2012;33:1635-1701.

[39] Eckart RE, Shry EA, Stevenson WG. Sudden death in young adults: an autopsy-based series of a population undergoing active surveillance. J Am Coll Cardiol. 2011;58:1254-1261.

[40] Patton KK, Sotoodehnia N, Kronmal RA. N-terminal pro-B-type natriuretic peptide is associated with sudden cardiac death risk: the Cardiovascular Health Study. Heart Rhythm. 2011;8(2):228-233.

[41] Korngold EC, Januzzi JL, Albert CM. Amino-terminal pro-B type natriuretic peptide and hsCRP as predictors of sudden cardiac death among women. Circulation. 2009;119(22):2868-2876.

[42] Antzelevitch C, Dumaine R. Electrical heterogeneity in the heart: physiological, pharmacological and clinical implications. In: Fozzard HA, Solaro RJ, editors. The Cardiovascular System. 1st ed. New York: Oxford University Press; 2002. p. 654-692.

[43] Antzelevitch M. Cells in the human heart. Circ Res. 2010;106(5):815-817.

[44] Sicouri S, Antzelevitch C. Electrophysiologic characteristics of M cells in the canine left ventricular free wall. J Cardiovasc Electrophysiol. 1995;6:591-603.

[45] Liu DW, Antzelevitch C. Characteristics of the delayed rectifier current (IKr and IKs) in canine ventricular epicardial, midmyocardial and endocardial myocytes. A weaker IKs contributes to the longer action potential of the M cell. Circ Res. 1995;76:351-365.

[46] Pall A, Czifra A, Szabo Z. Pathophysiological and clinical approach to cirrhotic cardiomyopathy. J Gastrointestin Liver Dis. 2014;23(3):301-310.

[47] Malik M, Batchvarov VN. Measurement, interpretation and clinical potential of QT dispersion. J Am Coll Cardiol. 2000;36(6):1749.

[48] Salvi V, Karnad DR, Narula D. Comparison of 5 methods of QT interval measurements on electrocardiograms from a thorough QT/QTc study: effect on assay sensitivity and categorical outliers. J Eletrocardiol. 2011;44(2):96-104.

[49] Moss AJ. QTc prolongation and sudden cardiac death. The association is in the detail. J Am Coll Cardiol. 2006;47:368-369.

[50] Sovari AA, Assasdi R, Rottman JN. Long QT Syndrome [Internet]. [Updated: 2015.12.31.]. Available from: http://emedicine.medscape.com/article/157826-overview#a4 [Accessed: 2016.05.05].

[51] Davey P. QT interval and mortality from coronary artery disease. Prog Cardiovasc Dis. 2000;42:359-384.

[52] Lorincz I, Matyus J, Kakuk G. QT dispersion in patients with end-stage renal failure and during hemodialysis. J Am Soc Nephrol. 1999;10:1297-1302.

[53] Rossing P, Breum L, Parving HH. Prolonged QTc interval predicts mortality in patients with type diabetes mellitus. Diabet Med. 2001;18(3):199-205.

[54] Sawiczki PT, Dahne R, Berger M. Prolonged QT interval as a predictor of mortality in diabetic nephropathy. Diabetologia. 1996;39:77-81.

[55] Maule S, Veglio M, Perin PC. Autonomic neuropathy and QT interval in hemodialysed patients. Clin Auton Res. 2004;14:233-239.

[56] Yap YG, Camm J. Risk of torsades de pointes with non-cardiac drugs. Doctors need to be aware that many drugs can cause QT prolongation. BMJ. 2000;320(7243):1158-1159.

[57] Gilotra NA, Chow GV, Cingolani OH. Cardiac amyloidosis presenting with prolonged QT interval and recurrent polymorphic ventricular tachycardia. Tex Heart Inst J. 2013;40(2):193-195.

[58] Uyarel H, Uslu N, Dayi SU. QT dispersion in sarcoidosis. Chest. 2005;128(4):2619-2625.

[59] Fox DJ, Khattar RS. Carcinoid heart disease: presentation, diagnosis and management. Heart Br Card Soc. 2004;90(10):1224-1228.

[60] Lee NR, Park JH, Rhee KS. Acquired long QT syndrome and sudden cardiac death due to secondary hemochromatosis with multitransfusions for severe aplastic anaemia. Ann Hematol. 2008;87(11):933-935.

[61] Cardoso C, Salles G, Siqueira-Filho AG. Clinical determinants of increased QT dispersion in patients with diabetes mellitus. Int J Cardiol. 2001;79(2-3):253-262.

[62] Ishizaki F, Harada T, Nakamura S. Prolonged QTc intervals in Parkinson's disease–relation to sudden death and autonomic dysfunction. No To Shinkei. 1996;48(5): 443-448.

[63] Straus SM, Kors JA, De Bruin ML. Prolonged QTc interval and risk of sudden cardiac death in a population of older adults. J Am Coll Cardiol. 2006;47:362-367.

[64] Moss AJ. Measurement of the QT interval and the risk associated with QTc interval prolongation. Am J Cardiol. 1993;72(6):23B-25B.

[65] Szabo Z, Harangi M, Paragh G. Effect of hyperlipidemia on QT dispersion in patients without ischemic heart disease. Can J Cardiol. 2005;21(10):847-850.

[66] Barta K, Czifra A, Szabo Z. Hemodiafiltration beneficially affects QT interval duration and dispersion compared to hemodialysis. Clin Exp Nephrol. 2014;18(6):952-959.

[67] Berger RD, Kasper EK, Tomaselli GF. Beat-to-beat QT interval variability: novel evidence for repolarization lability in ischemic and nonischemic dilated cardiomyopathy. Circulation. 1997;96:1557-1565.

[68] Piccirillo G, Magnanti M, Matera S. Age and QT variability index during free breathing, controlled breathing and tilt in patients with chronic heart failure and healthy control subjects. Transl Res. 2006;148:72-78.

[69] Murabayashi T, Fetics B, Berger RD. Beat-to-beat QT interval variability associated with acute myocardial ischemia. J Electrocardiol. 2002;35:19-25.

[70] Piccirillo G, Germano G, Quaglione R. QT interval variability and autonomic control in hypertensive subjects with left ventricular hypertrophy. Clin Sci. 2002;102:363-371.

[71] Bilchick K, Viitasalo N, Oikarinen L. Temporal repolarization lability differences among genotyped patients with the long QT syndrome. Am J Cardiol. 2004;94:1312-1316.

[72] Yeragani VK, Pohl R, Srinivasan K. Increased QT variability in patients with panic disorder and depression. Psychiatry Res. 2000;93:225-235.

[73] Haikney MC, Zareba W, Gentlesk PJ. QT interval variability and spontaneous ventricular tachycardia or fibrillation in the Multicentre Automatic Defibrillator Implantation Trial (MADIT) II patients. J Am Coll Cardiol. 2004;44:1481-1487.

[74] Piccirillo G, Magri D, Matera S. QT variability strongly predicts sudden cardiac death in asymptomatic subjects with mild or moderate left ventricular systolic dysfunction: a prospective study. Eur Heart J. 2007;28:1344-1350.

[75] Yeragani VK, Pohl R, Igell G. Effect of posture and isoproterenol on beat-to-beat heart rate and QT variability. Neuropsychobiology. 2000;41:113-123.

[76] Starc V, Schlegel TT. Real-time multichannel system for beat-to-beat QT interval variability. J Electrocardiol. 2006;39(4):358-367.

[77] Boriani G, Biffi M, Martignani C. Short QT syndrome and arrhythmogenic cardiac diseases in the young: the challenge of implantable cardioverter defibrillator therapy for children. Eur Heart J. 2006;27(20):2382-2384.

[78] Wolpert C, Schimpf R, Dumaine R. Further insights into the effect of quinidine in short QT syndrome caused by a mutation in HERG. J Cardiovasc Electrophysiol. 2005;16:54-58.

[79] Gaita F, Giustetto C, Wolpert C. Short QT syndrome: pharmacological treatment. J Am Coll Cardiol. 2004;43(8):1494-1499.

[80] Schimpf R, Bauersfeld U, Wolpert C. Short QT syndrome: successful prevention of sudden cardiac death in an adolescent by implantable cardioverter-defibrillator treatment for primary prophylaxis. Heart Rhythm. 2005;2:416-417.

[81] Derval N, Shah A, Jais P. Definition of early repolarization: a tug of war. Circulation. 2011;124(20):2185-2186.

[82] Gussak I, Antzelevitch C. Early repolarization syndrome: a decade of progress. J Electrocardiol. 2013;46(2):110-113.

[83] Yan GX, Antzelevitch C. Cellular basis for the electrocardiographic J wave. Circulation. 1996;93:372.

[84] Antzelevitch C. Genetic, molecular and cellular mechanisms underlying the J wave syndromes. Circ J. 2012;76:1054.

[85] Noseworthy PA, Tikkanen JT, Porthan K. The early repolarization pattern in the general population clinical correlates and heritability. J Am Coll Cardiol. 2011;57:2284.

[86] Haissaguerre M, Derval N, Sacher F. Sudden cardiac arrest associated with early repolarization. N Engl J Med. 2008;358:2016.

[87] Wellens HJ. Early repolarization revisited. N Engl J Med. 2008;358:2063.

[88] Nan GB, Kim YH, Antzelevitch C. Augmentation of J waves and electrical storms in patients with early repolarization. N Engl J Med. 2008;358:2078.

[89] Wilde AA, Friedman PA, Ackerman MJ, editors. Electrical Diseases of the Heart: Genetics, Mechanisms, Treatment, Prevention. 1st ed. London: Springer Verlag; 2008. 968 p.

[90] Junttila MJ, Sager SJ, Myerburg RJ. Clinical significance of variance of J points and J waves: early repolarization patterns and risk. Eur Heart J. 2012;33:2639.

[91] Antzelevitch C, Yan GX. J wave syndromes. Heart Rhythm. 2010;7:549.

[92] Watanabe H, Makiyama T, Koyama T. High prevalence of early repolarization in short QT syndrome. Heart Rhythm. 2010;7:647.

[93] Nam GB, Ko KH, Kim J. Mode of onset of ventricular fibrillation in patients with early repolarization pattern vs Brugada syndrome. Eur Heart J. 2010;31:330.

[94] Rosso R, Glikson E, Belhassen B. Distinguishing "benign" from "malignant" early repolarization: the value of the ST-segment morphology. Heart Rhythm. 2012;9:225.

[95] Tikkanen JT, Wichmann V, Junttila MJ. Association of early repolarization and sudden cardiac death during an acute coronary event. Circ Arrhythm Electrophysiol. 2012;5:714.

[96] Myojo T, Sato N, Nimura A. Recurrent ventricular fibrillation related to hypokalemia in early repolarization syndrome. Pacing Clin Electrophysiol. 2012;35:e234.

[97] Tikkanen JT, Junttila MJ, Anttonen O. Early repolarization electrocardiographic phenotypes associated with favourable long-term outcome. Circulation. 2011;123:2666.

[98] Pei J, Li N, Gao Y. The J wave and fragmented QRS complexes in inferior leads associated with sudden cardiac death in patients with chronic heart failure. Europace. 2012;14:1180.

[99] Haissaguerre M, Sacher F, Nogami A. Characteristics of recurrent ventricular fibrillation associated with inferolateral early repolarization: role of drug therapy. J Am Coll Cardiol. 2009;53:612.

[100] Tsuchiya T, Ashikaga K, Arita M. Prevention of ventricular fibrillation by cilostazol, an oral phosphodiesterase inhibitor, in a patient with Brugada syndrome. J Cardiovasc Electrophysiol. 2002;13:698.

[101] Narayan S. T wave alternans and the susceptibility to ventricular arrhythmias. J Am Coll Cardiol. 2006;47:269-281.

[102] Lorincz I. Microvolt T wave alternans. Cardiol Hung. 2008;38:C50-55.

[103] Chow T, Kereiakes DJ, Chan PS. Microvolt T wave alternans identifies patients with ischemic cardiomyopathy who benefit from implantable cardioverter defibrillator therapy. J Am Coll Cardiol. 2007;49(1):50-58.

[104] Huikuri HV, Raatikainen MJ, Moerch-Joergensen R. Prediction of fatal or near-fatal cardiac arrhythmia events in patients with depressed left ventricular function after an acute myocardial infarction. Eur Heart J. 2009;30:689-698.

[105] Bloomfield DM, Steinman RC, Bigger JT. Microvolt T wave alternans distinguishes between patients likely and patients not-likely to benefit from implanted cardiac defibrillator therapy: a solution to the Multicentre Automatic Defibrillator Implantation Trial. Circulation. 2004;110:1885-1889.

[106] Nieminen T, Lehtimaki T, Kahonen M. T wave alternans predicts mortality in a population undergoing a clinically indicated exercise test. Eur Heart J. 2007;28(19): 2332-2337.

[107] Verrier R, Klingenheben T, Malik M. Microvolt T wave alternans: physiological basis, methods of measurement and clinical utility: consensus guideline by International Society for Holter and Non-invasive Electrocardiology. J Am Coll Cardiol. 2011;58:1309-1324.

[108] Turitto G, Caref EB, El-Attar G. Optimal target heart rate for exercise-induced T wave alternans. Ann Noninvasive Electrocardiol. 2001;6:123-128.

[109] Bloomfield DM, Hohnloser SH, Cohen RJ. Interpretation and classification of microvolt T wave alternans tests. J Cardiovasc Electrophysiol. 2002;13:502-512.

[110] Rosenbaum DS, Jackson LE, Cohen RJ. Electrical alternans and vulnerability to ventricular arrhythmias. N Engl J Med. 1994;330:235-241.

[111] Kors JA, Ritsema van Eck HJ, van Herpen G. The meaning of the Tp-Te interval and its diagnostic value. J Electrocardiol. 2008;41:575-580.

[112] Haarmark C, Hansen PR, Vedel-Larsen E. The prognostic value of the T peak-T end interval in patients undergoing primary percutaneous coronary intervention for ST-segment elevation myocardial infarction. J Electrocardiol. 2009;42:555-560.

[113] Haarmark C, Graff C, Kanters JK. Reference values of electrocardiogram repolarization variables in a healthy population. J Electrocardiol. 2010;43(1):31-39.

[114] Kilicaslan F, Tokatli A, Ozdag F. Tp-e interval, Tp-e/QT ratio and Tp-e/QTc ratio are prolonged in patients with moderate and severe obstructive sleep apnea. Pacing Clin Electrophysiol. 2012;35:966-972.

[115] Topilski I, Rogowski O, Rosso R. The morphology of the QT interval predict torsades de pointes during acquired bradyarrhythmias. J Am Coll Cardiol. 2007;49:320-328.

[116] Shimizu M, Ino H, Okeie K. T peak to T end interval may be a better predictor of high-risk patients with hypertrophic cardiomyopathy associated with a cardiac troponin I mutation than QT dispersion. Clin Cardiol. 2002;25:335-339.

[117] Yamaguchi M, Shimizu M, Ino H. T wave peak-to-end interval and QT dispersion in acquired long QT syndrome: a new index for arrhythmogenicity. Clin Sci. 2003;105:671-676.

[118] Porthan K, Viitasalo M, Oikarinen L. Predictive value of electrocardiographic T wave morphology parameters and T wave peak to T wave end interval for sudden cardiac death in the general population. Circ Arrhythm Electrophysiol. 2013;6(4):690-696.

Chapter 3

Echocardiography and Other Noninvasive Imaging Techniques in the Selection and Management of Patients with Cardiac Resynchronization Therapy

Silvia Lupu, Lucia Agoston-Coldea and
Dan Dobreanu

Additional information is available at the end of the chapter

http://dx.doi.org/10.5772/64594

Abstract

Cardiac resynchronization therapy has become a widely used procedure for the treatment of patients with heart failure and severely impaired systolic function who associate left bundle branch block and remain symptomatic, in New York Heart Association II to IV functional class, despite maximum tolerated medical therapy. Imaging evaluation of these patients is complex, aiming to provide an accurate and extensive assessment before and after implantation, although a standardized protocol is yet to be implemented. Extensive research has been conducted to assess the ability of different imaging techniques and parameters to identify and quantify mechanical dyssynchrony, assess myocardial remodeling, provide prognostic information, or help guide lead placement and pacing parameters optimization in this category of patients. For these purposes, ultrasound-based imaging techniques, as well as cardiac magnetic resonance imaging, multislice cardiac computed tomography and nuclear ventriculography have been and are currently used, for research, as well as for clinical purposes. The aim of the current paper was to provide some insights into the imaging assessment of candidates and patients who have undergone cardiac resynchronization therapy.

Keywords: cardiac resynchronization therapy, mechanical dyssynchrony, echocardiography, cardiac magnetic resonance imaging

1. The role of imaging techniques in assessing patients with cardiac resynchronization therapy: general considerations

During the last two decades, cardiac resynchronization therapy (CRT) has become a valuable therapeutic procedure for patients with heart failure (HF) due to dilated cardiomyopathy (DCM), improving prognosis, symptoms, quality of life, and ventricular function [1–6]. Current ESC guidelines on cardiac pacing and CRT recommend the procedure as a class I indication in HF patients with left bundle branch block (LBBB), QRS width ≥120 ms, and left ventricle ejection fraction (LVEF) ≤35%, who remain in New York Heart Association (NYHA) functional class II, III, and ambulatory IV despite optimal medical therapy [7].

According to these guidelines, patient selection mainly relies on clinical and electrocardiogram (ECG) characteristics, while the role of echocardiography is limited to determining LVEF. Despite this rather frugal approach, extensive research involving echocardiography and other imaging techniques has been conducted over the last few years, with the purpose of improving the selection and management of CRT candidates. Since CRT is still a rather expensive procedure [8–10], and not entirely risk-free [11], even if performed by experienced electrophysiologists, efforts were made to establish sound patient selection criteria, as well as to find accurate methods, techniques, algorithms, and tools for prognosis assessment and pacing optimization. As a consequence, a plethora of ultrasound imaging parameters for cardiac mechanics and dyssynchrony evaluation have been developed, and expert consensus statements were released [12, 13] in order to help clinicians choose the best therapeutic strategy.

Early studies on mechanical dyssynchrony parameters seemed somewhat promising. For instance, Yu et al. attempted to prove that CRT was beneficial in patients who had echocardiographic evidence of mechanical dyssynchrony, even if they had narrow QRS complexes. In their research, results were quite spectacular, raising hope that CRT indications might extend beyond the recommendations of the guidelines [14]. Regrettably, the results of the much larger Echocardiography Guided Cardiac Resynchronization Therapy (Echo-CRT) trial contradicted these findings, highlighting the deleterious effects of CRT in patients with evidence of mechanical dyssynchrony at echocardiography and narrow QRS complexes (QRS complex duration <130 ms) [15].

In addition to that, the Predictors of Response to CRT (PROSPECT) trial tested the sensitivity and specificity of 12 different echocardiography mechanical dyssynchrony parameters, yielding disappointing results. The sensitivity and specificity of the studied parameters were either too low or discordant, and, as consequence, none of them was acknowledged as being clinically useful [16]. Sanderson JE challenged the results of the PROSPECT trial, stating that this trial was rather a study of error and did not provide an accurate assessment of the reproducibility and clinical value of mechanical dyssynchrony parameters; according to this author, the results of the PROSPECT trial were justified by the fact that participating centers were more focused on electrophysiology and lacked the technical possibilities and/or the expertise for an appropriate echocardiographic assessment [17]. Bax and Gorcsan also found flaws in the PROSPECT study, pointing out that among selected patients, 20.2% had an LVEF >35% while 37.8% had end-diastolic dimensions <65 mm, and were therefore unlikely to develop spectacular reverse remodeling since there was little remodeling and systolic function impairment to begin with; in addition to that, they brought up technical issues, such as the fact that ultrasound machines that have been used for the study came from three different vendors, while also suggesting that the high interobserver variability in some parameters might have been justified by the lack of a systematic examination protocol [18].

As a consequence, there is currently not enough proof to either fully embrace or dismiss myocardial dyssynchrony parameters. In fact, some studies have suggested that the evaluation of cardiac mechanics by echocardiography may have quite an important role in optimizing pacing parameters [19], choosing the most appropriate site for lead placement [20], and assessing patient prognosis [21], particularly if advanced ultrasound imaging techniques, such as speckle tracking, are used.

Data on the preferences of clinical practitioners are currently scarce. In a relatively recent European survey, 68% of physicians in the responding centers declared that they only relied on guideline criteria for selecting CRT patients, but 66% acknowledged using echocardiography for pacing parameters optimization. Among these, 37% stated they used tissue Doppler imaging, 20% used speckle tracking-based techniques, and only 10% used three-dimensional echocardiography [22], with the latter two being less used, probably due to limited availability.

Besides that, it is important to remember that echocardiography examination of patients with CRT is not limited to mechanical dyssynchrony assessment and must include a thorough study of left ventricular (LV) systolic and diastolic dysfunction, mitral regurgitation, right chamber structure and function, or the possibility of pulmonary hypertension. All these topics will be further discussed in this chapter.

Beyond echocardiography, other imaging techniques, such as multislice detector computer tomography (MDCT) or cardiac magnetic resonance imaging (CMRI), can be very useful in the management of patients who are candidates for CRT. Evaluation by MDCT, for instance, can safely exclude significant coronary artery disease [23] and accurately describe coronary veins anatomy [24], which can facilitate lead placement. CMRI provides the advantages of very accurate LVEF determination, the ability to identify the extent and location of fibrosis by late gadolinium enhancement, and an extensive study of myocardial deformation and dyssynchrony by tagging techniques [25].

2. Echocardiography parameters for the assessment of patients with CRT

2.1. Examination of the left chambers. LV size, systolic function and diastolic function. Left atrial size and function

Echocardiographic assessment of left chamber dimensions and function in patients who are candidates for CRT or have already been submitted to the procedure is essential.

Conventional bidimensional echocardiography can be used for measuring LV end-diastolic (EDD) and end-systolic (ESD) diameters and, preferably, LV volumes, assessed by the biplane Simpson's modified method and indexed to body surface area [26]. To enhance the quality of endocardial delineation, contrast agents can also be used, particularly if an extremely accurate evaluation of regional myocardial motion is also desired [27, 28], while three-dimensional echocardiography increases the accuracy of volumetric measurements by reducing errors due to the foreshortening of the LV [26].

LV dimensions were previously shown to predict the response to CRT. In the Multicenter Automatic Defibrillator Trial-CRT (MADIT-CRT) for instance, an LV end-diastolic volume (LVEDV) indexed to body surface area (BSA) ≥125 mL/m^2 was associated with a favorable response to CRT [29].

In a substudy of the Multisite Stimulation in Cardiomyopathies (MUSTIC) trial, EDD and EDS were shown to decrease 3 months after CRT (7.3 ± 0.8–6.8 ± 0.8 cm, $p < 0.001$, and 6.2 ± 0.8–5.9 ± 0.8 cm, $p < 0.05$, respectively), with further reduction after 12 months since device implantation (by 8.4 ± 7.8 and 8.8 ± 7.8 mm, respectively, both $p < 0.001$), with better results in patients with idiopathic DCM vs. patients with ischemic cardiomyopathy (8.9 and 9.8 mm, $p < 0.01$) [30]. The Multicenter InSync Randomized Clinical Evaluation (MIRACLE) Study also yielded significant reductions in EDD and ESD, as well as in LV mass at 6-month follow-up [31]. By contrast, in the Multicenter InSync ICD Randomized Clinical Evaluation (MIRACLE ICD) trial, no significant changes were recorded in neither LV dimensions, nor in LVEF, despite improved quality of life scores and NYHA functional class [32]. However, most of the patients in this trial had ischemic cardiomyopathy (64% vs. 36% with idiopathic DCM in the CRT-D group and 75.8% vs. 26.4% in the implanted cardioverter-defibrillator group) [32], which is very likely to have confounded results, since ischemic etiology [29, 33, 34] and the presence of scar tissue [35] and non-viable myocardium [36] are known predictors of limited response to CRT and reverse remodeling.

As previously mentioned, LVEF is the single echocardiographic parameter that has been accepted as a CRT patients' selection criterion in current guidelines [7], and the cutoff value has been established at 35%. LVEF has proved to be one of the most important parameters for assessing the success of CRT in all major clinical trials, as well as smaller studies that addressed this issue [37–44]. In MADIT-CRT despite more reduction in LV dimensions in the LVEF >30% group, clinical outcomes were similar in patients with lower LVEF [45]. A subanalysis of data from the REVERSE trial revealed similar extents of reverse remodeling and clinical benefits in patients who had LVEF <30% vs. LVEF >30%, which may be justified by the fact that, unlike patients included in the MADIT-CRT trial, patients in REVERSE only had mild HF [38].

Interestingly, responders to CRT [38] and particularly super-responders in whom the LVEF becomes >50% [46] have an excellent prognosis, with a reduced number of ventricular tachyarrhythmias and good clinical progression at 2.2 years; the authors concluded that, in such patients, switching off the ICD function to prevent inadequate therapies from the device might be considered.

Highlighting regional kinetic abnormalities by echocardiography could also be an important issue, considering the fact that it may help identify patients with ischemic DCM, which is associated with poorer outcomes after CRT and less reverse remodeling [29–36, 47].

Moreover, diastolic function assessment is not less important in this category of patients, since it was shown to improve after CRT, in parallel with the LVEF [47] and particularly in responders [48]. Diastolic dysfunction has been previously assessed by either conventional echocardiography, including parameters such as transmitral flow waves velocities and E-wave deceleration time, diastolic myocardial velocities, the E/e' ratio, diastolic filling duration, or isovolumic relaxation time, evaluated by pulsed wave and tissue Doppler imaging [48, 49], or advanced techniques, such as speckle tracking [50, 51].

During the last decade, left atrium (LA) dimensions, particularly LA indexed volume (LAVI) [52] and LA function, have become an important part of LV diastolic function assessment and studies exploring the use of these parameters in CRT patients have recently been published [53–59]. For instance, the MADIT-CRT trial showed significant reductions in LAVI in CRT-D vs. ICD-only patients [53]. Major improvements in LAVI 3–6 months after CRT have also been reported by Yu [54], Aksoy [55], and D'Andrea et al., the latter also showing better results in patients with idiopathic DCM, by comparison with ischemic DCM patients [56]. In addition to that, MADIT-CRT results highlighted the value of LAVI <40 ml/m^2 as a predictor of clinical response [29], which is also endorsed by Yu et al. who reported lower LAVI in responders [54]. In both the MADIT-CRT trial [53] and in the research by Kloosterman et al., increased preimplantation LAVI was associated with increased risk of HF progression and death, independently of LV volumes [57]. Other studies approached LA myocardial strain assessment in patients with CRT, suggesting its prognostic value in assessing the risk for atrial fibrillation development [58] or the response to CRT [59].

2.2. Right ventricular size and function evaluation: pulmonary hypertension assessment by echocardiography

Although the assessment of left chambers is essential in patients who are candidates for CRT or have undergone the procedure already, right chamber evaluation should not be overlooked. Echocardiography-based studies on the topic are scarce, since bidimensional ultrasound imaging has to overcome the obstacles posed by the complex anatomy of the right ventricle (RV). Volumetric measurements can be flawed due to gross geometrical assumptions, since the anatomic shape of the RV hardly resembles any geometric figure, and trabeculations of the RV free wall can hinder adequate tracings of myocardial borders. Also, normal values have not been firmly established for some right chamber parameters, such as the right atrium (RA) volume, which currently remains, however, the preferred parameter for assessing RA size [60], replacing RA area [26].

Despite these caveats, right chamber evaluation by echocardiography, as well as pulmonary artery pressure estimation following current guidelines [61], can and should be performed in CRT patients, as evidence regarding these parameters has started to accumulate, and right chamber dilatation has been shown to associate with higher mortality in HF patients [62].

Data from radionuclide ventriculography studies suggest that impaired RV systolic function, with RV ejection fraction ≤20%, is an independent predictor of mortality and hospitalization due to HF [63], and that poorer systolic function is associated with a lower response rate after CRT [65], accordingly, the evaluation of right chambers may have a certain role in selecting patients for CRT. Moreover, increased RA area and impaired myocardial deformation of the AD were proven to be negative predictors of response to CRT, as were ischemic DCM and low intraventricular asynchrony [65].

In the MADIT-CRT trial, RV ejection fraction was considerably improved, and patients with the highest values had the lowest rate of adverse events at one year [66].

2.3. Mitral regurgitation assessment

Mitral regurgitation is another target for echocardiographic assessment in chronic HF patients, since it has been shown to alter prognosis [67, 68]. In DCM, mitral regurgitation is usually functional, developing as a consequence of mitral annulus dilatation, but mostly due to the change of balance between tethering forces, pulling the leaflets towards the LV, and the forces that favor normal closure of the mitral valve. Tethering forces are amplified by LV remodeling and dilatation which result in an increased sphericity index and papillary muscle displacement. In addition to that, the normal closure of the mitral valve is impaired by the reduction of myocardial contractility and by ventricular contraction dyssynchrony [69], particularly in the presence of LBBB [70].

Quantifying mitral regurgitation in these patients can be challenging, since the regurgitation jet is often eccentric and should include measurements of vena contracta, the tenting area, as well as of the area of regurgitant orifice and the regurgitation volume by the proximal isovelocity surface area (PISA) method, when it is feasible. The extensive evaluation of mitral regurgitation should be completed by a thorough evaluation of the ventricular function and the asynchrony of contraction [71].

One study by Kanzaki et al. revealed the significant reduction of mitral regurgitation immediately after CRT [70], which was most likely caused by contraction synchrony recovery. Similar results have been reported by Breithardt et al. [72]. Moreover, LV reverse remodeling and diminished tethering forces were shown to contribute to reducing mitral regurgitation on the long term [73]. As far as short-term evolution is concerned, more data emerged supporting mitral regurgitation dependency on ventricular dyssynchrony, as one study proved its reduction after CRT, but also highlighted the fact that switching off the CRT device aggravates the regurgitation even if the event occurs six months after implantation [74]. A similar, although smaller study, also reported the reversal of mitral regurgitation, suggesting that CRT should be continued indefinitely [75]. For these reasons, it is reasonable to take into account mitral regurgitation reduction as a criterion for procedure success, particularly since it is associated with clinical response [76–77].

Mitral regurgitation assessment should be done carefully and accurately in non-responders, since some of these might benefit from further interventional treatment by MitraClip, which was shown to reduce symptoms and promote LV reverse remodeling [78], or by surgical mitral annuloplasty [79].

2.4. Dyssynchrony parameters evaluation

2.4.1. Clinical utility

Cardiac mechanics assessment by echocardiography is currently considered a challenge, and research in the field has been extensive and endorsed by newly emerging techniques. However, despite all research efforts, none of the explored dyssynchrony parameters had proved to be solid and reproducible enough for predicting the response to CRT, and, thus, for helping in patients' selection. Data from the CARE-HF study supported the use of echocardiographic dyssynchrony parameters, showing that patients who had altered values responded better to CRT [80], and had more reverse remodeling [81, 82]. In addition to that, Penicka et al., for instance, proved that both the parameters for interventricular and intraventricular dyssynchrony, assessed by tissue Doppler, were predictors of reverse remodeling and functional recovery of the LV [83].

As previously mentioned, the PROSPECT trial challenged the accuracy of echocardiographic dyssynchrony parameters [16] and was challenged in its turn by some authors [17, 18].

More recent and elaborate techniques motivated researchers to go further in the attempt to find the optimal parameters for dyssynchrony quantification. Suffoletto et al. explored the advantages of the speckle tracking technique, showing that radial dyssynchrony assessed by this method predicted the response to CRT on long and short term [84]. The evaluation of global strain [85], as well as the evaluation of longitudinal, circumferential, and radial strain by tissue Doppler, also provided encouraging results [86]. However, these methods are costly, not available in many clinical centers and time-consuming, requiring strenuous offline analysis.

More available methods, such as tissue Doppler, are, unfortunately, hindered by lower reproducibility in DCM patients, by comparison with normal individuals, probably due to the complex contraction movements of the dilated heart and the method's lack of standardization [87].

The controversy regarding the echocardiographic evaluation of ventricular dyssynchrony extends over their use for optimizing pacing parameters in CRT patients. Some electrophysiologists prefer out-of-the-box settings and only adjust delays if the patients are non-responders. This attitude is endorsed by the quite large SMART-AV (The SmartDelay Determined AV Optimization: A Comparison to Other AV Delay Methods Used in Cardiac Resynchronization Therapy) trial in which 1014 patients were enrolled; in this study, the ECG-based SmartDelay optimization algorithm, as well as echocardiography, did not show any benefit for optimization by comparison with the out-of-the box approach in which a standard atrio-ventricular delay of 120 msec was established [88]. Similar results emerged from smaller studies, such as the one by Sawhney et al. who compared the effects of pacing with out-of-the-box delays with those chosen after Doppler echocardiography, revealing quality of life and functional NYHA class improvement, without significant changes in LVEF and 6-minute walk test distance [89]. In a larger study, on 215 patients, delay adjustments only provided additional benefit in a low number of patients [90]. Vidal et al. also approached this issue, reporting minimal benefits in patients with optimized parameters [91]. A retrospective analysis of multicentric trials endorses the use of adaptive CRT, based on ambulatory measurements of intrinsic conduction, in addition to conventional echocardiographic assessment, for optimization [92].

Although there is no consensus regarding the correct approach on the necessity and benefit of optimization, or the appropriate means to perform it, American guidelines for the echocardiographic assessment of CRT patients released by the American Society of Echocardiography, endorsed by the Heart Rhythm Society, recommends considering echocardiography for pacing parameters adjustment [12]. Accordingly, for adjustment of atrio-ventricular delays, the guidelines suggest the evaluation of the transmitral flow by pulsed wave Doppler, based on the premises that a long delay can lead to E and A wave fusion, diastolic mitral regurgitation, and exposes the patient to the risk of native conduction that may lead to loss of resynchronization. On the other hand, an abnormally short atrio-ventricular delay can result in a truncated A wave, as a consequence of premature closure of the mitral valve [12]. The Ritter method and the iterative method are suggested as optimization algorithms [12, 92, 93]. For ventriculo-ventricular delay adjustment, the guidelines recommend measurements of the aortic velocity time integral after modifying the delay by 20 ms, starting with the maximal pre-excitation of the LV [12].

For adjusting both delays, a fast algorithm was suggested—QuickOpt—available on St Jude Medical devices, that was proved inferior to echocardiographic evaluation [94].

2.4.2. Cardiac mechanics evaluation parameters

Echocardiographic dyssynchrony evaluation protocols may differ from center to center according to logistics, the available ultrasound machines and softwares, as well as the experience of the examiners and the number of hospitalized CRT patients. Since dyssynchrony evaluation methods are not perfectly standardized, the choice of assessment parameters can be influenced by the examiner's opinion or the particularities of the case.

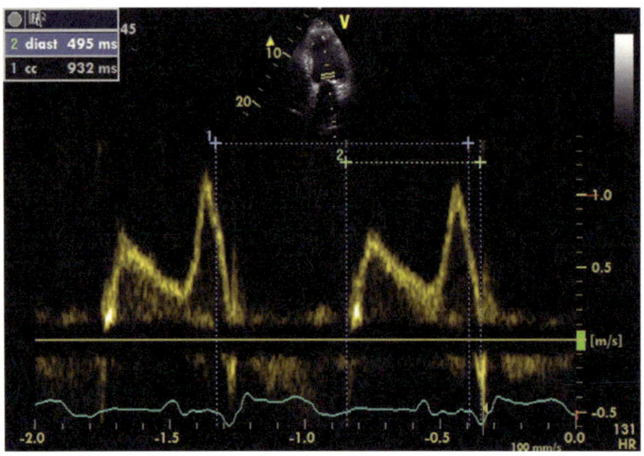

Figure 1. Transmitral flow assessment. Measurements of diastole and cardiac cycle duration.

Atrio-ventricular dyssynchrony criteria [12, 13]:

- duration of diastole—duration of diastolic filling measured on the pulsed wave Doppler transmitral flow, from the onset of the E wave until the end of the A wave, at a sweep speed of 100 cm/s;

http://dx.doi.org/10.5772/64594

- duration of the cardiac cycle—measured using identical tags on successive QRS complexes;
- duration of diastole to cardiac cycle ratio; values <40% suggest atrio-ventricular dyssynchrony (**Figure 1**);
- assessment of fusion of the E and A waves on the transmitral flow or the truncated A wave [12, 13].

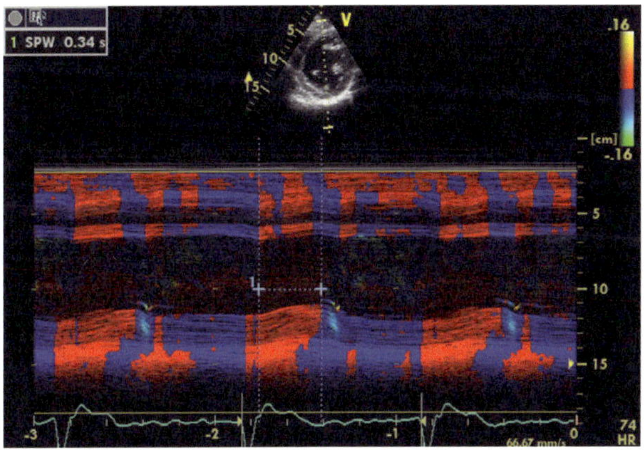

Figure 2. Septal-to-posterior wall motion delay measurement, using color M-mode imaging, from the parasternal short-axis view at papillary muscle level.

Intraventricular dyssynchrony criteria

- SPWMD (septal-to-posterior wall motion delay)—the delay between the maximal contraction of the posterior wall and the maximal contraction of the septum or anterior wall (**Figure 2**); SPWMD can be measured using either M-mode, or, preferably, color M-mode, from the parasternal short-axis view; values ≥130 msec suggest intraventricular dyssynchrony [12, 13]; Pitzalis et al. demonstrated the utility of this parameter as a predictor of remodeling after CRT [95].
- Q-MI: the time interval from the onset of the QRS complex to the onset on the transmitral flow, assessed by pulsed wave Doppler at a sweep speed of 100 cm/s [12, 96];
- Q-PW: the time interval from QRS onset until the maximum contraction of the LV posterior wall, evaluated by color M-mode, at a sweep speed of 100 cm/s [12, 96];
- The (Q-PW)—(Q-Mi) difference—negative values are considered normal (in the absence of intraventricular dyssynchrony, the maximum contraction of the LV posterior wall occurs before mitral valve opening) (**Figure 3**) [96];
- Aortic pre-ejection time (A-PEP)—measured from the onset of the QRS complex until the onset of the aortic flow, evaluated by pulsed wave Doppler from the apical five-chamber view at a sweep speed of 100 cm/s; values above 140 ms suggest intraventricular dyssynchrony [96];

- Measurements of delayed mechanical activity by tissue Doppler analysis of opposing walls motion (interventricular septum, lateral wall; anterior wall, inferior wall) using the apical two- and four-chamber views (**Figure 4**); measurements should be performed on minimum 3–5 cardiac cycles and in post-expiratory apnea; differences ≥65 ms predict the acute hemodynamic response post-CRT [83, 97, 98];
- Spectral tissue Doppler assessment of contraction delay between opposing LV walls; images are acquired from the apical two- and four-chamber views; the sample volume is placed 1 cm below the mitral annular plane, guided by color tissue Doppler, with narrow sector; the time interval from the onset of the QRS complex until maximal systolic myocardial motion (peak of the S-wave) is measured, at a sweep speed of 100 cm/s; maximum differences ≥65 ms and the septum to lateral wall difference ≥65 ms suggest intraventricular dyssynchrony [98, 99]. Although the method is widely available, it is hindered by the fact that analysis of the delays is performed in different cardiac cycles and is strictly limited to the basal area of LV walls; moreover, the method is time-consuming and measurements are performed online, being, thus, dependant, on translational movements of the heart. All these obstacles may result in low accuracy measurements.
- Tissue synchronization imaging

  Tissue synchronization imaging is performed by the offline analysis of bidimensional images from the apical four-, three- and two-chambers views with overlaid color tissue Doppler, using specialized software. To acquire appropriate images, pulse repetition frequencies, color gain, and sector depth and width should be optimized, to ensure the highest frame rate frequency [100].

  Tissue synchronization imaging allows the automatic and color-coded calculus of the time interval from QRS onset until maximum myocardial velocity in different points. The algorithm uses as reference points the onset of the QRS complex, either automatically identified by the echocardiograph, or manually adjusted by the examiner, as well as the onset and end point of the pulsed wave Doppler recording of the aortic flow, as surrogates of systole beginning and ending. The objective of the analysis is to assess post-systolic myocardial shortening in 2, 6, or 12 segments [101, 102]. The method requires a high degree of training, dedicated acquisition and analysis software, which is seldom available in many centers and is time-consuming. Yu et al. reported low interobserver and intra-observer variability of 5.9% and 4.2%, respectively [100]; however, in their study, measurements were most likely performed by highly skilled echocardiographers and might not be reproducible by less experienced examiners.
- Septal flash

  In the presence of LBBB, the interventricular septum has a particular two-phase active contraction pattern, with a leftward motion occurring in the pre-ejection phase, followed by a second excursion later in ventricular systole [103]. This particular inward/outward movement called septal flash (**Figure 5**) is visible by conventional bidimensional imaging, but is better assessed by M-mode or, preferably, by color M-mode, from the parasternal long-axis view [104].

http://dx.doi.org/10.5772/64594

Although apparently simplistic, as it does not require elaborate measurements or advanced technology, septal flash assessment is reliable, reproducible, and a proven good predictor of response to CRT [104], even in patients with atrial fibrillation [105] in which other imaging mechanical dyssynchrony parameters may sometimes be difficult to assess.

- Apical rocking

Apical rocking refers to the transverse movement of the apex, due to LV enlargement and asynchronous contraction of the interventricular septum and LV lateral wall. It can be visually assessed from the apical four-chamber view or can be quantified using specialized software and imaging techniques. The latter has proven superior to classical parameters of dyssynchrony quantification in terms of identifying dyssynchrony and predicting the response to CRT [106, 107].

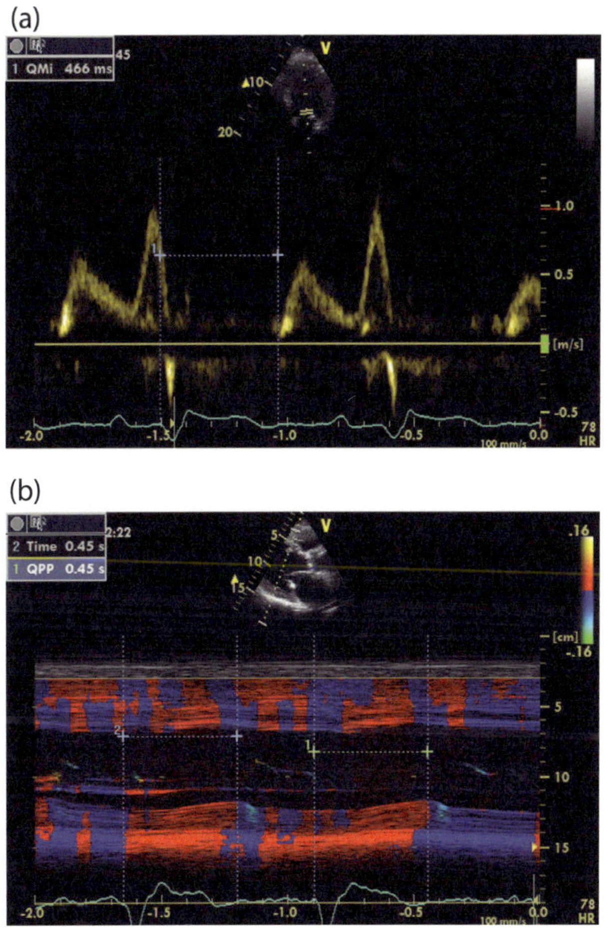

Figure 3. Assessment of left intraventricular dyssynchrony. (a) Q-Mi measurement, on the pulsed wave Doppler transmitral flow. Q-PW measurement, using M-mode, from the parasternal long-axis view.

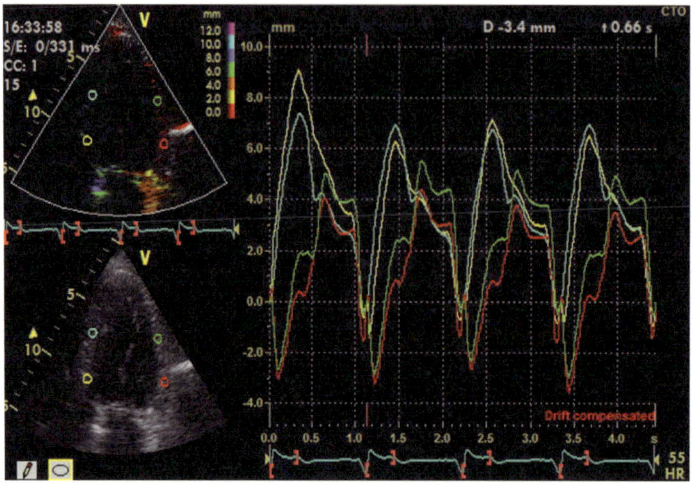

Figure 4. Assessment of left intraventricular dyssynchrony by color tissue Doppler, from the apical four-chamber view. Maximum contraction of the left ventricle lateral wall is significantly delayed by comparison with septal contraction.

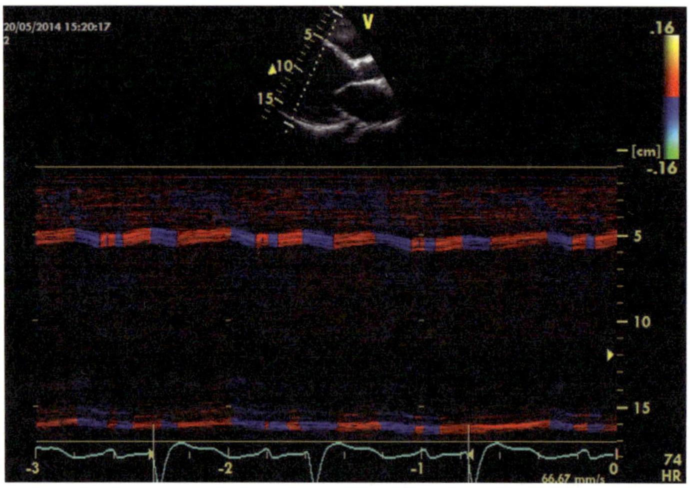

Figure 5. Septal flash evaluation by color M-mode from the parasternal long-axis view.

Interventricular dyssynchrony criteria

- A-PEP—aortic pre-ejection time, measured from QRS onset until the onset of the aortic flow analyzed by pulsed wave Doppler, with the sample volume placed in the LV outflow tract in the apical five-chamber view; values ≥140 ms are considered a criterion of intraventricular dyssynchrony [96].
- P-PEP—pulmonary pre-ejection time, measured from the onset of the QRS complex to the onset on the pulmonary artery flow measured from the RV outflow tract, in the parasternal

http://dx.doi.org/10.5772/64594

short-axis view; for measuring both parameters, as well as all other time-related measurements, a sweep-speed of 100 cm/s should be used;

- Interventricular motion delay—the delay between the contraction of the RV and the LV, assessed by the difference in the two pre-ejection times; values ≥40 msec suggest interventricular dyssynchrony (**Figure 6**); Ghio et al. suggested an association between IVMD and ventricular remodeling after CRT [81].

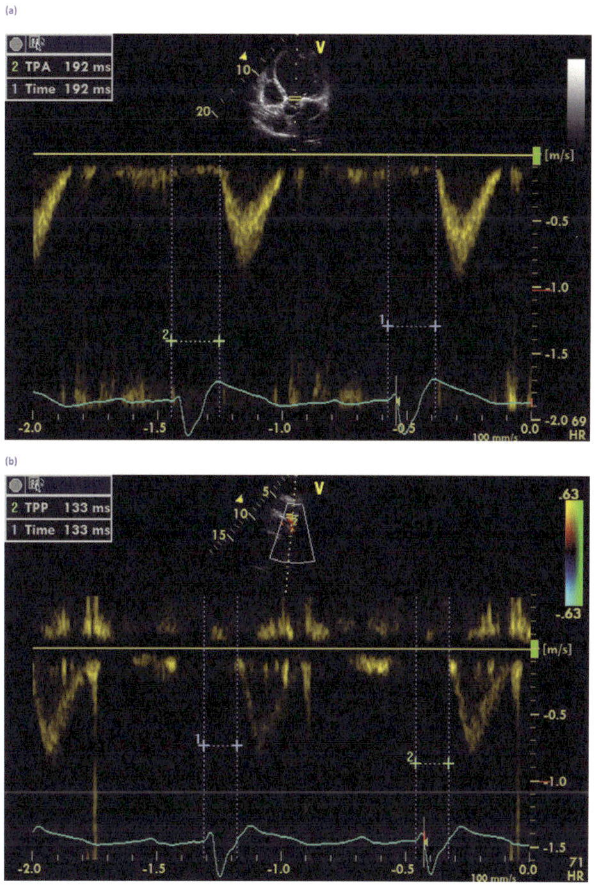

Figure 6. Interventricular dyssynchrony evaluation. (a) A-PEP measurement by pulsed wave Doppler from the parasternal short-axis-view. (b) P-PEP measurement by pulsed wave Doppler from the apical five-chamber view.

3. Multimodality imaging in the assessment of CRT patients

In CRT, procedural success depends on optimal lead placement, with reasonable stimulation thresholds and impedances in the absence of complications such as lead displacement, infection, coronary sinus dissection, or phrenic nerve stimulation.

The Resynchronization Reverse Remodeling in Systolic Left Ventricular Dysfunction (REVERSE) [108, 109] and SEPTAL-CRT [110] trials provided evidence that RV lead placement is not essential for procedure success, as similar results have been reported for both apical and mid-septal positions. However, when placing the coronary sinus lead, the optimal site for stimulation should be chosen, provided that venous anatomy is favorable. The importance of coronary sinus lead placement has been highlighted by several major trials. In the MADIT-CRT study, apical placement of the LV lead was associated with poorer outcomes [111], while in REVERSE, lead placement in the basal area of the LV posterolateral wall was associated with more LV reverse remodeling and longer intervals until either death or first hospitalization for HF [108].

Initially, the exact placement of the coronary sinus lead did not seem to be utterly important, as shown by the MADIT-CRT trial [111]. However, the Targeted Left Ventricular Lead Placement to Guide Cardiac Resynchronization Therapy (TARGET) study presented evidence that survival was increased if LV pacing occurred in the area of maximum contraction delay, provided there was no scar tissue on site [112]. Similar results have been reported in a smaller study [113].

Considering the results of these large trials, imaging techniques for identifying the area of maximal delay, the presence and location of scar tissue, and for describing venous anatomy could be helpful. In both the TARGET trial and another smaller study, speckle tracking was used to identify the area of maximum mechanical delay [112, 113].

Beyond cardiac ultrasonography, other imaging techniques have proved their use for targeting the areas for optimal lead placement. CMRI, for instance, can help identify the area of maximum mechanical delay by myocardial tagging techniques [114, 115], while also providing data on scar location [116, 117] and scar burden [118] by late gadolinium enhancement imaging, as well as an accurate quantification of LV and RV dimensions and systolic function [119, 120]. Also, although MDCT is more widely used for this purpose, CMRI scans with ECG-triggered respiratory-navigated three-dimensional SSFP after the injection of dimeglumine gadobenate and ECG-triggered inversion recovery assessment can be used for venous sinus anatomy visualization [117] (**Figure 7**).

Cardiac magnetic resonance imaging has been compared against speckle tracking echocardiography, yielding reasonable limits of agreement [121]. Some authors suggest the additive value of echocardiographic assessment of myocardial delays by speckle tracking and CMRI for identifying scarred areas in order to identify the best area for lead placement [122].

Although the efficiency of CMRI in assessing the response to CRT has been proved in some studies [114, 118], its routine clinical use in patients who have already undergone the implant procedure is somewhat hindered by the fact that, in most cases, CMRI-safe leads and devices are not available. Also, patients with CRT-D are exposed to the risk of inappropriate shocks.

MDCT is also a reliable method in the assessment of candidates for CRT, by being able to safely exclude significant coronary artery lesions [123], and, implicitly, the ischemic etiology of the DCM, as well as by offering a detailed and accurate description of venus anatomy that can help electrophysiologists in preparing the implant procedure [124, 125]; a keen study of venous

http://dx.doi.org/10.5772/64594

anatomy (**Figure 8**), combined with the identification of the area of maximum contraction delay by either echocardiography or CMRI, contributes to choosing the appropriate strategy before starting the implant procedure. As a consequence, during the intervention, the electrophysiologist can concentrate on the operation itself, rather than worrying over choosing the appropriate site for stimulation.

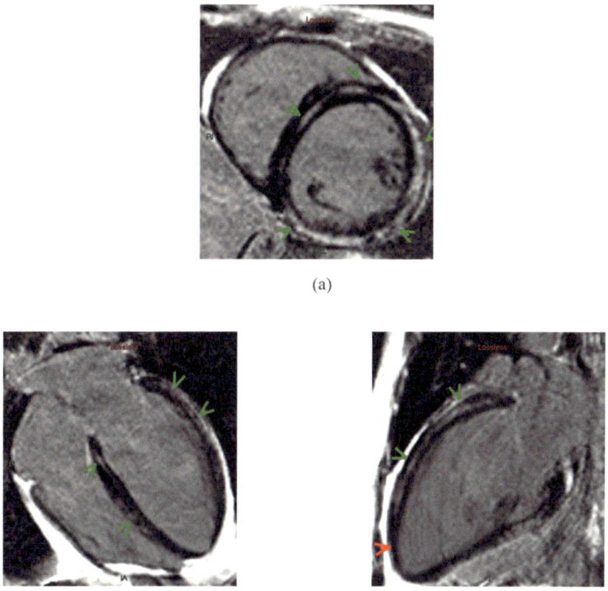

(a) (b) (c)

Figure 7. Late enhancement image in a patient with clinical presentation of myocarditis; midwall late gadolinium enhancement is present in the interventricular septum and diffuse subepicardial enhancement is visible on the lateral wall (arrows) in short-axis CMR views (a), four-chamber CMRI views (b) and two-chamber CMRI views (c).

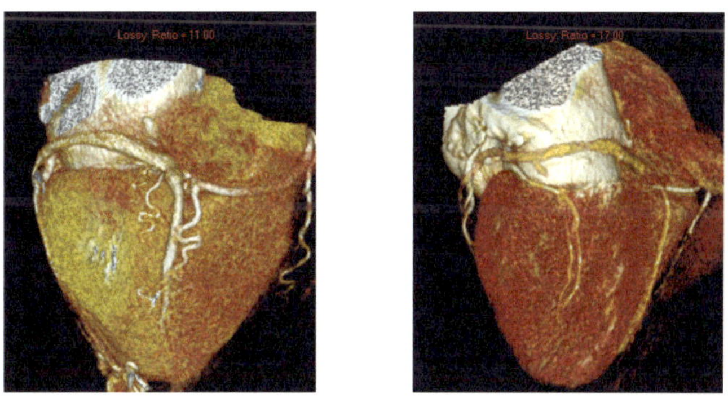

(a) (b)

Figure 8. Coronary venous anatomy using 3D volume rendered reconstructions.

The ongoing Imaging CRT trial aims to evaluate the benefits of multimodality imaging by speckle tracking echocardiography, single-photon emission computed tomography, and cardiac computed tomography in identifying the optimal positions for lead placement [126].

The extensive research conducted in this field proves the interest and necessity for developing evidence-based protocols in order to get optimum CRT results.

4. Conclusion

Despite the fact that areas of controversy still exist regarding the imaging assessment of patients with CRT, it is undisputed that it will always have an essential role in this type of patients. The extensive research on the topic, the fast progress and development of new imaging techniques, as well as the possibility of skill improvement in interested examiners, are likely to contribute to a more and more accurate assessment of the patients, thus improving management.

Author details

Silvia Lupu[1*], Lucia Agoston-Coldea[2] and Dan Dobreanu[1,3]

*Address all correspondence to: sil_lupu@yahoo.com

1 University of Medicine and Pharmacy of Târgu Mureş, Târgu Mureş, Romania

2 2nd Department of Internal Medicine, Iuliu Haţieganu University of Medicine and Pharmacy, Cluj-Napoca, Romania

3 Cardiovascular Disease and Transplant Institute, University of Medicine and Pharmacy, Târgu Mureş, Romania

References

[1] Cleland JGF, Freemantle N, Erdmann E, Gras D, Kappenberger L, Tavazzi L, Daubert JC. Long-term mortality with cardiac resynchronization therapy in the Cardiac Resynchronization-Heart Failure (CARE-HF) trial. Eur J Heart Fail. 2012;14:628–34. DOI: 10.1093/eurjhf/hfs055

[2] Cleland JGF, Freemantle N, Erdmann E, Gras D, Kappenberger L, Tavazzi L, Daubert JC. Longer-term effects of cardiac resynchronization therapy on mortality in heart

failure [the Cardiac RE synchronization-Heart Failure (CARE-HF) trial extension phase. Eur Heart J. 2006;27:1928–32. DOI:10.1093/eurheartj/ehl141

[3] Bristow MR, Saxon LA, Boehmer J, Krueger S, Kass DA, De Marco T, et al. Cardiac-resynchronization therapy with or without an implantable defibrillator in advanced chronic heart failure. N Engl J Med. 2004;350:2140–50. DOI: 10.1056/NEJMoa032423

[4] Moss JA, Hall WJ, Cannom DS, Klein H, Brown MW, Daubert JP, et al. Cardiac-resynchronization therapy for the prevention of heart-failure events. N Engl J Med. 2009;361:1329–38. DOI: 10.1056/NEJMoa0906431

[5] Tang ASL, Wells GA, Talajic M, Arnold MO, Sheldon R, et al. Cardiac resynchronization therapy for mild-to-moderate heart failure. N Engl J Med. 2010;363:2385–95. DOI: 10.1056/NEJMoa1009540

[6] Linde C, Abraham WT, Gold M, Sutton M, Ghio S, Daubert C. Randomized trial of cardiac resynchronization in mild symptomatic heart failure patients and in asymptomatic patients with left ventricular dysfunction and previous heart failure symptoms. J Am Coll Cardiol. 2008;52:1834–43. DOI: 10.1093/eurheartj/ehq408

[7] Auricchio A, Baron-Esquivias G, Bordachar P, Boriani G, Breithardt OA, Cleland J, et al. 2013 ESC Guidelines on cardiac pacing and cardiac resynchronization therapy. Eur Heart J. 2013;34:2281–329. DOI:10.1093/eurheartj/eht150

[8] Noyes K, Veazie P, Hall WJ, Zhao H, Buttaccio A, Thevenet-Morrison K, Moss AJ. Cost-effectiveness of cardiac resynchronization therapy in the MADIT-CRT trial. J Cardiovasc Electrophysiol. 2013;24:66–74. DOI: 10.1111/j.1540-8167.2012.02413.x

[9] Feldman AM, de Lissovoy G, Bristow MR, Saxon LA, De Marco T, Kass DA, et al. Cost effectiveness of cardiac resynchronization therapy in the Comparison of Medical Therapy, Pacing, and Defibrillation in Heart Failure (COMPANION) trial. J Am Coll Cardiol. 2005;46:2311–21. DOI:10.1016/j.jacc.2005.08.033

[10] Neyt M, Stroobandt S, Obyn C, Camberlin C, Devriese S, De Laet C, Van Brabandt H. Cost-effectiveness of cardiac resynchronisation therapy for patients with moderate-to-severe heart failure: a lifetime Markov model. BMJ Open. 2011;1:e000276. DOI: 10.1136/bmjopen-2011-000276

[11] Landolina M, Gasparini M, Lunati M, Iacopino S, Boriani G, Bonanno C, et al; Cardiovascular Centers Participating in the Clinical Service Project. Long-term complications related to biventricular defibrillator implantation: rate of surgical revisions and impact on survival: insights from the Italian Clinical Service Database. Circulation. 2011;123:2526–35. DOI: 10.1161/CIRCULATIONAHA.110.015024

[12] Gorcsan J 3rd, Abraham T, Agler DA, Bax JJ, Derumeaux G, Grimm RA, et al. Echocardiography for cardiac resynchronization therapy: recommendations for perform-

ance and reporting – a Report from the American Society of Echocardiography Dyssynchrony Writing Group Endorsed by the Heart Rhythm Society. J Am Soc Echocardiogr. 2008;21:191–213. DOI: 10.1016/j.echo.2008.01.003

[13] Mor-Avi V, Lang RM, Badano LP, Belohlavek M, Cardim NM, Derumeaux G, et al. Current and evolving echocardiographic techniques for the quantitative evaluation of cardiac mechanics: ASE/EAE consensus statement on methodology and indications endorsed by the Japanese Society of Echocardiography. J Am Soc Echocardiogr. 2011;24:277–313. doi: 10.1016/j.echo.2011.01.015

[14] Yu AM, Chan YS, Zhang Q, Yip GW, Chan CK, Kum LC, et al. Benefits of cardiac resynchronization therapy for heart failure patients with narrow QRS complexes and coexisting systolic asynchrony by echocardiography. J Am Coll Cardiol. 2006;48:2251–57. DOI:10.1016/j.jacc.2006.07.054

[15] Ruschitzka F, Abraham WT, Singh JP, Bax JJ, Borer JS, Brugada J, et al. Cardiac-resynchronization therapy in heart failure with a narrow QRS complex. N Engl J Med. 2013;369:1395–405. DOI: 10.1056/NEJMoa1306687

[16] Chung ES, Leon AR, Tavazzi L, Sun JP, Nihoyannopoulos P, Merlino J, et al. Results of the predictors of response to CRT (PROSPECT) Trial. Circulation. 2008;117:2608–16. DOI: 10.1161/CIRCULATIONAHA.107.743120

[17] Sanderson JE. Echocardiography for cardiac resynchronization therapy selection. J Am Coll Cardiol. 2009;53:1960–4. DOI: 10.1016/j.jacc.2008.12.071

[18] Bax JJ, Gorcsan J 3rd. Echocardiography and noninvasive imaging in cardiac resynchronization therapy results of the PROSPECT (Predictors of Response to Cardiac Resynchronization Therapy) Study in perspective. J Am Coll Cardiol. 2009;53:1933–43. DOI: 10.1016/j.jacc.2008.11.061

[19] Kamdar R, Frain E, Warburton F, Richmond L, Mullan V, Berriman T, et al. A prospective comparison of echocardiography and device algorithms for atrioventricular and interventricular optimization in cardiac resynchronization therapy. Europace. 2010;12:84–91. DOI: 10.1093/europace/eup337

[20] Saba S, Marek J, Schwartzman D, Jain S, Adelstein E, White P, et al. Echocardiography-guided left ventricular lead placement for cardiac resynchronization therapy: results of the Speckle Tracking Assisted Resynchronization Therapy for Electrode Region (STARTER) Trial. Circ Heart Fail. 2013;6:427–34. DOI: 10.1161/CIRCHEARTFAILURE.112.000078

[21] Tanaka H, Nesser HJ, Buck T, Oyenuga O, Janosi RA, Winter S, et al. Dyssynchrony by speckle-tracking echocardiography and response to cardiac resynchronization therapy: results of the Speckle Tracking and Resynchronization (STAR) study. Eur Heart J. 2010:31:1690–700. DOI: 10.1093/eurheartj/ehq213

[22] Dobreanu D, Dagres N, Svendsen JH, Marinskis G, Bongiorni MG, Blomström-Lundqvist C. Approach to cardiac resynchronization therapy. Europace. 2012;14:1359–32. DOI: 10.1093/europace/eus260

[23] Yang X, Gai LY, Li P, Chen YD, Li T, Yang, L. Diagnostic accuracy of dual-source CT angiography and coronary risk stratification. Vasc Health Risk Manag. 2010;6:935–41. DOI: 10.2147/VHRM.S13879

[24] Sun JP, Yang XS, Lam YY, Garcia MJ, Yu CM. Evaluation of coronary venous anatomy by multislice computed tomography. World J Cardiovasc Surg. 2012;2:91–5. DOI: 10.4236/wjcs.2012.24018

[25] Bilchick KC, Dimaano V, Wu KC, Helm RH, Weiss RG, Lima JA, et al. Cardiac magnetic resonance assessment of dyssynchrony and myocardial scar predicts function class improvement following cardiac resynchronization therapy. J Am Coll Cardiol Img. 2008;1:561–68. DOI:10.1016/j.jcmg.2008.04.013

[26] Lang RM, Badano LP, Mor-Avi V, Afilalo J, Armstrong A, Ernande L, et al. Recommendations for cardiac chamber quantification by echocardiography in adults: an update from the American Society of Echocardiography and the European Association of Cardiovascular Imaging. J Am Soc Echocardiogr. 2015;28:1–39.e14. DOI: 10.1016/j.echo.2014.10.003

[27] Mulvagh SL, Rakowski H, Vannan MA, Abdelmoneim SS, Becher H, Bierig SM, et al. American Society of Echocardiography Consensus Statement on the Clinical Applications of Ultrasonic Contrast Agents in Echocardiography. J Am Soc Echocardiogr. 2008;21:1179–201 DOI: 10.1016/j.echo.2008.09.009

[28] Porter TR, Abdelmoneim S, Belcik JT, McCulloch ML, Mulvagh SL, Olson JJ, et al. Guidelines for the cardiac sonographer in the performance of contrast echocardiography: a focused update from the American Society of Echocardiography. J Am Soc Echocardiogr. 2014;27:797–810. DOI: 10.1016/j.echo.2014.05.011

[29] Goldenberg I, Moss AJ, Hall WJ, Foster E, Goldberger JJ, Santucci P, et al; MADIT-CRT Executive Committee. Predictors of response to cardiac resynchronization therapy in the Multicenter Automatic Defibrillator Implantation Trial with Cardiac Resynchronization Therapy (MADIT-CRT). Circulation. 2011;124:1527–36. DOI: 10.1161/CIRCULATIONAHA.110.014324

[30] Duncan A, Wait D, Gibson D, Daubert JC. Left ventricular remodelling and haemodynamic effects of multisite biventricular pacing in patients with left ventricular systolic dysfunction and activation disturbances in sinus rhythm: sub-study of the MUSTIC (Multisite Stimulation in Cardiomyopathies) trial. Eur Heart J. 2003;24:430–41. DOI: 10.1016/S0195-668X(02)00475-X

[31] St John Sutton MG, Plappert T, Abraham WT, Smith AL, DeLurgio DB, Leon AR, et al; Multicenter InSync Randomized Clinical Evaluation (MIRACLE) Study Group. Effect

of cardiac resynchronization therapy on left ventricular size and function in chronic heart failure. Circulation. 2003;107:1985–90. DOI: 10.1161/01.CIR.0000065226.24159.E9

[32] Young JB, Abraham WT, Smith AL, Leon AR, Lieberman R, Wilkoff B, et al; for The Multicenter InSync ICD Randomized Clinical Evaluation (MIRACLE ICD) Trial Investigators. Combined cardiac resynchronization and implantable cardioversion defibrillation in advanced chronic heart failure. The MIRACLE ICD Trial. JAMA. 2003;289:2685–694. DOI:10.1001/jama.289.20.2685

[33] Cleland J, Freemantle N, Ghio S, Fruhwald F, Shankar A, Marijanowski M, et al. Predicting the long-term effects of cardiac resynchronization therapy on mortality from baseline variables and the early response. J Am Coll Cardiol. 2008;52:438–45. DOI: 10.1016/j.jacc.2008.04.036

[34] Richardson M, Freemantle N, Calvert MJ, Cleland JG, Tavazzi L; CARE-HF Study Steering Committee and Investigators. Predictors and treatment response with cardiac resynchronization therapy in patients with heart failure characterized by dyssynchrony: a pre-defined analysis from the CARE-HF trial. Eur Heart J. 2007;28:1827–34. DOI: 10.1093/eurheartj/ehm192

[35] Mele D, Agricola E, Monte AD, Galderisi M, D'Andrea A, Rigo F, et al. Pacing transmural scar tissue reduces left ventricle reverse remodeling after cardiac resynchronization therapy. Int J Cardiol. 2013;167:94–101. DOI: 10.1016/j.ijcard.2011.12.006

[36] Ypenburg C, Schalij MJ, Bleeker GB, Steendijk P, Boersma E, Dibbets-Schneider P, et al. Impact of viability and scar tissue on response to cardiac resynchronization therapy in ischaemic heart failure patients. Eur Heart J. 2007;28:33–41. DOI:10.1093/eurheartj/ehl379

[37] Solomon SD, Foster E, Bourgoun M, Shah A, Viloria E, Brown MW, et al; MADIT-CRT Investigators. Effect of cardiac resynchronization therapy on reverse remodeling and relation to outcome: multicenter automatic defibrillator implantation trial: cardiac resynchronization therapy. Circulation. 2010;122:985–92. DOI: 10.1161/CIRCULATIONAHA.110.955039

[38] Linde C, Daubert C, Abraham WT, St John Sutton M, Ghio S, Hassager C, et al; REsynchronization reVErses Remodeling in Systolic left vEntricular dysfunction (REVERSE) Study Group. Impact of ejection fraction on the clinical response to cardiac resynchronization therapy in mild heart failure. Circ Heart Fail. 2013;6:1180–89. DOI: 10.1161/CIRCHEARTFAILURE.113.000326

[39] Brambatti M, Guerra F, Matassini MV, Cipolletta L, Barbarossa A, Urbinati A, et al. Cardiac resynchronization therapy improves ejection fraction and cardiac remodelling regardless of patients' age. Europace. 2013;15:704–10. DOI: 10.1093/europace/eus376

[40] Kron J, Aranda JM Jr, Miles WM, Burkart TA, Woo GW, Saxonhouse SJ, et al. Benefit of cardiac resynchronization in elderly patients: results from the Multicenter InSync

Randomized Clinical Evaluation (MIRACLE) and Multicenter InSync ICD Randomized Clinical Evaluation (MIRACLE-ICD) trials. J Interv Card Electrophysiol. 2009;25:91–6. DOI: 10.1007/s10840-008-9330-2

[41] Higgins SL, Hummel JD, Niazi IK, Giudici MC, Worley SJ, Saxon LA, et al. Cardiac resynchronization therapy for the treatment of heart failure in patients with intraventricular conduction delay and malignant ventricular tachyarrhythmias. J Am Coll Cardiol. 2003;42:1454–59. DOI:10.1016/S0735-1097(03)01042-8

[42] Abraham WT, Fisher WG, Smith AL, Delurgio DB, Leon AR, Loh E, et al; MIRACLE Study Group. Multicenter InSync Randomized Clinical Evaluation. Cardiac resynchronization in chronic heart failure. N Engl J Med. 2002;346:1845–53. DOI: 10.1056/NEJMoa013168

[43] Abraham WT, Young JB, León AR, Adler S, Bank AJ, Hall SA, et al; Multicenter InSync ICD II Study Group. Effects of cardiac resynchronization on disease progression in patients with left ventricular systolic dysfunction, an indication for an implantable cardioverter-defibrillator, and mildly symptomatic chronic heart failure. Circulation. 2004;110:2864–8. DOI: 10.1161/01.CIR.0000146336.92331.D1

[44] Linde C, Leclercq C, Rex S, Garrigue S, Lavergne T, Cazeau S, et al; on behalf of the MUltisite STimulation In Cardiomyopathies (MUSTIC) Study Group. Long-Term Benefits of Biventricular Pacing in Congestive Heart Failure: Results from the MUltisite STimulation In Cardiomyopathy (MUSTIC) Study. J Am Coll Cardiol. 2002;40:111–8. DOI:10.1016/S0735-1097(02)01932-0

[45] Kutyifa V, Kloppe A, Zareba W, Solomon SD, McNitt S, Polonsky S, et al. The influence of left ventricular ejection fraction on the effectiveness of cardiac resynchronization therapy: MADIT-CRT (Multicenter Automatic Defibrillator Implantation Trial with Cardiac Resynchronization Therapy). J Am Coll Cardiol. 2013;61:936–44. DOI: 10.1016/j.jacc.2012.11.051

[46] Eickholt C, Siekiera M, Kirmanoglou K, Rodenbeck A, Heussen N, Schauerte P, et al. Improvement of left ventricular function under cardiac resynchronization therapy goes along with a reduced incidence of ventricular arrhythmia. PLoS One. 2012; 7: e48926. DOI: 10.1371/journal.pone.0048926

[47] Ruwald MH, Solomon SD, Foster E, Kutyifa V, Ruwald AC, Sherazi S, et al. Left ventricular ejection fraction normalization in cardiac resynchronization therapy and risk of ventricular arrhythmias and clinical outcomes: results from the Multicenter Automatic Defibrillator Implantation Trial with Cardiac Resynchronization Therapy (MADIT-CRT) trial. Circulation. 2014;130:2278–86. DOI: 10.1161/CIRCULATIONAHA.114.011283

[48] St John Sutton M, Ghio S, Plappert T, Tavazzi L, Scelsi L, Daubert C, et al; REsynchronization reVErses Remodeling in Systolic left vEntricular dysfunction (REVERSE) Study Group. Cardiac resynchronization induces major structural and functional

reverse remodeling in patients with New York Heart Association class I/II heart failure. Circulation. 2009;120:1858–65. DOI: 10.1161/CIRCULATIONAHA.108.818724

[49] Waggoner AD, Faddis MN, Gleva MJ, de las Fuentes L, Dávila-Román VG. Improvements in left ventricular diastolic function after cardiac resynchronization therapy are coupled to response in systolic performance. J Am Coll Cardiol. 2005;46:2244–49. DOI: 10.1016/j.jacc.2005.05.094

[50] Doltra A, Bijnens B, Tolosana JM, Gabrielli L, Castel MÁ, Berruezo A, et al. Effect of cardiac resynchronization therapy on left ventricular diastolic function: implications for clinical outcome. J Card Fail. 2013;19:795–801. DOI:10.1016/j.jacc.2005.05.094

[51] Shanks M, Antoni ML, Hoke U, Bertini M, Ng AC, Auger D, et al. The effect of cardiac resynchronization therapy on left ventricular diastolic function assessed with speckle-tracking echocardiography. Eur J Heart Fail. 2011;13:1133–39. DOI:10.1093/eurjhf/hfr115

[52] Nagueh SF, Smiseth OA, Appleton CP, Byrd BF 3rd, Dokainish H, Edvardsen T, et al. Recommendations for the evaluation of left ventricular diastolic function by echocardiography: an update from the American Society of Echocardiography and the European Association of Cardiovascular Imaging. J Am Soc Echocardiogr. 2016;29:277–314. DOI: 10.1016/j.echo.2016.01.011

[53] Kuperstein R, Goldenberg I, Moss AJ, Solomon S, Bourgoun M, Shah A, et al. Left atrial volume and the benefit of cardiac resynchronization therapy in the MADIT-CRT trial. Circ Heart Fail. 2014;7:154–60. DOI: 10.1161/CIRCHEARTFAILURE.113.000748

[54] Yu CM, Fang F, Zhang Q, Yip GW, Li CM, Chan JY, et al. Improvement of atrial function and atrial reverse remodeling after cardiac resynchronization therapy for heart failure. J Am Coll Cardiol. 2007;50:778–85. DOI:10.1016/j.jacc.2007.04.073

[55] Aksoy H, Okutucu S, Kaya EB, Deveci OS, Evranos B, Aytemir K, et al. Clinical and echocardiographic correlates of improvement in left ventricular diastolic function after cardiac resynchronization therapy. Europace. 2010;12:1256–61. DOI: 10.1093/europace/euq150

[56] D'Andrea A, Caso P, Romano S, Scarafile R, Riegler L, Salerno G, et al. Different effects of cardiac resynchronization therapy on left atrial function in patients with either idiopathic or ischaemic dilated cardiomyopathy: a two-dimensional speckle strain study. Eur Heart J. 2007;28:2738–48. DOI:10.1093/eurheartj/ehm443

[57] Kloosterman M, Rienstra M, Mulder BA, Van Gelder IC, Maass AH. Atrial reverse remodelling is associated with outcome of cardiac resynchronization therapy. Europace. 2015. pii:euv382. DOI:10.1093/europace/euv382

[58] Sade LE, Atar I, Özin B, Yüce D, Müderrisoğlu H. Determinants of new-onset atrial fibrillation in patients receiving CRT: mechanistic insights from speckle tracking imaging. JACC Cardiovasc Imaging. 2016;9:99–111. DOI: 10.1016/j.jcmg.2015.05.011

[59] Feneon D, Behaghel A, Bernard A, Fournet M, Mabo P, Daubert JC, et al. Left atrial function, a new predictor of response to cardiac resynchronization therapy? Heart Rhythm. 2015;12:1800–6. DOI: 10.1016/j.hrthm.2015.04.021

[60] Rudski LG, Lai WW, Afilalo J, Hua L, Handschumacher MD, Chandrasekaran K, et al. Guidelines for the echocardiographic assessment of the right heart in adults: a report from the American Society of Echocardiography endorsed by the European Association of Echocardiography, a registered branch of the European Society of Cardiology, and the Canadian Society of Echocardiography. J Am Soc Echocardiogr. 2010;23:685–713. DOI: 10.1016/j.echo.2010.05.010

[61] Galiè N, Humbert M, Vachiery JL, Gibbs S, Lang I, Torbicki A, et al. ESC/ERS Guidelines for the diagnosis and treatment of pulmonary hypertension: The Joint Task Force for the Diagnosis and Treatment of Pulmonary Hypertension of the European Society of Cardiology (ESC) and the European Respiratory Society (ERS): Endorsed by: Association for European Paediatric and Congenital Cardiology (AEPC), International Society for Heart and Lung Transplantation (ISHLT). Eur Respir J. 2015;46:903–75. DOI: 10.1093/eurheartj/ehv317

[62] Bourantas CV, Loh HP, Bragadeesh T, Rigby AS, Lukaschuk EI, Garg S, et al. Relationship between right ventricular volumes measured by cardiac magnetic resonance imaging and prognosis in patients with chronic heart failure. Eur J Heart Fail. 2011;13:52–60. DOI: 10.1093/eurjhf/hfq161

[63] Meyer P, Filippatos GS, Ahmed MI, Iskandrian AE, Bittner V, Perry GJ, et al. Effects of right ventricular ejection fraction on outcomes in chronic systolic heart failure. Circulation. 2010;121:252–8. DOI: 10.1161/CIRCULATIONAHA.109.887570

[64] Burri H, Domenichini G, Sunthorn H, Fleury E, Stettler C, Foulkes I, et al. Right ventricular systolic function and cardiac resynchronization therapy. Europace. 2010;12:389–94. DOI: 10.1093/europace/eup401

[65] D'Andrea A, Scarafile R, Riegler L, Salerno G, Gravino R, Cocchia R, et al. Right atrial size and deformation in patients with dilated cardiomyopathy undergoing cardiac resynchronization therapy. Eur J Heart Fail. 2009;11:1169–77. DOI: 10.1093/eurjhf/hfp158

[66] Campbell P, Takeuchi M, Bourgoun M, Shah A, Foster E, Brown MW, et al; for the Multicenter Automatic Defibrillator Implantation Trial with Cardiac Resynchronization Therapy (MADIT-CRT) Investigators. Right ventricular function, pulmonary pressure estimation, and clinical outcomes in cardiac resynchronization therapy. Circ Heart Fail. 2013;6:435–42. DOI: 10.1161/CIRCHEARTFAILURE.112.000127

[67] Trichon BH, Felker GM, Shaw LK, Cabell CH, O'Connor CM. Relation of frequency and severity of mitral regurgitation to survival among patients with left ventricular systolic dysfunction and heart failure. Am J Cardiol. 2003;91:538–43. DOI:10.1016/S0002-9149(02)03301-5

[68] Andrea Rossi A, Dini FL, Faggiano P, Agricola E, Cicoira M, Simioniuc A, et al. Independent prognostic value of functional mitral regurgitation in patients with heart failure. A quantitative analysis of 1256 patients with ischaemic and non-ischaemic dilated cardiomyopathy. Heart. 2011;97:1675–80. DOI: 10.1136/hrt.2011.225789

[69] Lancellotti P, Moura L, Pierard LA, Agricola E, Popescu BA, Tribouilloy C, et al. European Association of Echocardiography recommendations for the assessment of valvular regurgitation. Part 2: mitral and tricuspid regurgitation (native valve disease). Eur J Echocardiogr. 2010;11:307–32. DOI: 10.1093/ejechocard/jeq031

[70] Kanzaki H, Bazaz R, Schwartzman D, Dohi K, Sade LE, Gorcsan J 3rd. A mechanism for immediate reduction in mitral regurgitation after cardiac resynchronization therapy insights from mechanical activation strain mapping. J Am Coll Cardiol. 2004;44:1619–25. DOI:10.1016/j.jacc.2004.07.036

[71] Donal E, De Place C, Kervio G, Bauer F, Gervais R, Leclercq C, et al. Mitral regurgitation in dilated cardiomyopathy: value of both regional left ventricular contractility and dyssynchrony. Eur J Echocardiogr. 2009;10:133–8. DOI: 10.1093/ejechocard/jen188

[72] Breithardt OA, Sinha AM, Schwammenthal E, Bidaoui N, Markus KU, Franke A, et al. Acute effects of cardiac resynchronization therapy on functional mitral regurgitation in advanced systolic heart failure. J Am Coll Cardiol. 2003;41:765–70. DOI:10.1016/S0735-1097(02)02937-6

[73] Solis J, McCarty D, Levine RA, Handschumacher MD, Fernandez-Friera L, Chen-Tournoux A, et al. Mechanism of decrease in mitral regurgitation after cardiac resynchronization therapy: optimization of the force-balance relationship. Circ Cardiovasc Imaging. 2009;2:444–50. DOI: 10.1161/CIRCIMAGING.108.823732

[74] Ypenburg C, Lancellotti P, Tops LF, Bleeker GB, Holman ER, Piérard LA, et al. Acute effects of initiation and withdrawal of cardiac resynchronization therapy on papillary muscle dyssynchrony and mitral regurgitation. J Am Coll Cardiol. 2007;50:2071–7. DOI: 10.1016/j.jacc.2007.08.019

[75] Brandt RR, Reiner C, Arnold R, Sperzel J, Pitschner HF, Hamm CW. Contractile response and mitral regurgitation after temporary interruption of long-term cardiac resynchronization therapy. Eur Heart J. 2006;27:187–92. DOI:10.1093/eurheartj/ehi558

[76] Di Biase L, Auricchio A, Mohanty P, Bai R, Kautzner J, Pieragnoli P, et al. Impact of cardiac resynchronization therapy on the severity of mitral regurgitation. Europace. 2011;13:829–38. DOI: 10.1093/europace/eur047

[77] Cabrera-Bueno F, Molina-Mora MJ, Alzueta J, Pena-Hernandez J, Jimenez-Navarro M, Fernandez-Pastor J, et al. Persistence of secondary mitral regurgitation and response to cardiac resynchronization therapy. Eur J Echocardiogr. 2010;11:131–7. DOI: 10.1093/ejechocard/jep184

[78] Auricchio A, Schillinger W, Meyer S, Maisano F, Hoffmann R, Ussia GP, et al; on behalf of the PERMIT-CARE Investigators. Correction of mitral regurgitation in nonrespond-

ers to cardiac resynchronization therapy by MitraClip improves symptoms and promotes reverse remodeling. J Am Coll Cardiol. 2011;58:2183–9. DOI: 10.1016/j.jacc.2011.06.061

[79] Kainuma S, Taniguchi K, Toda K, Funatsu T, Kondoh H, Nishino M, et al. Restrictive Mitral annuloplasty for functional mitral regurgitation – acute hemodynamics and serial echocardiography. Circ J. 2011;75:571–9. DOI:10.1253/circj.CJ-10-0759

[80] Richardson M, Freemantle N, Calvert MJ, Cleland JG, Tavazzi L on behalf of the CARE-HF Study Steering Committee and Investigators. Predictors and treatment response with cardiac resynchronization therapy in patients with heart failure characterized by dyssynchrony: a pre-defined analysis from the CARE-HF trial. Eur Heart J. 2007;28:1827–34. DOI:10.1093/eurheartj/ehm192

[81] Ghio S, Freemantle N, Scelsi L, Serio A, Magrini G, Pasotti M, et al. Long-term left ventricular reverse remodelling with cardiac resynchronization therapy: results from the CARE-HF trial. Eur J Heart Fail. 2009;11:480–8. DOI: 10.1093/eurjhf/hfp034

[82] Stockburger M, Fateh-Moghadam S, Nitardy A, Celebi O, Krebs A, Habedank D, et al. Baseline Doppler parameters are useful predictors of chronic left ventricular reduction in size by cardiac resynchronization therapy. Europace. 2008;10:69–74. DOI:10.1093/europace/eum269

[83] Penicka M, Bartunek J, De Bruyne B, Vanderheyden M, Goethals M, De Zutter M, et al. Improvement of left ventricular function after cardiac resynchronization therapy is predicted by tissue Doppler imaging echocardiography. Circulation. 2004;109:978–83. DOI: 10.1161/01.CIR.0000116765.43251.D7

[84] Suffoletto MS, Dohi K, Cannesson M, Saba S, Gorcsan J 3rd. Novel speckle-tracking radial strain from routine black-and-white echocardiographic images to quantify dyssynchrony and predict response to cardiac resynchronization therapy. Circulation. 2006;113:960–8. DOI: 10.1161/CIRCULATIONAHA.105.571455

[85] Mele D, Pasanisi G, Capasso F, De Simone A, Morales MA, Poggio D, et al. Left intraventricular myocardial deformation dyssynchrony identifies responders to cardiac resynchronization therapy in patients with heart failure. Eur Heart J. 2006;27:1070–8. DOI:10.1093/eurheartj/ehi814

[86] Bertola B, Rondano E, Sulis M, Sarasso G, Piccinino C, Marti G, et al. Cardiac dyssynchrony quantitated by time-to-peak or temporal uniformity of strain at longitudinal, circumferential, and radial level: implications for resynchronization therapy. J Am Soc Echocardiogr. 2009;22:665–71. DOI: 10.1016/j.echo.2009.03.010

[87] Mandysova E, Mráz T, Táborský M, Niederle P. Reproducibility of tissue Doppler parameters of asynchrony in patients with advanced LV dysfunction. Eur J Echocardiogr. 2008;9:509–15. DOI:10.1016/j.euje.2007.08.005

[88] Ellenbogen KA, Gold MR, Meyer TE, Fernandez Lozano I, Mittal S, Waggoner AD, et al. Primary Results from the SmartDelay Determined AV optimization: a

comparison to other AV Delay Methods Used in Cardiac Resynchronization Therapy (SMART-AV) Trial. A randomized trial comparing empirical, echocardiography-guided, and algorithmic atrioventricular delay programming in cardiac resynchronization therapy. Circulation. 2010;122:2660–8. DOI: 10.1161/CIRCULATIONAHA.110.992552

[89] Sawhney NS, Waggoner AD, Garhwal S, Chawla MK, Osborn J, Faddis MN. Randomized prospective trial of atrioventricular delay programming for cardiac resynchronization therapy. Heart Rhythm. 2004;1:562–7. DOI:10.1016/j.hrthm.2004.07.006

[90] Kedia N, Ng K, Apperson-Hansen C, Wang C, Tchou P, Wilkoff BL, et al. Usefulness of atrioventricular delay optimization using Doppler assessment of mitral inflow in patients undergoing cardiac resynchronization therapy. Am J Cardiol. 2006;98:780–5. DOI:10.1016/j.amjcard.2006.04.017

[91] Vidal B, Sitges M, Marigliano A, Delgado V, Díaz-Infante E, Azqueta M, et al. Optimizing the programation of cardiac resynchronization therapy devices in patients with heart failure and left bundle branch block. Am J Cardiol. 2007;100:1002–6. DOI:10.1016/j.amjcard.2007.04.046

[92] Singh JP, Abraham WT, Chung ES, Rogers T, Sambelashvili A, Coles JA Jr, et al. Clinical response with adaptive CRT algorithm compared with CRT with echocardiography optimized atrioventricular delay: a retrospective analysis of multicentre trials. Europace. 2013;15:1622–8. DOI: 10.1093/europace/eut107

[93] Waggoner AD, Faddis MN, Osborn J, Reagan J, Heuerman S, Davila-Roman VG. AV delay programming and cardiac resynchronization therapy: Left ventricular diastolic function and relation to stroke volume. J Am Coll Cardiol. 2005;45 Suppl 1:99A

[94] Kamdar R, Frain E, Warburton F, Richmond L, Mullan V, Berriman T, et al. A prospective comparison of echocardiography and device algorithms for atrioventricular and interventricular interval optimization in cardiac resynchronization therapy. Europace. 2010 Jan;12(1):84–91. doi: 10.1093/europace/eup337.

[95] Pitzalis MV, Iacoviello M, Romito R, Massari F, Rizzon B, Luzzi G, et al. Cardiac resynchronization therapy tailored by echocardiographic evaluation of ventricular asynchrony. J Am Coll Cardiol. 2002;40:1615–22. DOI:10.1016/S0735-1097(02)02337-9

[96] Cleland JG, Daubert JC, Erdmann E, Freemantle N, Gras D, Kappenberger L, et al, On behalf of The CARE-HF study Steering Committee and Investigators. The CARE-HF study CArdiac REsynchronisation in Heart Failure study: rationale, design and end-points. Eur J Heart Fail. 2001;3:481–9. DOI: 10.1016/S1388-9842(01)00176-3

[97] Bax JJ, Marwick TH, Molhoek SG, Bleeker GB, van Erven L, Boersma E, et al. Left ventricular dyssynchrony predicts benefit of cardiac resynchronization therapy in patients with end-stage heart failure before pacemaker implantation. Am J Cardiol. 2003;92:1238–40. DOI:10.1016/j.amjcard.2003.06.016

[98] Bax JJ, Bleeker GB, Marwick TH, Molhoek SG, Boersma E, Steendijk P, et al. Left ventricular dyssynchrony predicts response and prognosis after cardiac resynchronization therapy. J Am Coll Cardiol. 2004;44:1834–40. DOI:10.1016/j.jacc.2004.08.016

[99] Bader H, Garrigue S, Lafitte S, Reuter S, Jaïs P, Haïssaguerre M, et al. Intra-left ventricular electromechanical asynchrony. A new independent predictor of severe cardiac events in heart failure patients. J Am Coll Cardiol. 2004;43:248–56. DOI:10.1016/j.jacc.2003.08.038

[100] Yu CM, Zhang Q, Fung JW, Chan HC, Chan YS, Yip GW, et al. A novel tool to assess systolic asynchrony and identify responders of cardiac resynchronization therapy by tissue synchronization imaging. J Am Coll Cardiol. 2005;45:677–84. DOI:10.1016/j.jacc.2004.12.003

[101] Yu CM, Lin H, Zhang Q, Sanderson JE. High prevalence of left ventricular systolic and diastolic asynchrony in patients with congestive heart failure and normal QRS duration. Heart. 2003;89:54–60. DOI:10.1136/heart.89.1.54

[102] Yu CM, Chau E, Sanderson JE, Fan K, Tang MO, Fung WH, et al. Tissue Doppler echocardiographic evidence of reverse remodeling and improved synchronicity by simultaneously delaying regional contraction after biventricular pacing therapy in heart failure. Circulation. 2002;105:438–45. DOI: 10.1161/hc0402.102623

[103] Gjesdal O, Remme EW, Opdahl A, Skulstad H, Russell K, Kongsgaard E, et al. Mechanisms of abnormal systolic motion of the interventricular septum during left bundle-branch block. Circ Cardiovasc Imaging. 2011;4:264–73. DOI: 10.1161/CIRCIMAGING.110.961417

[104] Parsai C, Bijnens B, Sutherland GR, Baltabaeva A, Claus P, Marciniak M, et al. Toward understanding response to cardiac resynchronization therapy: left ventricular dyssynchrony is only one of multiple mechanisms. Eur Heart J. 2009;30:940–9. DOI: 10.1093/eurheartj/ehn481

[105] Gabrielli L, Marincheva G, Bijnens B, Doltra A, Tolosana JM, Borràs R, et al. Septal flash predicts cardiac resynchronization therapy response in patients with permanent atrial fibrillation. Europace. 2014;16:1342–9. DOI: 10.1093/europace/euu023

[106] Szulik M, Tillekaerts M, Vangeel V, Ganame J, Willems R, Lenarczyk R, et al. Assessment of apical rocking: a new, integrative approach for selection of candidates for cardiac resynchronization therapy. Eur J Echocardiogr. 2010;11:863–9. DOI: 10.1093/ejechocard/jeq081

[107] Voigt JU, Schneider TM, Korder S, Szulik M, Gürel E, Daniel WG, et al. Apical transverse motion as surrogate parameter to determine regional left ventricular function inhomogeneities: a new, integrative approach to left ventricular asynchrony assessment. Eur Heart J. 2009;30:959–68. DOI: 10.1093/eurheartj/ehp062

[108] Thébault C, Donal E, Meunier C, Gervais R, Gerritse B, Gold MR, et al; REVERSE study group. Sites of left and right ventricular lead implantation and response to cardiac

resynchronization therapy observations from the REVERSE trial. Eur Heart J. 2012;33:2662–71. DOI: 10.1093/eurheartj/ehr505

[109] Khan FZ, Salahshouri P, Duehmke R, Read PA, Pugh PJ, Elsik M, et al. The impact of the right ventricular lead position on response to cardiac resynchronization therapy. Pacing Clin Electrophysiol. 2011;34:467–74. DOI: 10.1111/j.1540-8159

[110] Leclercq C, Sadoul N, Mont L, Defaye P, Osca J, Mouton E, et al; SEPTAL CRT Study investigators. Comparison of right ventricular septal pacing and right ventricular apical pacing in patients receiving cardiac resynchronization therapy defibrillators: the SEPTAL CRT Study. Eur Heart J. 2016;37:473–83. DOI: 10.1093/eurheartj/ehv422

[111] Singh JP, Klein HU, Huang DT, Reek S, Kuniss M, Quesada A, et al. Left ventricular lead position and clinical outcome in the Multicenter Automatic Defibrillator Implantation Trial–Cardiac Resynchronization Therapy (MADIT-CRT) Trial. Circulation. 2011;123:1159–66. DOI: 10.1161/CIRCULATIONAHA

[112] Kydd AC, Khan FZ, Watson WD, Pugh PJ, Virdee MS, Dutka DP. Prognostic benefit of optimum left ventricular lead position in cardiac resynchronization therapy: follow-up of the TARGET Study Cohort (Targeted Left Ventricular Lead Placement to guide Cardiac Resynchronization Therapy). JACC Heart Fail. 2014;2:205–12. Doi: 10.1016/j.jchf.2013.11.010

[113] Becker M, Kramann R, Franke A, Breithardt OA, Heussen N, Knackstedt C, et al. Impact of left ventricular lead position in cardiac resynchronization therapy on left ventricular remodelling. A circumferential strain analysis based on 2D echocardiography. Eur Heart J. 2007;28:1211–20. DOI: http://dx.doi.org/10.1093/eurheartj/ehm034

[114] Marsan NA, Westenberg JJ, Ypenburg C, van Bommel RJ, Roes S, Delgado V, et al. Magnetic resonance imaging and response to cardiac resynchronization therapy: relative merits of left ventricular dyssynchrony and scar tissue. Eur Heart J. 2009;30:2360–7. DOI: 10.1093/eurheartj/ehp280

[115] Westenberg JJ, Lamb HJ, van der Geest RJ, Bleeker GB, Holman ER, Schalij MJ, et al. Assessment of left ventricular dyssynchrony in patients with conduction delay and idiopathic dilated cardiomyopathy: head-to-head comparison between tissue Doppler imaging and velocity-encoded magnetic resonance imaging. J Am Coll Cardiol. 2006;47:2042–8. DOI:10.1016/j.jacc.2006.01.058

[116] Duckett SG, Ginks M, Shetty A, Kirubakaran S, Bostock J, Kapetanakis S, et al. Adverse response to cardiac resynchronisation therapy in patients with septal scar on cardiac MRI preventing a septal right ventricular lead position. J Interv Card Electrophysiol. 2012;33:151–60. DOI: 10.1007/s10840-011-9630-9

[117] Duckett SG, Chiribiri A, Ginks MR, Sinclair S, Knowles BR, Botnar R, et al. Cardiac MRI to investigate myocardial scar and coronary venous anatomy using a slow infusion of

dimeglumine gadobenate in patients undergoing assessment for cardiac resynchronization therapy. J Magn Reson Imaging. 2011;33:87–95. DOI: 10.1002/jmri.22387

[118] White JA, Yee R, Yuan X, Krahn A, Skanes A, Parker M, et al. Delayed enhancement magnetic resonance imaging predicts response to cardiac resynchronization therapy in patients with intraventricular dyssynchrony. J Am Coll Cardiol. 2006;48:1953–60. DOI: 10.1016/j.jacc.2006.07.046

[119] Hoffmann R, von Bardeleben S, ten Cate F, Borges AC, Kasprzak J, Firschke C, et al. Assessment of systolic left ventricular function: a multi-centre comparison of cineventriculography, cardiac magnetic resonance imaging, unenhanced and contrast-enhanced echocardiography. Eur Heart J. 2005;26:607–16. DOI: http://dx.doi.org/10.1093/eurheartj/ehi083

[120] Alpendurada F, Guha K, Sharma R, Ismail TF, Clifford A, Banya W, et al. Right ventricular dysfunction is a predictor of non-response and clinical outcome following cardiac resynchronization therapy. J Cardiovasc Magn Reson. 2011;13:68. DOI: 10.1186/1532-429X-13-68.

[121] Onishi T, Saha SK, Ludwig DR, Onishi T, Marek JJ, Cavalcante JL, et al. Feature tracking measurement of dyssynchrony from cardiovascular magnetic resonance cine acquisitions: comparison with echocardiographic speckle tracking. J Cardiovasc Magn Reson. 2013;15:95. DOI: 10.1186/1532-429X-15-95

[122] Bakos Z, Ostenfeld E, Markstad H, Werther-Evaldsson A, Roijer A, Arheden H, et al. A comparison between radial strain evaluation by speckle-tracking echocardiography and cardiac magnetic resonance imaging, for assessment of suitable segments for left ventricular lead placement in cardiac resynchronization therapy. Europace. 2014;16:1779–86. DOI: 10.1093/europace/euu167

[123] Mark DB, Berman DS, Budoff MJ, Carr JJ, Gerber TC, Hecht HS, et al. Expert Consensus Document on Coronary Computed Tomographic Angiography. J Am Coll Cardiol 2010;23:2663–2699. DOI: 10.1016/j.jacc.2010;23:2663–99.

[124] Ricapito Mde L, Conde D, Theriault MM, Rivera S, Badra-Verdu MG, Roux JF, et al. Multidetector cardiac tomography: a useful tool before cardiac resynchronization therapy. Cardiol J. 2015;22:590–6. DOI: 10.5603/CJ.a2015.0011

[125] Catanzaro JN, Makaryus JN, Jadonath R, Makaryus AN. Planning and guidance of cardiac resynchronization therapy-lead implantation by evaluating coronary venous anatomy assessed with multidetector computed tomography. Clin Med Insights Cardiol. 2015;8:43–50. DOI: 10.4137/CMC.S18762.

[126] Sommer A, Kronborg MB, Poulsen SH, Böttcher M, Nørgaard BL, Bouchelouche K, et al. Empiric versus imaging guided left ventricular lead placement in cardiac resynchronization therapy (ImagingCRT): study protocol for a randomized controlled trial. Trials. 2013;14:113. DOI: 10.1186/1745-6215-14-113

Chapter 4

Multimodality Echocardiographic Assessment of Patients Undergoing Atrial Fibrillation Ablation

Mariana Floria and Maria Daniela Tanase

Additional information is available at the end of the chapter

http://dx.doi.org/10.5772/64723

Abstract

Atrial fibrillation (AF) is most common sustained arrhythmia in clinical practice. The new treatment standard in paroxysmal and persistent AF is the catheter ablation. Echocardiography plays a key role in risk stratification and management of patients with AF and is critical in the assessment of candidates for AF ablation, providing both anatomic and hemodynamic information. Echocardiography is crucial for patient selection, preprocedural left atrial appendage thrombus excluding, intraprocedural guidance, and detection and monitoring for early and late ablation related complications. Transthoracic echocardiography allows rapid and comprehensive assessment of cardiac anatomical structure and function. Transoesophageal echocardiography also provides accurate information about the presence of a thrombus in the atria and thromboembolic risk, making safe the ablation procedure by immediately detection of the complications related procedure. Intracardiac echocardiography has emerged as a popular and useful tool in the everyday practice of interventional electrophysiology, being very useful only during the ablation procedure. This paper presents the role of echocardiography in all these steps concerning AF ablation procedure, and also (1) delineates the role of echocardiographic techniques in guiding the procedure, (2) discusses the critical echocardiographic aspects of this procedure, and (3) underlines the strengths and limitations of various echocardiographic modalities.

Keywords: atrial fibrillation, ablation, transthoracic echocardiography, transoesophageal echocardiography, intracardiac echocardiography

1. Introduction

The most common sustained cardiac arrhythmia, nonvalvular atrial fibrillation (AF), has an increasing prevalence and incidence in association with increased age and medical comorbidities. Nonvalvular AF is defined as AF in the absence of prosthetic mechanical heart valves, or haemodynamically significant mitral stenosis (moderate or severe) [1]. Evaluation of patients with AF requires an assessment of cardiac structure and function by echocardiography. Such an assessment complements the clinical evaluation and helps decision-making regarding rhythm strategy (rhythm control vs. rate control), stroke risk stratification, and prognosis. Currently approved AF therapies are only partially effective and are associated with substantial morbidity and mortality. The new treatment standard in this arrhythmia, AF catheter ablation, requires a multidisciplinary team approach involving interventional cardiologists and imaging specialists. For AF ablation, there is a need to identify individualized mechanism-based ablation targets (defined as mapping), located especially in left atrium (LA). Achieving durable pulmonary vein isolation as first step in AF ablation therapy remains technically challenging. AF substrate ablation (by targeting LA myocardium attaint by fibrosis due to the LA structural remodelling), in addition to pulmonary vein isolation, may prevent AF recurrence if pulmonary veins reconnect or nonpulmonary vein triggers emerge. Intrinsic cardiac autonomic nerve activity precedes the onset of AF. Autonomic activity is mediated by discrete ganglionated plexi localized on the LA posterior epicardium. It promotes LA electrical remodelling. Targeting these ganglionated plexi is another method for AF ablation. New approaches to mapping and ablation may target regions of oscillating action potential duration (especially in the LA myocardium) that can cause wave breaks leading to AF [2]. Recently, European Association of Cardiovascular Imaging and the European Heart Rhythm Association published evidences available on the role of imaging techniques (including echocardiography) and their applications in patients with AF, and provided recommendations for their use in clinical practice [3]. Echocardiography is critical in the assessment of candidates for AF ablation, providing both anatomic and haemodynamic information; it offers the potential for improved safety of AF ablation. Echocardiography is very useful at each step of the procedure: before AF ablation (by patient selection and pre-procedural LA appendage thrombus exclusion), intraprocedural guidance, and after AF ablation for detection and monitoring for early and late ablation-related complications, and also atrial reverse remodelling occurrence after obtaining stable sinus rhythm.

2. Echocardiography before atrial fibrillation ablation

Transthoracic echocardiography (TTE) allows rapid and comprehensive assessment of cardiac anatomical structure and function. It plays a central role in each of identifying comorbidities and identification of suitable candidates for AF catheter ablation. Pulmonary vein flow monitoring using echocardiography has the potential to an increasing role in the evaluation of cardiac diastolic function directly related to LA remodelling. Transoesophageal echocardiography (TOE) also provides accurate information about the presence of a thrombus in the atria or LA appendage (which is an absolute contraindication for AF ablation) and thromboembolic risk. The novel technique of intracardiac echocardiography (ICE) has emerged as a popular and useful tool in AF ablation during the procedure.

http://dx.doi.org/10.5772/64723

2.1. Echocardiography Assessment of Left Atrial Size, Anatomy and Function

LA dilatation (structural remodelling) can occur in a broad spectrum of cardiovascular diseases including hypertension, left ventricular dysfunction, mitral valve disease, and AF. In general, two major conditions are associated with LA dilatation: pressure overload and volume overload. TTE has an important role to diagnose all these diseases in patients with AF. The LA size has an incremental value of overconventional risk factors. However, LA size has also prognostic value for long-term outcome. The current guidelines on management of patients with AF recommend a standard two-dimensional (2D) TTE and Doppler echocardiogram, with assessment of LA *size and function*, in the clinical evaluation of all patients with AF (not only before AF ablation) [2].

LA size in addition to LA anatomy and function are the parameters mandatory to be assessed before deciding to include a patient for AF ablation procedure. The LA anterior-posterior diameter was one of the first standardized echocardiographic parameters for assessment of *LA* size. LA enlargement may result in an asymmetrical geometry of the LA. LA anterior-posterior diameter assessed in the parasternal long-axis view by 2D or M-mode echocardiography may underestimate LA size [4]. Anterior-posterior linear dimension should not be used as the sole measure of LA size [4]. Optimal assessment of LA size should include LA volume or LA area (preferably indexed) measurements [4]. LA dimensions can be assessed in the apical four- and two-chamber views. LA dimensions should be measured at end-ventricular systole, at maximal LA size. Each view must be optimized in order to avoid: an underestimation of LA size by foreshortening of the major length of the LA, inaccurate assumption of the mitral annulus boundary, loss of lateral resolution of the LA wall in the apical view, or dropout of the interatrial septum or anterior wall [4]. LA area is easy to assess and closer to LA size than anterior-posterior diameter. Various methods for the assessment of LA volume with 2D echocardiography are available, including the cubical method, area-length method, ellipsoid method, and modified Simpson's rule [4]. Because it is theoretically more accurate than the area-length method, the biplane disk summation technique, which incorporates fewer geometric assumptions, should be the preferred method to measure LA volume in clinical practice. For LA volume assessment, the same views as LA area are indicated (**Figure 1**). In

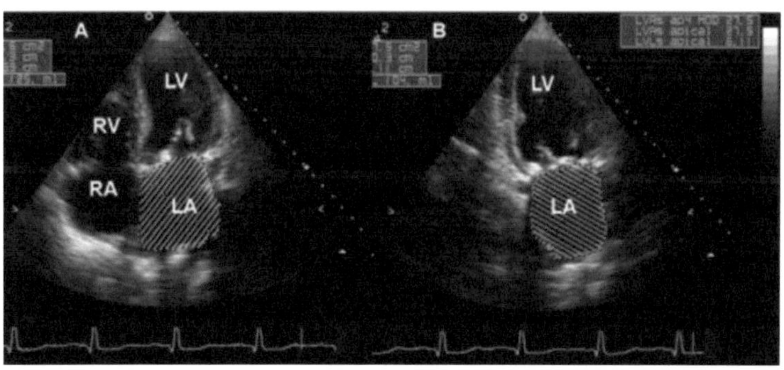

Figure 1. Biplane left atrial volume measurement by disk summation method in apical 4-chamber (A) and apical 2-chamber (B) views of bidimensional transthoracic echocardiography. LA: left atrium, LV: left ventricle, RA: right atrium, RV: right ventricle.

addition, the same precautions must to be respected. LA appendage and pulmonary veins should be avoided to be included as LA cavity. LA long diameter is recommended to be considered the shorter value of this length assessed in the two views specified above. The measurement of LA length is considered appropriate if the difference between the two values (in apical two- and four-chamber views) is not higher than 5 mm.

Alternatively, LA volume can be calculated using the disk summation technique by adding the volume of a stack of cylinders and area calculated by orthogonal minor and major transverse axes assuming an oval shape.

LA volume enables accurate assessment of the asymmetric structural remodelling of the LA and is a more robust predictor of cardiovascular events than linear or area measurements. However, the cornerstone of LA volume assessment is geometric assumptions about LA shape (as an ellipsoid shape).

The upper normal limit for 2D echocardiographic LA volume is 34 mL/m^2 for both genders. Single-plane apical four-chamber indexed LA volumes are typically 1–2 mL/m^2 smaller than apical two-chamber volumes. Apical four- and two-chamber linear measurements and nonindexed LA area and volume measurements are not recommended for routine clinical use [4].

In conclusion, TTE is the recommended approach for assessing LA size [4]. LA size should be measured at end-ventricular systole, at maximal LA size, with precautions to not underestimate or overestimate LA dimensions [4]. TOE slightly underestimates LA size; it provides good correlation with TTE. Although TOE permits good views on the LA and the LA appendage, it should not be used to assess LA size [4].

Recently has been demonstrated the feasibility of three-dimensional (3D) TTE for the assessment of LA volumes [5]. 3D echocardiography has the advantage that no geometrical assumption about LA shape has to be made and it seems to be more accurate when compared to 2D measurements. In addition, this echocardiographic method has a lower intraobserver and interobserver variability as compared to 2D echocardiography [5]. However, there still remain some technical limitations: The spatial and temporal resolution is low, depends on adequate image quality, and requires patient's cooperation; in addition, there are limited data on normal values [4].

LA size and volumes throughout the cardiac cycle can be acquired more precise with magnetic resonance image or computer tomography. Because the longitudinal axes of the left ventricle and LA frequently lie in different planes, dedicated acquisitions of the LA from the apical approach should be obtained for optimal LA volume measurements. However, these imaging methods are more expensive, sometimes with limited accessibility and more invasive (X-ray irradiation for computer tomography and potential kidney complications for both image techniques).

ICE is only used during AF catheter ablation procedure [6]. Therefore, no standardized measurements of LA size or volume are available. Although ICE is limited by the monoplane character and the lack of standardized measurements of LA size, it is a valuable tool for guidance ablation procedure.

http://dx.doi.org/10.5772/64723

The assessment of *LA anatomy* is important in the setting of catheter ablation procedures for AF [6]. Because of the complex anatomy of the LA and the variability in pulmonary vein anatomy, a detailed roadmap is mandatory to be known before the ablation procedure. The various imaging modalities that are available for assessment of LA and pulmonary vein anatomy in catheter ablation procedures include multislice computed tomography, magnetic resonance imaging, ICE, and electroanatomical mapping systems. Patients referred for AF ablation often have highly variable pulmonary vein anatomy, which could influence the procedure technique [6]. Four discrete pulmonary veins are present in the minority of patients with paroxysmal AF undergoing pulmonary vein isolation [6]. Anatomical variations include a single insertion or common antrum of the ipsilateral pulmonary veins, and an additional pulmonary vein. Assessment of LA and pulmonary vein anatomy by cardiac magnetic resonance or computed tomography before AF ablation is mandatory before the procedure. Pulmonary vein anatomy may in part explain the variable outcome to electrical isolation in patients with paroxysmal AF, although there is still debate concerning the best ablation strategy and the optimal lesion set. This information might aid in planning procedural strategies, and reducing unexpected procedural complications in AF ablation [6]. Among echocardiographic methods, only ICE (not TTE and TOE) has the capacity to assess a detailed pulmonary vein anatomy and morphology [7–9]. The interest in LA anatomy increases with AF ablation techniques developing [7–9]. New image integration systems have become available for AF catheter ablation procedures [8].

In patients in sinus rhythm LA has three important functions: the reservoir, the conduit, and the booster pump function. The change in the *LA function* in different phases can be evaluated noninvasively by echocardiography, utilizing not only usual methods including transmitral flow and changes in LA area and volume.

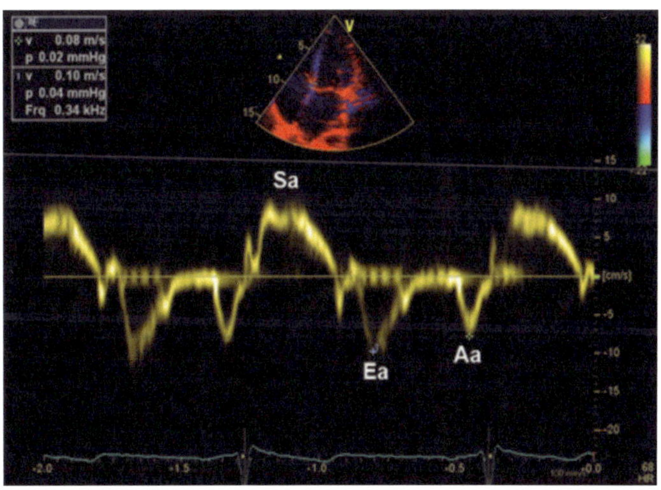

Figure 2. Tissue Doppler Imaging study (at the level of basal segment of septal interventricular wall) in apical four-chamber view of transmitral inflow in a patient with paroxysmal atrial fibrillation during sinus rhythm. Sa represents systolic myocardial velocity of left ventricle; Ea represents early diastolic filling myocardial velocity of left ventricle; Aa represents late diastolic filling myocardial velocity of left ventricle.

Pulsed-wave Doppler permits the assessment of late diastolic filling wave (A) on transmitral inflow pattern as marker of LA mechanical function. Both peak velocity and time-velocity integral of the mitral A wave could be used. However, in AF patients A wave is absent, so cannot be used for LA mechanical function assessment [5].

New echocardiographic techniques, such as Tissue Doppler Imaging (TDI) and speckle tracking (strain and strain rate) imaging, allow noninvasive measurement of regional function of the myocardium (including LA). TDI allows the quantification of the low-velocity, high-amplitude, long-axis intrinsic myocardial velocities in both systole and diastole, and provides a relatively load-independent measure of both left ventricle systolic and diastolic function (**Figure 2**).

The similar parameter of peak A velocity measured by TDI (Aa) is a myocardial velocity (not flow velocity) and could be also used as an atrial function parameter. It correlates with other parameters of atrial function as atrial fraction and atrial ejection force. In addition, it seems that Aa velocity assessed by TDI correlates with LA fractional area and volume change [5].

However, regional LA function is not routinely assessed, and therefore, no standardized parameters for regional LA functions are yet available [5]. A strong limitation for current using of this parameter is LA walls, which are thin and therefore difficult to be measured during wall moving. Improvement of LA regional function as marker of atrial electromechanical remodelling is an important outcome in patients that underwent AF catheter ablation.

Total electromechanical activity of the atria could be calculated by the interval between the onsets of the P-wave on the electrocardiogram to the end of the Aa wave on the TDI. However, TDI evaluation of regional LA function is the angle dependent. Therefore, careful adjustment of the beam and gain settings should be made to avoid aliasing and to allow reliable measurement of tissue velocities of the LA.

Another brand new technique, namely speckle tracking, is based on myocardial deformation assessment. Strain and strain rate are the two parameters that measure myocardial tissue velocity gradient by speckle tracking. This technique has some major advantages comparing with TDI: It is independent of wall movements and could differentiate between active and passive motion [5].

All TDI-derived parameters of the LA, including tissue velocities, strain and strain rate, were significantly reduced in patients with AF. Using TDI and/or strain imaging techniques, the decreased compliance of LA walls, the impairment of the reservoir and conduit function of LA, and the loss of the booster pump function in patients with AF were found.

After catheter ablation of AF, decreasing of these parameters means a possible criterion of do not interrupt the antiarrhythmic and anticoagulation treatment even in sinus rhythm due to the AF recurrences [5].

All changes in left ventricle diastolic function reflect on pulmonary venous flow morphology assessed by pulsed-wave Doppler [5]. In patients with AF due to LA pressure and functions (mainly the reservoir function), the following changes are possible: The wave of atrial reverse flow is absent due to the active LA mechanical function disappearance; peak velocity of systolic flow decreases and is related to the LA appendage dysfunction and thromboembolic risk; peak diastolic velocity higher than peak systolic velocity; an early systolic reverse flow is present [5]. In patients with AF catheter ablation pulmonary venous flow monitoring is important to assess LA mechanical function recovering. Preserved reservoir function of LA during AF is predictive of satisfactory recovery of mechanical function after pulmonary vein isolation [4, 5].

Pulmonary venous diastolic deceleration time is very useful to predict diastolic left ventricle filling pressure, as estimated by pulmonary capillary wedged pressure in AF [9]. This parameter is easy to be assessed after pulmonary venous flow registration by pulsed-wave Doppler. It is defined as duration between peak diastolic velocity and the upper deceleration slope extrapolated to the baseline.

According to the current guidelines, all these measurements should be taken on 5–10 cardiac cycles during a heart rate of 60–80 beats/min.

It seems that pulmonary venous deceleration time correlates better with pulmonary capillary wedged pressure than transmitral deceleration time in patients with AF [10]. Pulmonary venous deceleration time ≤150 ms could predict pulmonary capillary wedged pressure ≥18 mm Hg with 100% sensitivity and 96% specificity in patients with AF [10].

Patients with larger LA size, reduced LA function, and increased LA fibrosis (as marker of advanced electrical and structural remodelling) content are more likely to experience AF recurrences after ablation. The new echocardiography techniques have an emerging role in assessment of atrial fibrosis in patients with AF [7]. The appropriate selection of patients is mandatory for better outcomes in AF ablation; less fibrosis (that means less structural remodelling) seems to translate in better outcomes. Until now, there are not known imaging techniques able to predict AF ablation rate success tailored to each patient undergoing this treatment. However, there are some useful clinical tools (risk scores such as CHADS2, CHA2DS2-VASc, or APPLE scores) to identify patients with low, intermediate, or high risk of AF recurrence after AF ablation. However, echocardiography is very useful to detect and monitor LA reverse remodelling and improvement in atrial or ventricular function after AF ablation.

Atrial cardiomyopathies may provide the basis for the development of atrial fibrillation. The molecular alterations may also contribute to the occurrence of atrial thrombi. Thus, the concept of thrombogenic endocardial remodelling was introduced. In the future, echocardiography might be useful in this new type of atrial remodelling assessment.

2.2. Echocardiography Assessment of Left Atrial or Left Atrial Appendage Thrombus

The presence of LA appendage or LA thrombi is an absolute contraindication for AF ablation. Therefore, echocardiography assessment of thrombi presence is mandatory before AF ablation procedure. 2D TTE has a low sensitivity for detection of thrombi in LA and especially LA appendage. 2D or 3D TOE provides excellent visualization of posterior cardiac structures because of the anatomic relationship of these structures to the oesophagus. TOE is one of the modality of choice for detecting LA or LAA thrombi (**Figure 3A**).

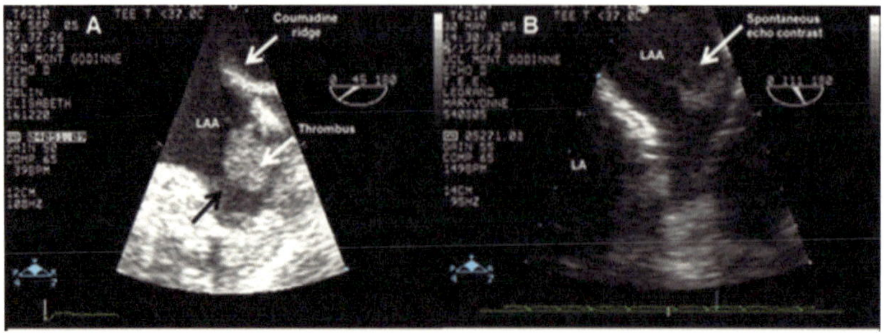

Figure 3. Two-dimensional transesophageal echocardiogram, midoesophageal view, allowing the identification of a left atrial appendage thrombus (A); zoom of the left atrial appendage illustrating the presence of a dense spontaneous echo contrast with swirling movements in the left atrial appendage (B).

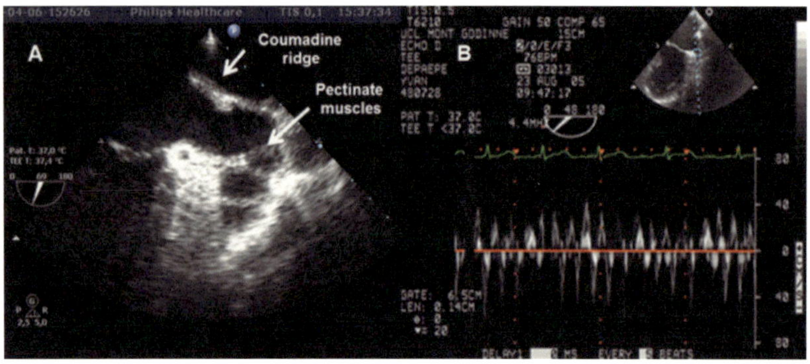

Figure 4. (A) Two-dimensional transesophageal echocardiogram, midoesophageal view, shows left atrial appendage with muscular ridge, namely coumadin ridge and pectinate muscles which could be misinterpreted as clots. (B) Pulsed-wave Doppler of the left atrial appendage demonstrates the decreased emptying and filling velocities in patients with atrial fibrillation.

It can detect thrombi with a high degree of sensitivity and specificity varying from 93% to 100% [5]. LA appendage has a very complex anatomy with variable shape, size, and orientation, with the possibility of several lobes and branches; therefore, thrombi assessment can be challenging. The muscular ridges and pectinate muscles (**Figure 4A**) must be carefully observed, because they can be misinterpreted as clots. Also ICE is very useful during AF ablation procedure to make the difference between muscular ridges and pectinate muscles (**Figure 5**). However, 3D TOE could make a better distinction between the pectinate muscles and thrombi, comparing with 2D TOE [11]. In addition, TOE is helpful in assessment of LA appendage velocities by pulsed-wave Doppler (**Figure 4B**). Usually, in patients in sinus rhythm without history of AF the average LA appendage filling velocity is 40–50 cm/s and correlates well with the LA appendage contraction velocity; the average LA appendage contraction velocity is 50–60 cm/s. Low LA appendage emptying flow velocities (defined as <20 cm/s) in AF correlate strongly with the presence of spontaneous echo contrast and thrombus formation. For patients with AF, TOE risk factors for thromboembolism associated with high risk of stroke include at least one of the following factors: LA appendage thrombus, severe spontaneous echo contrast, low flow velocities at LA appendage ostium, and complex aortic plaques [3].

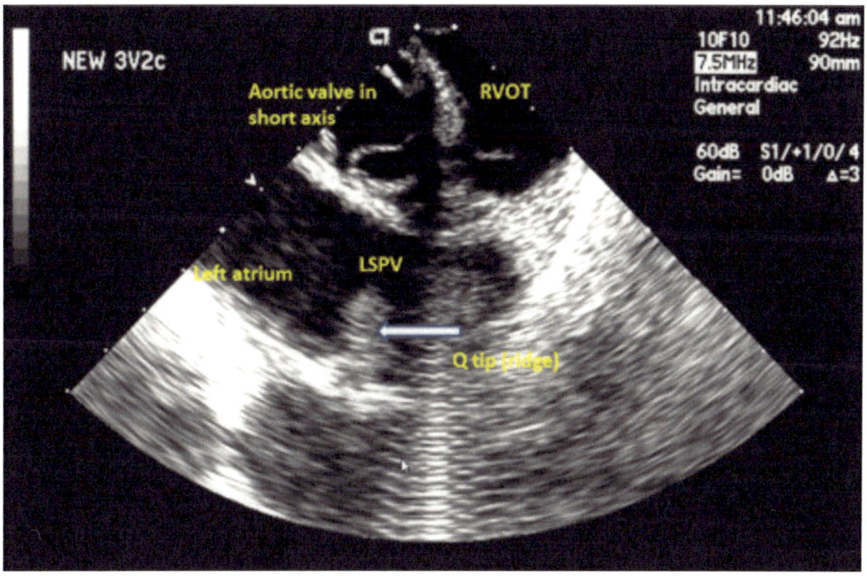

Figure 5. Intracardiac echocardiography shows very clearly anatomic structures during ablation procedure. This image was offered by courtesy of the editor. RVOT: right ventricle outflow tract; LSPV: left superior pulmonary vein.

Thrombus identification is also challenging even if the appendage is visualized adequately. In the absence of formed thrombi, a dense spontaneous echo contrast (**Figure 3B**) has been demonstrated to be strong a predictor of thromboembolism. Spontaneous echo contrast can be classified into four groups (1 to 4+), depending on the intensity, location, and presence of the swirling movement [12]. It seems that patients under anticoagulation and with thromboembolic risk scores (CHADS2 and CHA2DS2-VASc) <2 have a negative predictive value approaches to 100%; therefore, TOE before catheter ablation of AF might be avoided [13].

Sometimes it is difficult to distinguish small thrombi from artefacts, including prominent trabecular structures, duplication artefacts, and adipose tissue within the transverse sinus. It is necessary to attempt to differentiate any suspicious abnormalities from thrombus in multiple views. The mechanical function of LA appendage is best assessed with TOE utilizing pulsed-wave Doppler measurement of LA appendage emptying and filling velocities.

In addition to LA appendage Doppler assessment, measuring LA appendage area and ejection fraction (evaluated through vector velocity imaging), TDI, and 3D TOE are less validated and less frequently performed parameters associated with cerebrovascular events and the formation of LA appendage thrombus [11]. Pre-procedural multislice computed tomography may also identify the presence of thrombi in the LA appendage, but the gold standard is TOE [11]; in addition to the anatomy of the LA and pulmonary veins, it also provides detailed information on surrounding structures, such as the oesophagus and coronary arteries.

3. Echocardiography-Guided Ablation of Atrial Fibrillation

According to the new theories of AF physiopathology, some ablation strategies were elaborated; however, none is known as golden standard of this therapy. Depending on ablation technique, LA anatomy and pulmonary vein morphology are of essential importance to be well known during the ablation procedure. The veno-atrial junctions and anatomical structures of the LA, such as Coumadin ridge or the ridge between the left superior pulmonary vein and LA appendage, are critical for a safe and successful procedure.

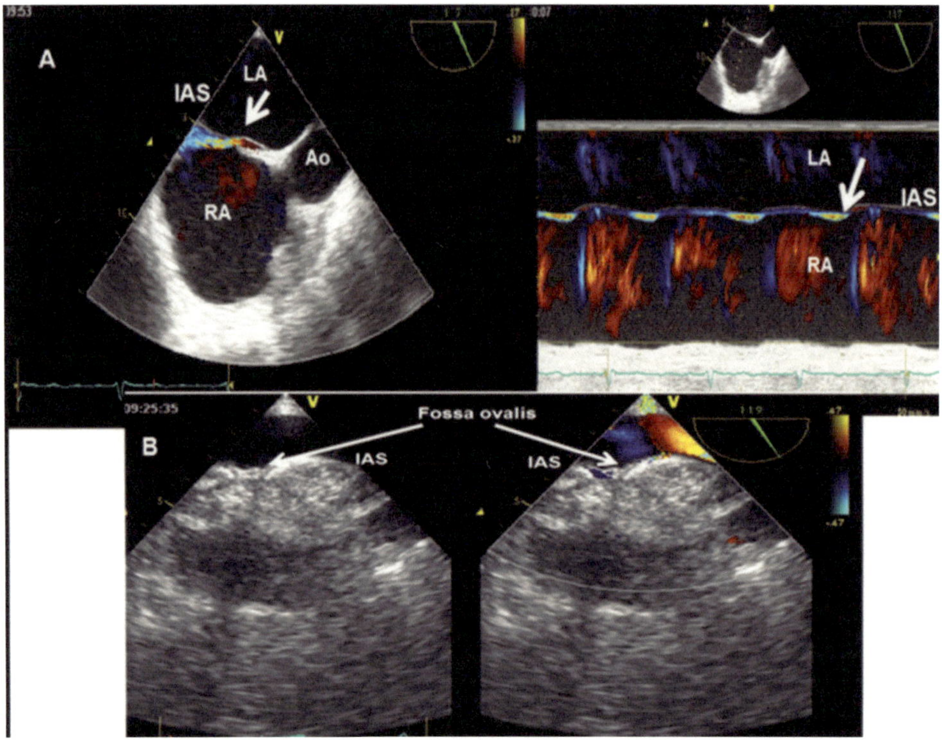

Figure 6. Two-dimensional transesophageal echocardiogram, midoesophageal view, shows (A) interatrial septum with left-right shunt in colour Doppler through patent foramen oval and (B) lipomatous interatrial septum. Ao: aorta; IAS: interatrial septum; LA: left atrium; RA: right atrium.

For pulmonary vein isolation or LA substrate ablation, it is mandatory to puncture the interatrial septum to gain left atrial posterior wall and pulmonary veins. If the patient has a patent foramen oval (**Figure 6A**), some operators say that transseptal puncture could be avoided. However, this is arguable, because accessibility to LA to gain pulmonary veins is difficult through a patent foramen oval. During TOE, a microbubble test under Valsalva manoeuvre could unmask a patent foramen oval. Rarely, TTE in subxiphoid view could identify the presence of a patent foramen oval. However, TOE has better sensibility to diagnose patent foramen oval before AF ablation. In patients with the lipomatous hypertrophy of the interatrial septum (**Figure 6B**), transseptal puncture could be difficult, without echocardiographic guidance.

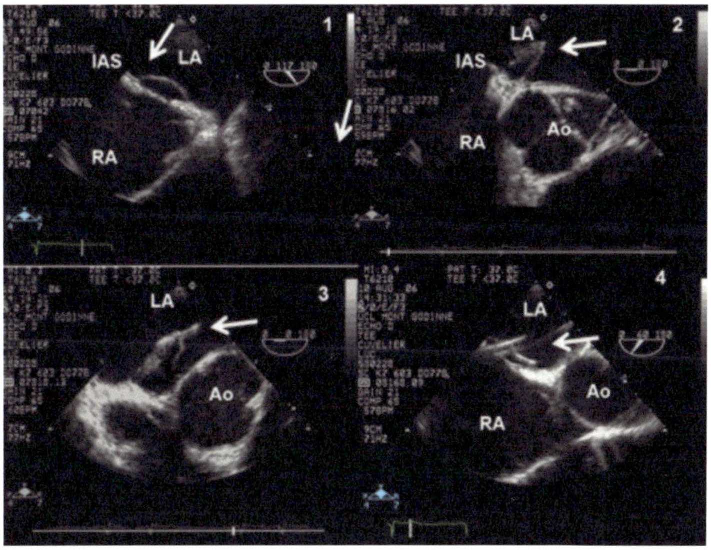

Figure 7. Transseptal puncture guided by bidimensional TOE shows direct visualization of the transseptal catheter and its relationship to the fossa ovalis and the ascending aorta. Ao: aorta; IAS: interatrial septum; LA: left atrium; RA: right atrium.

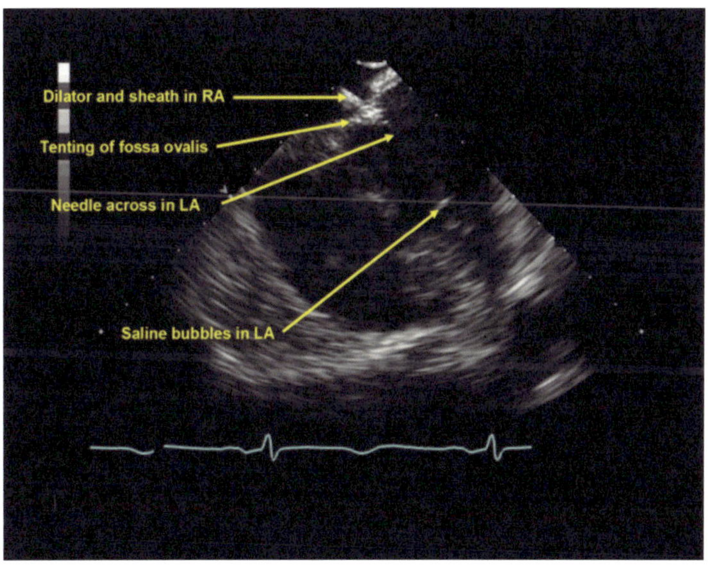

Figure 8. Uses of ICE for transseptal puncture guidance. LA: left atrium; RA: right atrium. This image was offered by courtesy of the editor.

Transseptal puncture allows procedural access to the LA. Anatomic structures are not directly visualized during transseptal puncture by fluoroscopic guidance. TTE and especially TOE may be helpful in performing this procedure by allowing direct visualization of the transseptal catheter and its relationship to the fossa ovalis. Anatomic variability in the position and orientation of the fossa ovalis and its surrounding structures may be challenging to even those interventional cardiologists with significant transseptal experience. However, echocardiography imaging offers increased safety to the operator, by avoiding the puncture of the intrapericardial aorta, a serious complication of transseptal puncture. In addition, radiation minimizes the fluoroscopy time required for the procedure, being very important during the learning curve. It was shown that TOE is of great value in performing transseptal punctures in AF ablation procedures. TTE can delineate the aorta and interatrial septum, and the characteristic bulging (or tenting) of the fossa ovalis and saline contrast echocardiography with TTE may help confirm needle position in the right atrium before puncture and in the LA after puncture (**Figure 7**). Anatomical variations in interatrial septum such as aneurismal septum, double-membrane septum, patent foramen oval, and others make this process complicated. Because TTE does not always offer sufficient imaging resolution, TOE and more recently ICE are preferably (**Figure 8**).

ICE could be useful only during the ablation procedure. It enables visualization of anatomical particularities of LA, being mostly important in transseptal puncture guidance and circular Lasso catheter positioning [14]. ICE enables to visualize the tenting of the interatrial septum due to the transseptal sheath tip during the puncture. It is important to be correctly placed in the posterior region of the fossa ovalis to avoid potential life-threatening complications such as aortic root perforation or LA lateral wall penetrating. For an appropriate mapping and ablation lesions, a good placement of Lasso catheter at the pulmonary vein antrum is mandatory. It could avoid important complications such as acute thrombus formation or early or late pulmonary vein stenosis by power, impedance, and temperature monitoring during energy delivery. Impedance increasing could be proceeding by microbubbles due to tissue superheating. ICE enables directly visualization of these microbubbles. In this case, immediate interruption of lesion creation is recommended to prevent severe complications such as cardiac tamponade by LA perforation, oesophageal injury or pulmonary vein stenosis. ICE is a useful tool also for the placement of mapping/ablation catheter according to anatomic landmarks and morphologic lesion changes monitoring for a safety and efficacy AF ablation procedure [7]. ICE has becoming a gold standard in complex AF ablation procedures by replacing fluoroscopy technique [14].

There has been a revival in the use of transseptal catheterization due to the increased use of radiofrequency ablation in the LA. Utilization of ICE in conjunction with fluoroscopy allows the electrophysiologist to clearly identify the interatrial septum and adjacent structures. ICE provides excellent views of the fossa ovalis and of the transseptal apparatus [7]. Life-threatening complications following inadvertent puncture of anatomic structures can be avoided under direct visualization. For electrophysiologist is important a direct visualization of the Brockenbrough needle and the Mullins sheath during the transseptal puncture. Sheath position in the LA could be verified by saline microbubbles or intravenous contrast injection.

The location of the Marshall vein, relevant in AF ablation, can also be identified from imaging of the "Q-tip" ridge, seen between the LA appendage and left pulmonary veins [7].

During AF ablation procedure, the mapping is followed by energy applications and lesion creation. Atrial myocardium suffers some alterations after energy application such as thickening, dimpling, and hyper-echogenicity. ICE enables identification of all myocardium sites transformed during ablation. The characteristics of lesions could be controlled by monitoring and titrating of energy parameters (temperature, impedance, and power). In addition, ICE allows identification of triggers sites such ligament of Marshall and to treat by applications under direct visualization. The applications on LA posterior wall could translate into fistula between anterior wall of the oesophagus and LA, a lethal complication of an extensive AF ablation procedure. Therefore, ICE is very useful during the procedure to titrate energy parameters to avoid this. In conclusion, ICE is used only during the ablation procedure; it allows better results of the procedure and lower risk of complications [15].

All echocardiography methods, TTE, TOE, or ICE, have the ability to detect early and avoid potential lethal complications during AF ablation [15]. Appropriate anticoagulation could prevent spontaneously thrombus formation and embolization during the procedure. Immediate detecting of thrombus by ICE allows prompting removal of catheters to avoid embolic complications.

Microbubbles visualization is most useful for prompting discontinuation of energy delivery when microbubbles are seen. Early detection of a pericardial effusion before cardiac tamponade (preferable before signs of haemodynamic compromise) and catheter-based treatment of the effusion are two facilitations allowed by TTE, TOE, or ICE. Pulmonary vein stenosis is a serious complication that can be detected early by visual tissue swelling and assessing severity with peak velocity measurements and colour flow parameters or pulsed-wave Doppler imaging, available with phased-array imaging [14].

During ablation procedure, ICE can accurately visualize LA anatomy and related structures and may guide transseptal catheterization and it is helpful in monitoring potential complications during catheter ablation procedures. In addition, it allows to establish a clear-cut relationship between the catheter tip and underlying tissue and to visualize the lesion formation; it can be performed with minimal additional patient risk and discomfort, without additional sedation or general anaesthesia; it does not need prolonged oesophageal intubation, accompanying patient discomfort, or the risk for aspiration. ICE offers imaging that is comparable with or superior to TOE and is an alternative to TOE in selected patients with absolute contraindications to TOE (oesophagectomy). This technique is quite safe with a negligible rate of complications and good patient tolerance. It allows improvement in success rate and decrease in complication when compared to fluoroscopic approach. ICE has been shown to improve patient comfort, shorten both procedure and fluoroscopy times, and offer comparable cost with TEE-guided interventions [5].

Comparing with TOE, ICE has some advantages: clearer image, reduced irradiation, and shorter duration of the procedure [16]. It has also some disadvantages such as: the shaft is thick without the possibility to have ports for pressure, therapeutic devices, and guide wires; the phased-array catheters are cost-ineffective (single use, higher costs); ICE offers only monoplane image views being difficult to obtain some sections as for TOE [10]. In addition, there are not still standard views for ICE as for other echocardiographic imaging modality such as TTE or TOE. In addition, in the literature there are described some potential risks of vascular lesion, cardiac perforation, arrhythmias, thromboembolism, and cutaneous nerve palsy [5]. However, it is expected to be used widely in clinical practice and even to become the standard for the transseptal catheterization.

4. Echocardiography after Atrial Fibrillation Ablation

Echocardiography is very useful after AF ablation for detection and monitoring for early and late related complications, and also for LA reverse remodelling assessment in patients with stable sinus rhythm.

Pulmonary veins flow monitoring is used to detect early pulmonary vein stenosis after AF ablation, which could occur in 1% to 3% of current series [17]. TOE allows the suspicion of a significant PV stenosis (**Figure 9**) by a combination of elevated peak pulmonary vein velocity (≥110 cm/s) with turbulence and little flow variation [17]. Although TOE has been used, it does not usually provide adequate assessment.

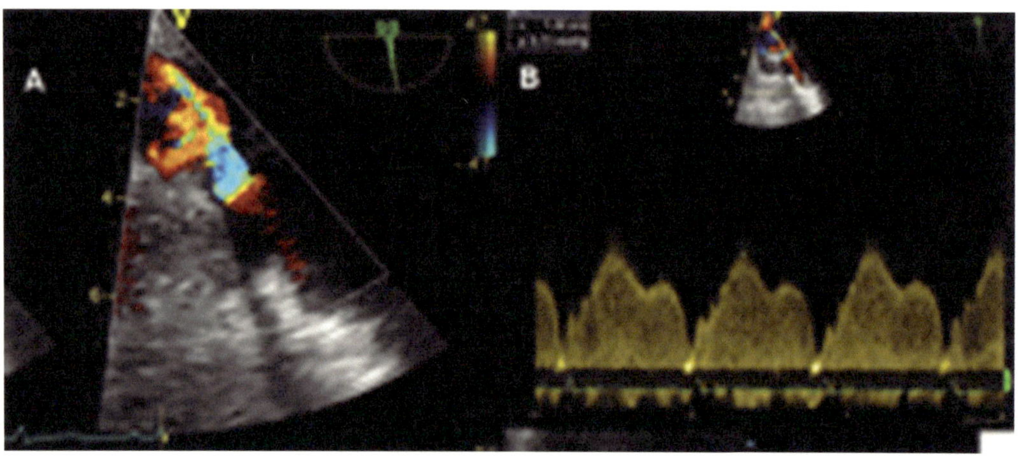

Figure 9. (A) Colour Doppler mode by transoesophageal echocardiography at the level of left superior pulmonary vein identify a significant pulmonary vein stenosis. (B) Pulsed-wave Doppler of left superior pulmonary vein inflow confirms haemodynamically significant stenosis. LA: left atrium, AO: aorta, LSPV: left superior pulmonary vein.

However, TTE or TOE are limited by its inability to image deeply into all four pulmonary veins and are less useful in establishing the extent and location of pulmonary vein stenosis. Diagnostic tests of value include magnetic resonance angiography and computed tomography. Progression of stenosis is unpredictable and may be rapid. Recurrent restenosis after angioplasty and stenting, as therapeutic solution of this complication, may occur in 30–50% of patients with pulmonary veins stenosis [17]. Follow-up of these patients typically involves computed tomography imaging to document restenosis.

Pulmonary vein stenosis could occur late after AF ablation. TOE could raise the suspicion by detection of high pulmonary vein velocities. Follow-up of these patients typically involves computed tomography or magnetic resonance imaging to document stenosis.

TOE and ICE allow early identification of complications related with procedure including damage to intracardiac structures, thrombus formation, pulmonary vein stenosis, and pericardial effusion during catheter ablation of AF.

A TOE performed 3–6 months after AF ablation can also evaluate thromboembolic risk and need for long-term anticoagulation, as echocardiographic risk factors may be present even if restoration of sinus rhythm is successful.

Catheter ablation has been demonstrated to be successful in the restoration of sinus rhythm and is performed in an increasing number of patients with symptomatic drug-refractory paroxysmal and persistent AF. It has been demonstrated that restoration and maintenance of sinus rhythm after catheter ablation is associated with a decrease in LA volumes (reverse structural LA remodelling), with subsequent improvement of LA function [5]. Using the new tissue Doppler-derived parameters, it was shown that in parallel with the improvement in LA function, both left ventricle systolic and diastolic function improved in the patients who maintained sinus rhythm [5]. In addition to LA reverse remodelling, even the area of the pulmonary venous ostia may decrease after successful catheter ablation procedures [5]. Post-procedural imaging to evaluate the extent of reverse LA remodelling after catheter ablation is critical to appropriate decisions regarding ongoing anti-arrhythmic therapy and long-term anticoagulation.

Conversion of AF and atrial flutter to sinus rhythm could result in a transient mechanical dysfunction of LA and LA appendage, termed atrial stunning [17]. Atrial stunning has been reported including after radiofrequency ablation. This phenomenon is well recognized with peak A velocity of transmitral inflow (by a very low value or absence) as well as TDI or strain imaging. Atrial stunning is at maximum immediately after procedure and improves progressively with a complete resolution within a few minutes to 4–6 weeks depending on the duration of the preceding AF, atrial size, and structural heart disease [18]. This suggests that a dissociation of electrical and mechanical recovery occurs after successful restoration of sinus rhythm, with a delay in gradual improvement of atrial mechanical function.

Stiff LA syndrome, defined as pulmonary hypertension with LA diastolic dysfunction, has regained attention in patients who had undergone catheter ablation for AF, especially after multiple ablation procedures [19]. This syndrome is a rare but potentially significant complication of AF ablation. Severe LA scarring, LA ≤45 mm, diabetes mellitus, obstructive sleep apnoea, and high LA pressure are clinical variables that predict the development of this syndrome [19]. The main echocardiographic findings include pulmonary hypertension in the absence of pulmonary vein stenosis or LA pressure tracings in the absence of mitral regurgitation. Pulmonary vein diastolic flow velocity (assessed by TTE or TOE) and E/Ea (by TTE using pulse wave Doppler and TDI) can be used as a noninvasive parameter predicting high

LA pressure peak (during sinus rhythm) in patients with AF [19]. Elevated LA pressure was closely associated with electroanatomical remodelling of the LA and was an independent predictor for recurrence after AF ablation [20, 21].

5. Conclusion

Multimodality echocardiography is needed at each step of AF ablation procedure. LA size, morphology, and function together with other cardiac parameters are mandatory for patient selection. 2D TTE allows rapid and comprehensive assessment of cardiac anatomical structure and function. 2D or 3D TOE provides accurate information about preprocedural LA appendage thrombus in the atria and thromboembolic risk and is very useful for intraprocedural guidance. The novel technique of ICE has emerged also as a popular and useful tool in the guidance of AF ablation procedure. TTE or TOE is need for early and late ablation-related complications detection and monitoring. In the future, echocardiography might be useful in thrombogenic endocardial remodelling assessment, a novel concept in atrial cardiomyopathies such as atrial fibrillation.

Author details

Mariana Floria* and Maria Daniela Tanase

*Address all correspondence to: floria_mariana@yahoo.com

Gr. T. Popa University of Medicine and Pharmacy, Iasi, Romania

References

[1] Van Wagoner DR, Piccini JP, Albert CM, Anderson ME, Benjamin EJ, Brundel B, Califf RM, Calkins H, Chen PS, Chiamvimonvat N, Darbar D, Eckhardt LL, Ellinor PT, Exner DV, Fogel RI, Gillis AM, Healey J, Hohnloser SH, Kamel H, Lathrop DA, Lip GY, Mehra R, Narayan SM, Olgin J, Packer D, Peters NS, Roden DM, Ross HM, Sheldon R, Wehrens XH: Progress toward the prevention and treatment of atrial fibrillation: a summary of the Heart Rhythm Society Research Forum on the Treatment and Prevention of Atrial Fibrillation, Washington, DC, 9–10 December 2013. Heart Rhythm 2015;12:e5–e29. doi: 10.1016/j.hrthm.2014.11.011.

[2] Camm AJ, Lip GY, De Caterina R, Savelieva I, Atar D, Hohnloser SH, Hindricks G, Kirchhof P: ESC committee for practice guidelines-CPG; document reviewers: 2012 focused update of the ESC guidelines for the management of atrial fibrillation: an

update of the 2010 ESC Guidelines for the management of atrial fibrillation. Europace 2012;14:1385–413.

[3] Donal E, Lip GY, Galderisi M, Goette A, Shah D, Marwan M, Lederlin M, Mondillo S, Edvardsen T, Sitges M, Grapsa J, Garbi M, Senior R, Gimelli A, Potpara TS, Van Gelder IC, Gorenek B, Mabo P, Lancellotti P, Kuck KH, Popescu BA, Hindricks G, Habib G, Cosyns B, Delgado V, Haugaa KH, Muraru D, Nieman K, Cohen A: EACVI/EHRA Expert Consensus Document on the role of multi-modality imaging for the evaluation of patients with atrial fibrillation. Eur Heart J Cardiovasc Imaging 2016;17:355–83. doi: 10.1093/ehjci/jev354.

[4] Lang RM, Badano LP, Mor-Avi V, Afilalo J, Armstrong A, Ernande L, Flachskampf FA, Foster E, Goldstein SA, Kuznetsova T, Lancellotti P, Muraru D, Picard MH, Rietzschel ER, Rudski L, Spencer KT, Tsang W, Voigt JU: Recommendations for cardiac chamber quantification by echocardiography in adults: an update from the American Society of Echocardiography and the European Association of Cardiovascular Imaging. Eur Heart J Cardiovasc Imaging 2015;16:233–70. doi:10.1093/ehjci/jev014.

[5] Tops LF, van der Wall EE, Schalij MJ, Bax JJ: Multi-modality imaging to assess left atrial size, anatomy and function. Heart 2007;93:1461–1470. doi:10.1136/hrt.2007.116467.

[6] Shigenaga Y, Okajima K, Ikeuchi K, Kiuchi K, Ikeda T, Shimane A, Yokoi K, Teranishi J, Aoki K, Chimura M, Yamada S, Taniguchi Y, Yasaka Y, Kawai H: Usefulness of non-contrast-enhanced MRI with two-dimensional balanced steady-state free precession for the acquisition of the pulmonary venous and left atrial anatomy pre catheter ablation of atrial fibrillation: Comparison with contrast enhanced CT in clinical cases. J Magn Reson Imaging 2016;43:495–503. doi:10.1002/jmri.24990.

[7] Longobardo L, Todaro MC, Zito C, Piccione MC, Di Bella G, Oreto L, Khandheria BK, Carerj S: Role of imaging in assessment of atrial fibrosis in patients with atrial fibrillation: state-of-the-art review. Eur Heart J Cardiovasc Imaging 2014;15:1–5. doi:10.1093/ehjci/jet116.

[8] McLellan AJ, Ling LH, Ruggiero D, Wong MC, Walters TE, Nisbet A, Shetty AK, Azzopardi S, Taylor AJ, Morton JB, Kalman JM, Kistler PM: Pulmonary vein isolation: the impact of pulmonary venous anatomy on long-term outcome of catheter ablation for paroxysmal atrial fibrillation. Heart Rhythm 2014;11:549–56. doi:10.1016/j.hrthm.2013.12.025.

[9] Kanaji Y, Miyazaki S, Iwasawa J, Ichihara N, Takagi T, Kuroi A, Nakamura H, Taniguchi H, Hachiya H, Iesaka Y: Pre-procedural evaluation of the left atrial anatomy in patients referred for catheter ablation of atrial fibrillation. J Cardiol 2016;67:115–21. doi:10.1016/j.jjcc.2015.02.016.

[10] Dravid SG, Hope B, McKinnie JJ: Intracardiac echocardiography in electrophysiology: a review of current applications in practice. Echocardiography 2008;25:1172–5. doi:10.1111/j.1540-8175.2008.00784.x.

[11] Providência R, Trigo J, Paiva L, Barra S: The role of echocardiography in thromboembolic risk assessment of patients with nonvalvular atrial fibrillation. J Am Soc Echocardiogr 2013;26:801–12. doi:10.1016/j.echo.2013.05.010.

[12] Fatkin D, Kelly RP, Feneley MP: Relations between left atrial appendage blood flow velocity, spontaneous echocardiographic contrast and thromboembolic risk *in vivo*. J Am Coll Cardiol 1994;23:961–9.

[13] Floria M, De Roy L, Xhaet O, Blommaert D, Jamart J, Gerard M, Dormal F, Deceuninck O, Ambarus V, Marchandise B, Schroeder E: Predictive value of thromboembolic risk scores before an atrial fibrillation ablation procedure. J Cardiovasc Electrophysiol 2013;24:139–45. doi:10.1111/j.1540-8167.2012.02442.x.

[14] Kadakia MB1, Silvestry FE, Herrmann HC: Intracardiac echocardiography-guided transcatheter aortic valve replacement. Catheter Cardiovasc Interv 2015;85:497–501. doi:10.1002/ccd.25409.

[15] Kim TS, Youn HJ: Role of Echocardiography in Atrial Fibrillation. J Cardiovasc Ultrasound 2011;19:51–61. doi:10.4250/jcu.2011.19.2.51.

[16] George JC, Varghese V, Mogtader A: Intracardiac echocardiography: evolving use interventional cardiology. J Ultrasound Med 2014;33:387–95. doi:10.7863/ultra.33.3.387.

[17] Holmes DR Jr, Monahan KH, Packer D: Pulmonary vein stenosis complicating ablation for atrial fibrillation: clinical spectrum and interventional considerations. JACC Cardiovasc Interv 2009;2:267–76. doi:10.1016/j.jcin.2008.12.014.

[18] Khan IA: Atrial stunning: basics and clinical considerations. Int J Cardiol 2003;92:113–28.

[19] Gibson DN, Di Biase L, Mohanty P, Patel JD, Bai R, Sanchez J, Burkhardt JD, Heywood JT, Johnson AD, Rubenson DS, Horton R, Gallinghouse GJ, Beheiry S, Curtis GP, Cohen DN, Lee MY, Smith MR, Gopinath D, Lewis WR, Natale A: Stiff left atrial syndrome after catheter ablation for atrial fibrillation: clinical characterization, prevalence, and predictors. Heart Rhythm 2011;8:1364–1371. doi:10.1016/j.hrthm.2011.02.026.

[20] Park J, Yang PS, Kim TH, Uhm JS, Kim JY, Joung B, Lee MH, Hwang C, Pak HN: Low left atrial compliance contributes to the clinical recurrence of atrial fibrillation after catheter ablation in patients with structurally and functionally normal heart. PLoS One 2015;10:e0143853. doi:10.1371/journal.pone.0143853.

[21] Park J, Joung B, Uhm JS, Young Shim C, Hwang C, Hyoung Lee M, Pak HN: High left atrial pressures are associated with advanced electroanatomical remodeling of left atrium and independent predictors for clinical recurrence of atrial fibrillation after catheter ablation. Heart Rhythm 2014;11:953–60. doi:10.1016/j.hrthm.2014.03.009.

Section 2

Echocardiography in Heart Failure

Speckle-Tracking Imaging, Principles and Clinical Applications: A Review for Clinical Cardiologists

Iacopo Fabiani, Nicola Riccardo Pugliese,
Veronica Santini, Lorenzo Conte and
Vitantonio Di Bello

Additional information is available at the end of the chapter

http://dx.doi.org/10.5772/64261

Abstract

Evaluation of myocardial mechanics, although complex, has now entered the clinical arena, thanks to the introduction of bedside imaging techniques, such as speckle-tracking echocardiography.

Overcoming the limitations of previous techniques, such as tissue Doppler Imaging (TDI), bi-dimensional (2D) and, only recently, three-dimensional (3D) speckle tracking, allows a fast, reproducible, and semi-automated description of myocardial deformation parameters, including strain, strain rate, velocity, displacement, torsion, and timing of contraction/relaxation. From research tool, speckle tracking has become a great help for clinicians, validated with respect to more complex, time-consuming, and expensive techniques.

Nowadays, further development in technology and image processing draws the attention of the cardiology community. This review intends to describe the fundamental aspects of the imaging technique, together with some recent innovations and clinical applications in this field.

Keywords: cardiac mechanics, deformation, strain, strain rate, speckle tracking

1. Introduction

Speckle-tracking imaging (STI) is a non-invasive ultrasound technique that allows an objective and quantitative evaluation of global and regional myocardial function, independently from the angle of insonation and partly from cardiac translational movements [1–4].

Technique	Advantage	Disadvantage
STI	• Analysis in 2D	• Temporal resolution
	• Tissue movement relative to adjacent segments	• Poor image quality
	• Angle independency	• Myocardial curvature
	• Spatial resolution	• Lower frame rates in tachycardia
	• Low noise	
	• Automated tracking system	
	• Lower interobserver variability	
TDI	• Adequate image quality	• Interobserver variability
	• Temporal resolution	• Time-consuming
		• Technically demanding
		• Low signal-noise ratio
		• Poor spatial resolution
		• Angle dependency
		• One dimension
		• Displacement in relation to transducer

2D, bi-dimensional; STI, speckle-tracking imaging; TDI, tissue Doppler imaging

Table 1. Advantage and disadvantage of different techniques for myocardial deformation analysis.

Echocardiographic estimation of segmental left ventricular contractility is routinely accomplished through visual interpretation of endocardial motion and myocardial thickening. This method is subjective and requires a relatively experienced observer. Quantitative analysis based on tracing of the endocardial border may also be hampered by endocardial "dropout" and trabeculations.

Tissue Doppler imaging (TDI) has been previously used in deriving myocardial velocities and assessing fundamental parameters of myocardial deformation (strain and strain rate) [5]. Myocardial tissue velocities represent the net effect of the contractile and elastic properties of the area under investigation and the motion caused by traction and tethering from other regions. In contrast, strain is a dimensionless index reflecting the total deformation of the ventricular myocardium during a cardiac cycle, as a percentage of its initial length. Strain rate is the rate of deformation or stretch. Strain techniques are, in principle, the optimal modalities for the assessment of regional myocardial function. The major limitation of TDI has been its angle dependency [5], requiring alignment of the ultrasound beam parallel to the direction of tissue movement. Thus, deformation study was substantially limited to the analysis of the tissue moving toward or away from the probe (**Table 1**).

STI is based on bi-dimensional (2D) echocardiographic technology, not limited by Doppler analysis [6–8]. Segments of myocardial tissue show a pattern of gray values in the ultrasound. This pattern, resulting from the spatial distribution of gray values, is commonly referred to as speckle pattern, characterizes the underlying myocardial tissue acoustically and is unique for each myocardial segment. Speckle tracking allows the measure of all in-plane components of the velocity vector, in all pixels [9]. More recently, the addition of the third dimension (3D) has partly expanded the scope of this technology.

2. Human myocardium

Human myocardium is made up of multiple layers [10–12]. According to the helical model described by Torrent-Guasp, a single myocardial muscle band folding upon itself creates varying orientations of fibers throughout the myocardium, with two principal loops, basal (transverse) and apical (oblique). Myocardium finally consists of three separate layers: transversely oriented circular fibers that wrap (around both ventricles), the inner oblique layer (clockwise rotation), and the outer oblique layer (counterclockwise rotation). Briefly, the myofiber geometry of the LV changes gradually from a right-handed helix in the subendocardium to a left-handed helix in the subepicardium.

The mechanics of the LV is complex, but three principal components contribute to systole: inward motion, longitudinal motion (base moving toward the apex), and differential rotation of the apex and base (twisting). Diastolic mechanics is the opposite of systolic motion. LV torsion (or twist) has an important role in cardiac systo-diastolic mechanics. During the cardiac cycle, there is a systolic twist and an early diastolic untwist around left ventricular long axis, due to opposite apical and basal rotations. Systolic apical rotation is counterclockwise and basal rotation is clockwise [13]. LV rotation is a sensitive indicator of changes in regional and global LV function.

2.1. Cardiac mechanics and limits of conventional indices

Cardiac function is the result of force development (inotropism: opening of the cardiac valves) and deformation (shortening of the myocytes: volume ejection) and can be evaluated globally (pump performance) or regionally [14]. Correct evaluation of systolic function should focus on the intrinsic properties of the fibers and myocytes that represent the real actors behind heart function as well as a pathologic process. The deformation of a myocardial segment during the cardiac cycle is a complex phenomenon and consists of normal deformation (longitudinal shortening/lengthening, radial thickening/thinning, and circumferential shortening/lengthening) and shear deformation (base-apex twisting, epi-endo circumferential shear, and epi-endo longitudinal shear). There is a clear gradient from base to apex in both velocity and displacement (stationary of the apex within the thorax while the base is moving toward it). In contrast, deformation is more or less homogenous throughout the (normal) myocardial wall.

It is important to understand the relation between intrinsic function (contractility) and the resulting motion/deformation. A myocardial segment develops a force but it is also subject to the forces developed by near segments. The intrinsic contractile force of the myocardium (inotropism) is the most important determinant of myocardial performance, but any segment of myocardium is part of a ventricle, with external forces acting up on it (mostly in the opposite direction of the contractile force) and resulting from local wall stress, caused by the intracavitary pressure (related to local geometry of the ventricle) and the interaction with neighboring contracting segments ("pulling" the segment itself). The relationship between acting forces and the resultant deformation is influenced by regional elasticity, which by itself is not a constant; due to the structure of the tissue, the more the myocardium is stretched, the more difficult it becomes to stretch it even further.

Regional myocardial deformation is thus the result of:

Active forces:

- Intrinsic contractility (influenced by tissue perfusion and electrical activation).

Passive forces:

- Intracavitary pressure (afterload/preload; ventricular geometry);
- Segment interaction.

Tissue elasticity:

- Myofibrillar architecture;
- Collagen amount (fibrosis).

Despite this pathophysiological insight, echocardiography is still mainly based on global and indirect indices such as ejection fraction, a volume-based parameter that does not reflect contractility, being based on geometric assumptions. For example, "supranormal" values of ejection fraction (EF) are often found in hypertrophied or volume-overloaded ventricles, thus not reflecting real changes in contractility. EF is also load dependent and, per se, is only a global index, without regional implications and not taking into account segmental interactions, which do not contribute to pump function. Moreover, indices for global functional assessment reflect mainly radial function, ignoring longitudinal function, which is usually altered long before changes occur in radial indices.

2.2. The concept of myocardial deformation

When two neighboring points of the myocardium move at different velocities, myocardium changes its shape (deforming). Otherwise, myocardium is moving but not deforming. When the velocity of the tissue is known, several other parameters can be derived.

Displacement is the integral of the velocity over time (Eq. (1)).

http://dx.doi.org/10.5772/64261

$$d = \int_{T_0}^{T} v(t)dt \tag{1}$$

Strain and strain rate are measures of changes in shape, that is, deformation.

For mono-dimensional deformations, that is, shortening or lengthening, the simplest measurement is conventional or Lagrangian strain (Eq. (2)).

$$\varepsilon(t) = \frac{L(t) - L_0}{L_0} \tag{2}$$

The Greek letter epsilon (ε) is commonly used as a symbol for conventional strain. The strain value is dimensionless and can be presented as a fractional number or as a percentage. For Lagrangian strain, a single reference length (L_0) is defined, against which all subsequent deformation ($L(t)$) will be measured. Strain is positive if L is major than L_0 (an object has lengthened) and negative if L is smaller than L_0 (shortening). If L equals L_0, the strain is thus zero.

Natural strain (ε') is defined as [15]:

$$\varepsilon' = \ln(\frac{L}{L_0}) \tag{3}$$

Natural strain employs a reference length that changes as the object deforms. It therefore describes the instantaneous length change and it is independent of reference times. Compared to that of conventional strain, the natural strain amplitude is smaller for positive strains and larger for negative strains. This concept applies in principle to all three one-dimensional (longitudinal, circumferential, and radial) displacement and strain components.

In two or three dimensions, we should also consider shear strain, i.e., measurement of deformation in angle. It is also mandatory to specify directions and magnitudes of maximal and minimal strain.

The strain rate is the temporal derivative of the strain (Eq. (4)).

$$\varepsilon' = \frac{d\varepsilon}{dt} \tag{4}$$

Whereas strain indicates the amount of deformation, strain rate indicates the rate of the deformation. The spatial gradient in myocardial velocities represents the rate of myocardial deformation, that is, the strain rate. The unit of the strain rate is normally 1/s or s^{-1}. Strain rate is more uniformly distributed along the different regions of the LV, whereas myocardial velocity decreases from base toward apical parts of the LV. Strain can subsequently be derived by temporal integration of the strain rate curve. Indeed, if the rate of deformation is known at each time instance during the cardiac cycle, the total amount of deformation can easily be calculated. A positive strain rate means that the length of the object is increasing, whereas a negative strain rate means that the length is decreasing. If the length is constant, the strain rate is zero. Therefore, whereas strain is a measurement of deformation relative to a reference state, strain rate is an instantaneous measurement. When the strain rate has been calculated for each time point during the deformation, the strain can be found as the temporal integral of the strain rate (Eq. (5)).

$$\varepsilon' = \int_{T_0}^{T} \varepsilon'(t)dt \tag{5}$$

2D strain comprises four measurements: two natural strains and two shear strains [6].

A 3D model allows the evaluation of three natural strain and six shear strain measurements along x, y, and z or azimuthal axes.

2.3. Fundamentals of speckle tracking

"Speckles" are small groups of myocardial pixels created by the interaction of ultrasonic beams and the myocardium, with specific gray scale characteristics. A speckle is commonly defined as the spatial distribution of gray values in the ultrasound image. The result of a speckle-tracking procedure (followed by regularization process) is an estimate of the in-plane velocity vector in all pixels in each of the frames of the ultrasound data set (dynamic velocity vector field). The spatial distribution of the gray values within the ultrasound image is due to constructive and destructive interference of reflections from the individual scatterers within the myocardium. Reflections occur at transitions between different types of tissues or at specific sites, and are much smaller than the wavelength. Constructive interference generates a high-amplitude signal, destructive a low-amplitude one. The exact scatter positions determine the speckle characteristics. Speckle-tracking technology offers the ability to identify and track the same speckle throughout the cardiac cycle [4].

In the ultrasound image, we see the speckle pattern occurring at a position further away from the transducer. To correctly detect speckles, the motion of the tissue should be slower than the motion of the ultrasound beam (image lines). Sound waves propagate through tissues at an average velocity of 1530 m/s, while myocardial tissue moves at velocities in the order of centimeters per second: the basic condition is thus clearly met [16].

There are different algorithms used by different vendors in tracking these speckles. Some speckle-tracking methods are based on so-called block matching, where a region in the image is selected (the kernel) and is followed in the next image frame by subsequently trying out different positions and by determining the similarity between the kernel and the pattern observed in that position. The position where the similarity between the kernel ("fingerprint") and the observed pattern is maximal is assumed to be the new position of the speckle pattern

[16]. Another common approach is based on conservation of gray value, that is, it is assumed that gray values do not change over time. Radio frequency (RF) speckle—used in block-matching method—is a high-frequency signal, so that small between-frame motion can be detected, whereas its corresponding gray-scale speckle—used in gray-scale tracking—is derived from lower-frequency signals, being less sensitive to small displacements. Importantly, speckle tracking of gray-scale images does not necessarily perform well on high frame-rate data [16]. Then, RF-based methods allow to obtain a higher spatial, temporal, and velocity resolution because they use a signal with a higher-frequency content; at the same time, these methods are more sensitive to decorrelation and noise, requiring more severe regularization, which in turn might limit their resolution. Because both RF and gray-scale approaches offer advantages, a hybrid method was recently proposed.

So far, it is possible to evaluate the direction of movement, the speed of movement, and the distance of such movement at any point in the myocardium, independently from the transducer, relative to adjacent segments. The semi-automated nature of speckle-tracking echocardiography guarantees good intra-observer and inter-observer reproducibility [4].

Given that the velocity vector field is known for all pixels within the image, the axes are known with minimal user interaction. The radial, longitudinal, or circumferential velocity profiles throughout the cardiac cycle can be reconstructed, independent of the angle between the ultrasound image line and the direction of motion as in the conventional Doppler imaging [16]. The process of correcting the initial velocity vector estimates by applying additional boundary conditions based on a priori knowledge about the characteristics of the velocity field is called regularization. Regularization can consist of median filtering, weighted smoothing, elastic model, and myocardial boundaries definition.

Velocity vector imaging is partly analogous to 2D STI as it too tracks the speckles using 2D echocardiography, but utilizes additional physiological information to more robustly track the speckle kernels [17]. Each vector is an expression of direction and the magnitude of the velocity. The qualitative evaluation of the velocity is determined by comparing vectors along the tracked contour. Longitudinal strain is the percentage decrease in the length of the myocardium during systole (movement of the base toward the apex). It is expressed as a percent negative value (decrease in length in systole) [18]. Longitudinal strain may be calculated as an endocardial strain, midline strain, epicardial strain, or averaged over the entire cardiac wall. There is currently insufficient evidence to favor one way over another. Radial strain refers to the thickening of the myocardial wall during inward motion of the ventricle, measured in the short-axis views. The value is traditionally defined as percent positive (thickening in systole). Circumferential strain represents the change in the length along the circular perimeter, by definition percent negative in systole. Strain parameters can be individualized for each myocardial segment or can be expressed as global strain (averaging of all segments). Strain rate (evaluated globally or for each segment) represents rate of longitudinal, radial, or circumferential deformation in time. It has a marked systolic negative peak (S) with two positive peak in early (E) and late diastole (A).

Relevant strain values along strain curves are, but are not limited to:

- End-systolic strain: the value at end-systole;
- Peak systolic strain: the peak value during systole;
- Positive peak systolic strain;
- Peak strain: the peak value during the entire heart cycle. The peak strain may coincide with the systolic or end-systolic peak, or may appear after aortic valve closure (AVC) (it may be described as "post-systolic strain") [19].

Modern software allows display of results in bull's eye (polar map) similar to single-photon emission computed tomography (SPECT). This is more familiar to cardiologists as it depicts single myocardial segments with relative values of strain, strain rate, and time to peak strain/strain rate (synchronicity). A more unfamiliar method to display results in a monoplane view is the so-called curved anatomic M-mode (CAMM) which depicts timely variation of single parameters evaluated for a specific segment of interests from base to the apex and from septal to lateral wall. This offers a unique opportunity for timing and recognizing precise phases of a cardiac cycle (relaxation) and for the evaluation of AVC. End-systole coincides with AVC and can be visualized in the parasternal or apical long-axis view or by detecting the closure click on the spectral tracing of the pulsed-wave Doppler of aortic valve flow [19].

Rotation is the measure of the rotational movement of the myocardium in relation to an imaginary long-axis line from apex to base drawn through the middle of LV cavity 4]. Clockwise rotation is defined as negative, while counterclockwise rotation has a positive value. Twist is the algebraic difference in rotation between the apex and the base. Torsion is the twist normalized for the length of the LV cavity (degrees per centimeter). LV rotation or twisting motion has an important role in LV systolic and diastolic function. Normal values for LV rotation and twist angle have shown high variability (technique used, location of the region of interest, age, and loading hemodynamics of the ventricle). The increase in LV twist angle with age observed in literature can be explained by less opposed apical rotation, resulting from a gradual decrease in subendocardial function with aging. Worsening of diastolic relaxation and reduced diastolic suction is, however, associated with an early reduced and delayed diastolic untwisting.

Myocardial strain and Strain Rate (SR) are sensitive parameters for the quantification of diastolic function. Diastolic SR signals can be recorded during isovolumic relaxation, during early filling, and in late diastole. The hemodynamic determinants of protodiastolic strain rate include LV relaxation, regional diastolic stiffness, systolic function, end-systolic wall stress, and filling pressures. In addition, protodiastolic strain rate can assess interstitial fibrosis and can be used to identify viable myocardium after stunning and infarction. Measurement of diastolic strain and strain rate may be useful for research applications but is presently not recommended for routine clinical use.

The detection of myocardial fibrosis and viability depends on the evaluation of myocardial characteristics and shape during the cardiac cycle. Fibrotic tissue may be focal (as occurs in patients with myocardial infarction [MI]) or diffuse (systemic or metabolic disturbances). Fibrosis is actually accurately identified using myocardial late enhancement or T-weighted mapping with cardiac magnetic resonance imaging (MRI), but speckle tracking (especially systolic and protodiastolic strain rate) has a good correlation with tissue fibrosis, evaluated via cardiac magnetic resonance or biopsy.

All these parameters can be measured not only for the LV but also for the right ventricle (RV) and left and right atria (LA and RA, respectively), but have not been fully validated and, still together, commercial applications to process these chambers do not exist.

Timing peak strain is pivotal in defining dyssynchrony as well as for the evaluation of ischemia (post-systolic thickening or shortening).

2.4. Image acquisition

Gated images are obtained during end-expiratory breath holding with stable electrocardiographic traces, avoiding foreshortening of the ventricle and proper visualization of endocardial border. Images acquired should be of high quality. Optimal frame rate should be 60–110 frames per second (FPS). The operator should keep the sector width and depth minimal to focus on the structure of interest. Usually, three consecutive cardiac cycles are obtained and the values averaged for the final processing. Low FPS limits tracking efficacy, while higher FPS "smooths" speckle pattern and the final quality of the analysis. Apical four-chamber, two-chamber, and three-chamber views are necessary for estimation of LV strain and strain rates by 2D STI. This finally offers global longitudinal strain (GLS) value, that is, the average of longitudinal strain for all segments in all views. Parasternal short-axis views (basal, papillary muscles, and apex) are necessary for radial and circumferential strains (finally averaged in global radial and circumferential strain) and strain rates as well as for rotation, twist, and torsion analysis. The ways myocardial segments are divided widely vary among vendors, but in general, a 16–18-segment LV model is used. Myocardium is divided into six segments: basal septal, mid septal, apical septal, apical lateral, mid lateral, and basal lateral. For the timing determination of cardiac events, mitral inflow and LV outflow velocities are recorded using pulsed-Doppler echocardiography and the aortic and mitral valve closure/opening (AVC/O and MVC/O, respectively) times are obtained, as well as visually (AVC in apical long-axis view) or semi-automatically (evaluation of CAMM). The recordings are analyzed offline using semi-automated computer software for estimation of strain and strain rate by 2D STI. A region of interest (ROI) has to be outlined manually, tracing the endocardium. The epicardium is automatically traced by the system, but the wall thickness can be manually adjusted.

The ROI is defined at end-diastole by [19]:

- Endocardial border;
- Epicardial border;
- Myocardial midline.

Each of these contours can be user defined or generated automatically.

Topographic definitions of the myocardial ROI in apical views are [19]:

- "Left/right base";
- "Midbase";
- "Apex";
- "Left/right ROIs."

Vendors have incorporated tools to help users identify tracking reliability. Various methods are utilized. Some vendors have introduced protocols that identify segments where tracking is suboptimal and is excluded from the final results. In addition, some vendors provide accuracy indices to guide the user in tracking performance estimates.

Longitudinal strain is more robust and reproducible than other parameters. The values tend to be partly different for different walls and segments. There is a gradient of longitudinal strain values from base to apex (higher values for apical segments) as well as from endo to epicardium (higher values of strain in the subendocardial region). **Table 2** depicts the recently published data on normal values for different strains of LV, while **Table 3** depicts the principal advantages and pitfalls of different strain imaging techniques [20].

Longitudinal Strain	**Circumferential Strain**	**Radial Strain**
Apical septal 21 ± 4	Anterior 24 ± 6	Anterior 39 ± 16
Mid septal 19 ± 4	Lateral 22 ± 7	Lateral 37 ± 18
Basal septal 17 ± 4	Posterior 21 ± 7	Posterior 37 ± 17
Apical lateral 21 ± 7	Inferior 22 ± 6	Inferior 37 ± 17
Mid lateral 19 ± 6	Septal 24 ± 6	Septal 37 ± 19
Basal lateral 19 ± 6	Anteroseptal 26 ± 11	Anterospetal 39 ± 15

Table 2. Mean percentage left ventricular strain values for strain in healthy adults.

A recent meta-analysis identified normal values for strain as (GLS) -19.7% (95% CI, −20.4 to −18.9%), global circumferential strain (GCS) −23.3% (95% CI, −24.6 to −22.1%), global radial strain (GRS) 47.3% (95% CI, 43.6–51.0%). Age, gender, body mass index, systolic blood pressure, frame rate, and equipment vendor were considered the variables most likely to influence GLS. In a general linear model, only mean blood pressure was independently associated with higher values of strain. The differences in each strain component are probably actually linked to technical motives: the superiority of longitudinal strain is linked to the reliability of measurements in the axial plane respective to azimuthal one; the variability of radial strain may reflect the limited amount of tissue to track in the short-axis view of the non-hypertrophied heart; the ROI, which is user defined, may affect the strain amplitude [21]. 2D strain parameters have been validated against tagged MRI studies and sonomicrometry studies [22–24]. 2D strain data correlate well with TDI-derived ones, although with higher strength and reproducibility [2].

	TDI	2D STI	3D STI
Feasibility	++	++	+
Reproducibility	++	++	+++
Temporal resolution (strain curves)	+++	+	–
Spatial resolution (strain curves)	++	+	+
Angle independency	–	+	++
Validation: simulated	+	+	+
Validation: in vitro	+(+)	+(+)	+
Validation: in vivo	++	++	++
Validation: other techniques in clinical scenario	++	+++	+
Defined normal values	+++	+++	–
Time sparing	–	++	++
Standardized software	–	+/-	–

2D, bi-dimensional; 3D, three-dimensional; STI, speckle-tracking imaging; TDI, tissue Doppler imaging.

Table 3. Tissue Doppler imaging, bi-dimensional and three-dimensional speckle-tracking imaging.

2.5. 3D strain

With developments in ultrasound transducer technology and both hardware and software computing, systems capable of acquiring real-time volumetric LV data are now widely available. Reasonable spatial and temporal resolution of 3D data sets can now be achieved. The ability to estimate true 3D myocardial motion and deformation using various STI approaches may provide cardiologists with a better view of regional myocardial mechanics, which may be important for diagnosis, prognosis, and therapy. These 3D approaches can measure all strain components in all LV segments from a single acquisition [25–27]. Furthermore, they are angle independent, do not suffer from strain estimation errors associated with out-of-plane motion, and may in theory allow more precise calculations of LV twist and assessment of shear strain components [28–31]. This tool is promising for the evaluation of deformation parameters, although only preliminary data are available. A single apical full-volume acquisition is performed, according to standard modalities, with an FPS between 18 and 25 (3D temporal resolution is lower than that obtained with 2D images) [32]. This avoids multiple acquisitions making readily and instantaneously available evaluation of strain parameters and torsion. The operator is able to limit foreshortening and properly identify walls and segments [33, 34]. 3D strain offers a combined assessment of longitudinal and circumferential strain [35]. To evaluate transmural (radial) deformation, due to image quality and tracking limitation, a derivative parameter, area strain, has been introduced. However, it is important to note that full volume is the result of a stitching process, which can limit tracking of speckles. Frame rate and lateral resolution can also limit good tracking.

2.6. Recent advances and consensus: need for standardization

Recognizing the critical need for standardization in strain imaging, in particular in order to derive a common standard for GLS, the most affordable parameter, in 2010, the European Association of Echocardiography and the American Society of Echocardiography (ASE) invited technical representatives from all interested vendors to participate in a concerted effort to reduce intervendor variability of strain measurement [36, 37]. In order to obtain a perfectly defined strain, synthetic ultrasound images simulated from mathematically modeled ventricles (phantoms) were developed. Jan D'hooge and colleagues from the University of Leuven generated cine loops mimicking normal, hypertrophied, and dysfunctional ventricles (**Figures 1–3**), and provided them to the vendors: after several attempts, results were similar for the principal vendors.

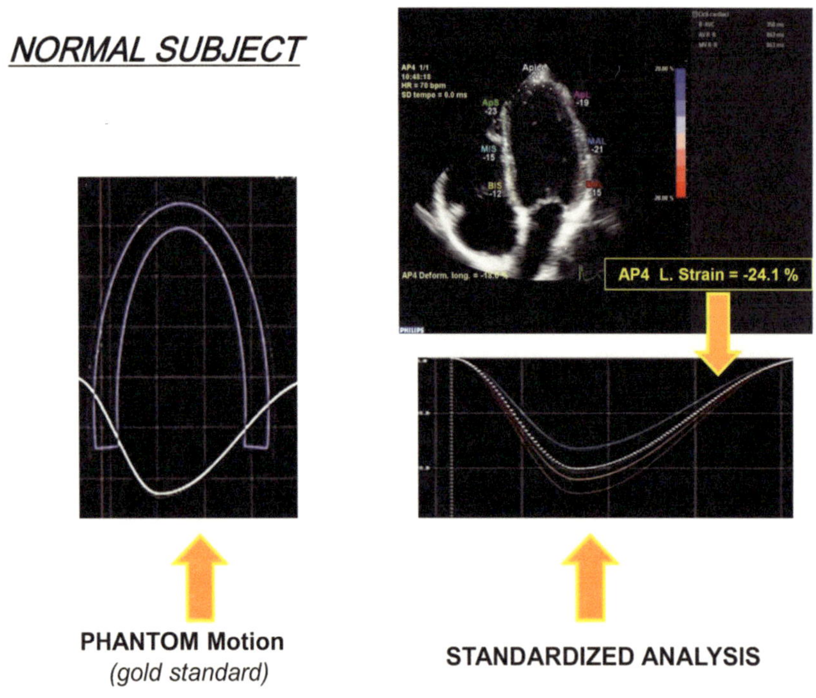

Figure 1. Global longitudinal strain calculation from phantom model (normal). AP4: apical four-chamber view; L. Strain: longitudinal strain.

http://dx.doi.org/10.5772/64261

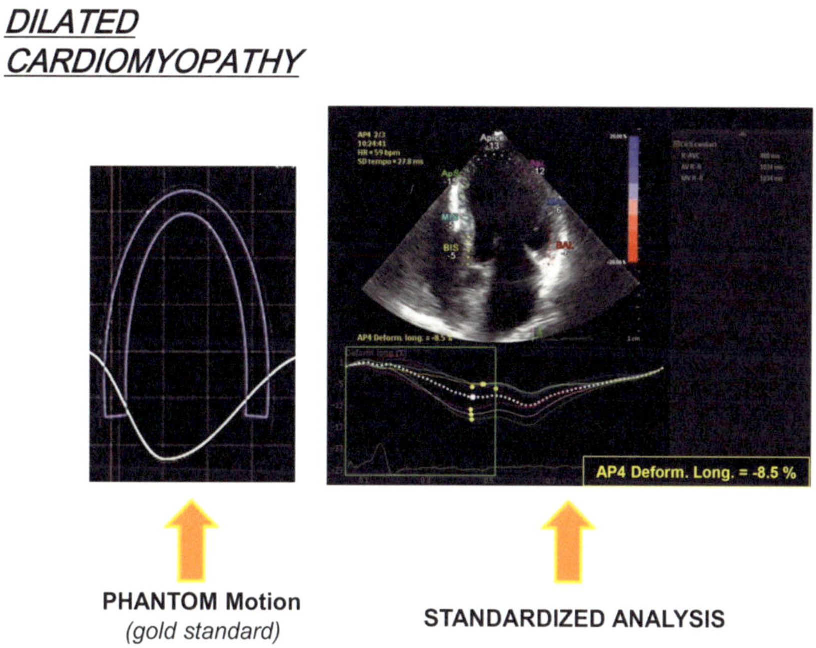

Figure 2. Global longitudinal strain from phantom model (dilated cardiomyopathy). AP4: apical four-chamber view; Deform. Long.: longitudinal deformation.

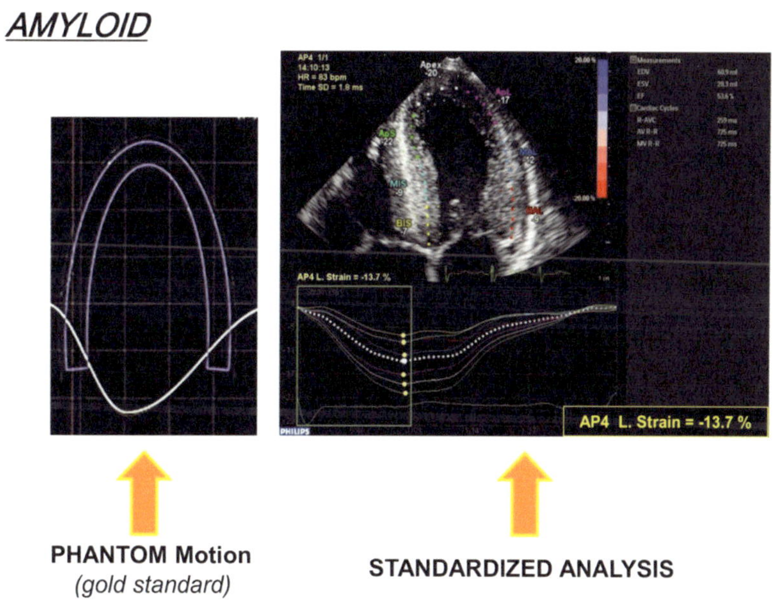

Figure 3. Global longitudinal strain from phantom model (amyloid). AP4: apical four-chamber view; L. Strain: longitudinal strain.

Moreover, a great effort has been made to standardize, speedup, and automatize (less subjective approach) GLS calculation, in order to offer immediate results to clinicians (bedside) and avoid errors in calculations (heart rate variability).

2.7. Clinical applications

2D STI has a wide field of clinical applications. We focus on main and novel fields of application (see also '**Table 4**') [38–48].

Field of Application	Explanation
Myocardial ischemia	Reduction in strain by 2D STI more objective than WMSI. Longitudinal, radial, and circumferential strain reduction in ischemia.
Myocardial infarction	Differentiation of transmural from subendocardial infarction. Remodeling.
Myocardial viability	Objective evaluation during stress echo. Differentiation of active contraction from passive tethering.
Heart failure with normal LVEF (HFnEF)	Twisting/untwisting.
Cardiac resynchronization therapy (CRT)	Longitudinal strain from TDI velocity with 2D STI radial strain. Longitudinal strain delay index. Radial strain and survival.
Takotsubo cardiomyopathy	Impaired longitudinal strain.
Restrictive cardiomyopathy	Impaired longitudinal deformation and twist.
Constrictive pericarditis	Impaired LV circumferential deformation and torsion.
Cardiotoxicity	Chemotherapy.
Detection of subclinical myocardial disease	Systemic hypertension, diabetes mellitus, systemic sclerosis, amyloidosis, and Duchenne's muscular dystrophy.
Valvular heart disease	Decreased radial, circumferential, and longitudinal strain in patients with severe aortic stenosis despite normal EF. Septal strain and mitral regurgitation.
Congenital heart disease	Right ventricular longitudinal strain and strain rate.

2D, bi-dimensional; 3D, three-dimensional; EF, ejection fraction; HFnEF, heart failure with normal ejection fraction; LV, left ventricle; STI, speckle-tracking imaging; TDI, tissue Doppler imaging; WMSI, wall motion score index.

Table 4. Principal clinical applications of speckle-tracking echocardiography.

Moreover, a recent meta-analysis presented the incremental value respective to EF retained by GLS [49]. It is essential to understand that technology development has today made available a fast, objective (automatized), and standardized definition of GLS, with final representation of bull's-eye plot of longitudinal strain value making it appealing, easily recognizable, and aligned with standardized segmentation of LV wall (**Figures 4** and **5**).

http://dx.doi.org/10.5772/64261

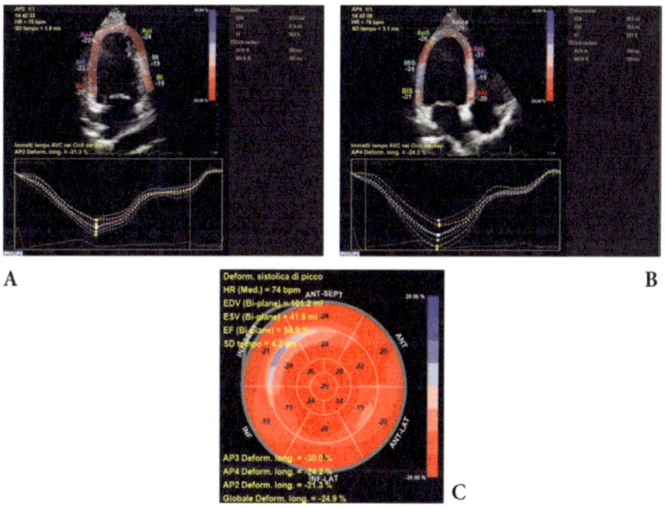

Figure 4. Global longitudinal strain calculation: on top showing tracking in four- (**B**) and two- (**A**) chamber view with strain curves; final bull's-eye plot (**C**) showing global results and superimposed regional values (Normal subject). AP2: apical two-chamber view; AP3: apical three-chamber view; AP4: apical four-chamber view; Deform. Long.: longitudinal deformation; EDV (bi-plane): end-diastolic volume (bi-plane); ESV (bi-plane): end-systolic volume (bi-plane); EF (bi-plane): ejection fraction (bi-plane); global Deform. Long. (GLS): global longitudinal strain; HR: heart rate.

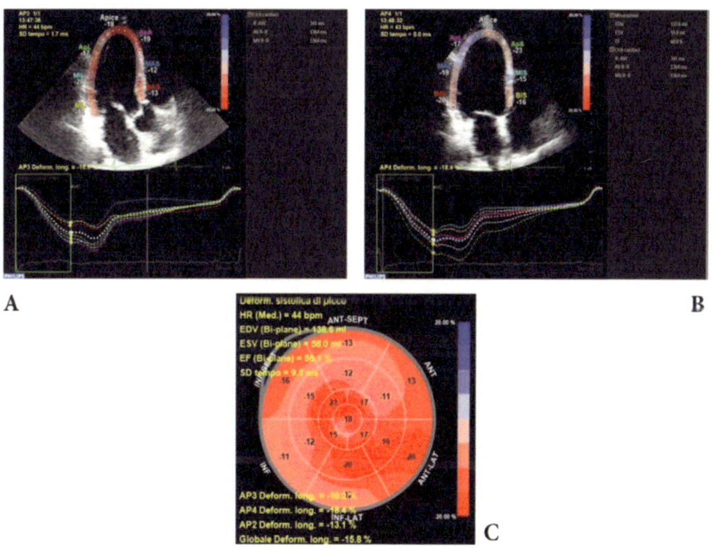

Figure 5. Global longitudinal strain calculation: on top showing tracking in three- (**A**) and four- (**B**) chamber view with strain curves; final bull's-eye plot (**C**) showing global results and superimposed regional values (dysfunctioning patient). AP2: apical two-chamber view; AP3: apical three-chamber view; AP4: apical four-chamber view; Deform. Long.: longitudinal deformation; EDV (bi-plane): end-diastolic volume (bi-plane); ESV (bi-plane): end-systolic volume (bi-plane); EF (bi-plane): ejection fraction (bi-plane); global Deform. Long. (GLS): global longitudinal strain; HR: heart rate.

2.7.1. Ischemic cardiomyopathy

In coronary artery disease, an assessment of myocardial ischemia other than simple visual wall motion score estimation (high inter-observer variability) has been invoked from a long time. Regional velocities (TDI) as well as peak systolic strain rate and systolic strain (TDI and STI) reduce linearly with a reduction in regional perfusion, time-delay prolongation to treatment, and the presence of fibrosis [14, 50, 51]. Subendocardial longitudinal fibers are the most vulnerable ones, resulting in an early deterioration of longitudinal strain, followed by radial and circumferential strains. Anyway, it's rather improper to consider a "radial function," because there are no myocardial fibers going in the radial direction. Actually, wall thickening measured by radial strain is a function of wall shortening, as the heart muscle is incompressible. At the same time, circumferential strain does not reflect circumferential fiber contraction because circumferential shortening is mainly due to the inward movement of mid-wall circumference as the wall thickens (inwards—as described by the eggshell model) [52–54]. Briefly, there would have been circumferential shortening even without circumferential fibers. These aspects, together with less standardized values than GLS, make GRS and GCS considerably reliable.

Dobutamine stress echocardiography is an important area of interest because in normal tissues an increased deformation occurs (continuously increasing strain/strain rate) as long as filling is not reduced by increased heart rate. On the contrary, acutely ischemic tissue during stress test shows less deformation and post-systolic deformation (PSD, thickening/shortening with radial/longitudinal strain, respectively), that is, the continued contraction of the myocardium after AVC. PSD is a common finding in myocardial ischemia. All these alterations are proportional to the severity of ischemia and persist in the experimental setting for up to 2 h after the ischemic insult resolution, with a peculiar time decay [55–57]. A noteworthy fact is that the stunned myocardium is characterized by decreased systolic deformation and PSD at rest, but almost normal systolic deformation and disappearance of PSD with dobutamine [50]. This behavior could be secondary to the heterogeneous contractile properties of the myocardium, probably linked to myofibrillar edema reducing the effective force myocardium can develop [58]. Furthermore, interstitial myocardial edema results in a sudden and temporary increase in end-diastolic wall thickness (this behavior is observed also in infarcted segments at the moment of reperfusion) [59, 60]. In chronic infarction, dobutamine is associated with low or no deformation increase, depending on the fibrosis extension (from subendocardial to transmurality involvement) [50].

2.7.2. Volume overload

Deformation is also closely related to ventricular geometry. Dilation is the end stage of most of the cardiomyopathies and heart valve diseases because for a given volume, the object with the smallest surface area is the sphere. This means that the same deformation (determined by the contractile force) can generate a larger stroke volume in a dilated heart. Similarly, in a dilated heart the same amount of stroke volume can be generated with less contractility and less deformation, that we can directly evaluate with strain(-rate) [14]. Remodeling in the long term will lead to irreversible damage to the heart muscle and finally ventricular dysfunction, but there is no specific diagnostic method to detect subclinical changes in systolic function. STI and TDI might potentially be useful in detecting subclinical changes in cardiac function [60].

Mitral regurgitation (MR) is a typical volume overload condition. Primary MR leads to cardiac remodeling, increased left ventricular filling pressure, pulmonary arterial hypertension, and myocardial dysfunction. Conventional 2D, M-mode, and Doppler examination play a critical role in the initial and longitudinal assessment; anyway, most variables are load dependent and both afterload and preload are altered during the disease course. TDI and STI provide new parameters to assess regional and global myocardial performance and may help in identifying asymptomatic patients and choosing the optimal time for surgical correction. It is worthy to note that patients with severe primary degenerative MR may have near-normal left ventricle ejection fractions (LVEFs) because of disproportionately higher compensation in GLS. Moreover, the higher the GLS, the higher the risk of substantial reduction in LVEF (>10%) during the immediate postoperative period [61]. On the contrary, in patients tested at 6 months after surgery, when LV reverse remodeling has already settled, LVEF reductions >10% were associated with lower baseline strains [62]. Chronic ischemic MR instead is not a valvular disease per se but is rather a "ventricular disease." In particular, inferior MI has been recognized as the most frequent cause of ischemic MR because of the geometric distortion in the papillary muscle-bearing segments [63]. Therefore, the site of MI might be a more important determinant of MR degree in LV dysfunction than the extent of post-MI LV remodeling. Under normal conditions, the basal rotation, which is determined mainly by inferior and posterior myocardial segments [64], shortens the distance between the mitral valve and the head of the papillary muscles, contributing to MVC and counterbalancing the tethering forces. When local remodeling occurs, as in patients with inferior-posterior MIs, the basal strain and basal rotation are significantly lower and fail to shorten the distance between the papillary muscles and the mitral valve. Interestingly, Zito et al. demonstrated that basal rotation but not basal strain was an independent predictor of the severity of MR [65].

2.7.3. Pressure overload

Considering pressure overload pathology, aortic stenosis (AS) is the most common valve lesion causing chronic pressure overload on the LV. The development of symptoms in AS heralds a malignant phase of the condition and prompt aortic valve replacement results in a clear reduction in mortality [66]. In contrast, the management of patients with severe AS in the absence of symptoms remains one of the most controversial and debated areas in modern cardiology [67, 68].

The increased afterload leads to left ventricular hypertrophy and the basal septal is the first to show changes, due to increased wall stress according to the Laplace law [69]. It first shows a decrease in strain(-rate) and the development of PSD is observed, as well as the development of localized hypertrophy (septal bulge) [70]. Recently, GLS has been shown to be an independent predictor of outcomes in patients with severe asymptomatic AS, incremental to other echocardiographic markers [71]. Not to forget, the role of exercise testing in asymptomatic AS is well established, and recommended by guidelines in equivocal cases [72].

2.7.4. Mechanical dyssynchrony

Searching for the presence of mechanical dyssynchrony to identify potentially recruitable function, rather than looking only for electrocardiogram (ECG) manifestations of ventricular conduction delay, could increase the rate of cardiac resynchronization therapy (CRT) responders [73]. Mitigation of intraventricular dyssynchrony is currently thought to be the primary mechanism of improved myocardial performance with CRT. Anyway, many patients eligible for CRT have dilated ventricles with complex motion, especially if infarcted areas are present. Moreover, in dilated hearts local motion is importantly influenced by other myocardial segments and even by right ventricular motion [74]. That's why to this day, M-mode, 2D e TDI analyses have expressed modest sensitivity and specificity in measuring dyssynchrony and improving patient selection for CRT [73].

STI-based methods, mostly assessing the time difference between maximal values form different myocardial segments (e.g. septal to posterior wall motion delay [75], septal rebound stretch [76], wasted work ratio) [77, 78], are promising, but they must be validated in multicenter randomized trials.

2.7.5. Diabetic cardiomyopathy

Another field of interest is represented by diabetes mellitus because studies showed that myocardial damage occurred in at least 30% diabetic patients when LV diameter and LVEF were normal [79]. Diabetic myocardial diastolic dysfunction seems to precede systolic dysfunction, but this might be explained by the insensitivity of techniques for detecting LV systolic function. In many but small studies, longitudinal dysfunction (segmental GLS) occurred in early stages of diabetes, while LV torsion increased compensatively [80–84].

2.7.6. Cancer therapeutics-related cardiac dysfunction

Cardiotoxicity from cancer therapy has become a leading cause of morbidity and mortality in survivors [85, 86]. A careful consideration of potential cardiotoxicity during therapy and a focus on early detection and intervention are developing. Echocardiography is the cornerstone in the cardiac imaging evaluation of patients in preparation for, during, and after cancer therapy because of its wide availability, repeatability, versatility, lack of radiation exposure, and safety. The most commonly used parameter for monitoring LV function with echocardiography is LVEF. In addition, the calculation of LVEF should be combined with assessment of the wall motion score index [87]. Anyway, 2D echocardiography appears to be reliable in the detection of differences close to 10% in LVEF [88]. Because this is the same magnitude of change used to adjudicate cancer therapeutics-related cardiac dysfunction, the sensitivity of LVEF has been questioned. Moreover, detecting a decreased LVEF after anthracyclines may be too late for treatment [89], suggesting that more sensitive parameters of LV dysfunction could be helpful. The prognostic value of early measurement of systolic deformation indices (above all ΔGLS) measured in the prediction of subsequent LV systolic function has been evaluated in several studies, both in animals [90] and in humans [91–94].

2.7.7. *Left atrium*

Speckle tracking was recently applied to study the myocardial mechanics of a thin-walled structure such as the LA [95–98]. For the analysis, apical views are obtained using conventional 2D gray-scale echocardiography, during a breath-hold, with a stable electrocardiographic recording. The frame rate is set between 60 and 80 frames/s, and recordings are processed using acoustic-tracking software. The LA mechanical indices are calculated by averaging values observed in all LA segments (global strain) with a 15-segment or a 12-segment model. The software generates longitudinal strain and strain rate curves for each atrial segment. The radial deformation cannot be calculated because the LA wall is thin and the spatial resolution is limited [99].

2.7.8. *Right ventricle*

A recent methodological study has reported the feasibility, the reference values, and the reproducibility of right ventricular longitudinal strain measured by STI in normal patients and in patients with RV dysfunction [100]. The technique is similar as for LV: global strain is the average of six single segments (ROI) traced semi-automatically and processed by software packages (today, a dedicated software for RV does not exist). The evaluation of right ventricular function with STI, considering the important limitations of other parameters and methods, could offer more detailed information about regional and global RV mechanics with important clinical implications for non-invasive evaluation of RV systolic function (subclinical RV dysfunction). Further prospective studies are necessary to define its role in the management of patients.

3. Limitations

Rotation, deformation, and out-of-plane motion can cause speckle patterns to change between acquisitions (decorrelation). Loss of tracking can be limited acquiring at a proper frame rate. Image artifacts should be avoided. In general, high-quality acquisition is a prerequisite for optimal speckle-tracking results [16].

Among limitations of the method, we should include:

- Lack of reproducibility: even if much less compared with TDI, every STI study should include an intra- and interobserver variability testing [101];
- Intervendor variability: lack of standardization results in changes in reference values [102];
- Oversimplification due to software processing algorithms: automatic tracking of epicardial border (assumption of uniform thickness of myocardium); averaging of parameters within a segment; drifting;
- 2D imaging limitations: image quality; artifacts; image dropout; frame rate (low frame: no tracking, as at high heart frequencies; high frame: limited lateral resolution); lateral resolu-

tion and depth; depth dependence of transverse tracking; out-of-plane motion in short axis limiting tracking of the same ROI; noise.

Evaluation of radial strain poses important technical challenges compared to longitudinal one.

This is due to:

- Measurements in the axial plane are more reliable than those that depend on lateral and elevation (or azimuthal) resolution;
- Limited amount of tissue to track in the short-axis view of the non-hypertrophied heart;
- Placement of the ROI is user defined;
- Intervendors' differences.

4. Conclusions

Speckle tracking is actually a reality in echocardiography. Simple protocols of acquisition and novel processing packages have made available deformation analysis in daily clinical arena.

Overcoming many of the previous limitations, thanks to technological development, including 3D introduction and STI, offers to the cardiologists the potential benefit of a solid, fast, easy, and reproducible quantization of myocardial mechanics [37].

Author details

Iacopo Fabiani[1*], Nicola Riccardo Pugliese[2], Veronica Santini[1], Lorenzo Conte[1] and Vitantonio Di Bello[1]

*Address all correspondence to: iacopofabiani@gmail.com

1 Dept. Section Universitary Cardio-Angiology, Surgical, Medical, Molecular and Critical Area Pathology Department, Pisa Univeristy, Pisa, Italy

2 Operative Unit Cardio-Vascular Disease Univ., Surgical, Medical, Molecular and Critical Area Pathology Department, Pisa Univeristy, Pisa, Italy

References

[1] Perk G, Tunick PA, Kronzon I. Non-Doppler two-dimensional strain imaging by echocardiography – from technical considerations to clinical applications. J Am Soc Echocardiogr. 2007;20:234–243. DOI: 10.1016/j.echo.2006.08.023

[2] Dandel M, Lehmkuhl H, Knosalla C, Suramelashvili N, Hetzer R. Strain and strain rate imaging by echocardiography – basic concepts and clinical applicability. Curr Cardiol Rev. 2009;5:133–148. DOI: 10.2174/157340309788166642

[3] Blessberger H, Binder T. NON-invasive imaging: two dimensional speckle tracking echocardiography: basic principles. Heart. 2010;96:716–722. DOI: 10.1136/hrt.2007.141002

[4] Blessberger H, Binder T. Two dimensional speckle tracking echocardiography: clinical applications. Heart. 2010;96:2032–2040. DOI: 10.1136/hrt.2010.199885

[5] Storaa C, Aberg P, Lind B, Brodin LA. Effect of angular error on tissue Doppler velocities and strain. Echocardiography. 2003;20:581–587. DOI: 10.1046/j.1540-8175.2003.01135

[6] Dandel M, Hetzer R. Echocardiographic strain and strain rate imaging – clinical applications. Int J Cardiol. 2009;132:11–24. DOI: 10.1016/j.ijcard.2008.06.091

[7] Dokainish H, Sengupta R, Pillai M, Bobek J, Lakkis N. Usefulness of new diastolic strain and strain rate indexes for the estimation of left ventricular filling pressure. Am J Cardiol. 2008;101:1504–1509. DOI: 10.1016/j.amjcard.2008.01.037

[8] Gorcsan J, 3rd, Tanaka H. Echocardiographic assessment of myocardial strain. J Am Coll Cardiol. 2011;58:1401–1413. DOI: 10.1016/j.jacc.2011.06.038

[9] Mor-Avi V, Lang RM, Badano LP, Belohlavek M, Cardim NM, Derumeaux G, et al. Current and evolving echocardiographic techniques for the quantitative evaluation of cardiac mechanics: ASE/EAE consensus statement on methodology and indications endorsed by the Japanese Society of Echocardiography. Euro J Echocardiogr. 2011;12:167–205. DOI: 10.1093/ejechocard/jer021

[10] Streeter DD, Jr., Spotnitz HM, Patel DP, Ross J, Jr., Sonnenblick EH. Fiber orientation in the canine left ventricle during diastole and systole. Circ Res. 1969;24:339–347. DOI: 10.1371/journal.pone.0132360

[11] Greenbaum RA, Ho SY, Gibson DG, Becker AE, Anderson RH. Left ventricular fibre architecture in man. Br Heart J. 1981;45:248–263. DOI: 10.1136/hrt.45.3.248

[12] Torrent-Guasp F, Buckberg GD, Clemente C, Cox JL, Coghlan HC, Gharib M. The structure and function of the helical heart and its buttress wrapping. I. The normal macroscopic structure of the heart. Semin Thorac Cardiovasc Surg. 2001;13:301–319. DOI: none

[13] Sun JP. Ventricular Torsion. In: Marwick TH, Yu CM, Sun JP. Myocardial Imaging Tissue Doppler and Speckle Tracking. Wiley-Blackwell; Hoboken, New Jersey, 2007. pp. 273–277. DOI: 10.1002/9780470692448.ch23

[14] Bijnens BH, Cikes M, Claus P, Sutherland GR. Velocity and deformation imaging for the assessment of myocardial dysfunction. Eur J Echocardiogr. 2009;10:216–226. DOI: 10.1093/ejechocard/jen323

[15] Heimdal A. Technical Principles of Tissue Velocity and Strain Imaging Methods. In: Marwick TH, Yu CM, Sun JP. Myocardial Imaging Tissue Doppler and Speckle Tracking. Wiley-Blackwell; Hoboken, New Jersey, 2007. pp. 3–16. DOI: 10.1002/9780470692448.ch1

[16] D'hooge J. Principles and Different Techniques for Speckle Tracking. In: Marwick TH, Yu CM, Sun JP. Myocardial Imaging Tissue Doppler and Speckle Tracking. Wiley-Blackwell; Hoboken, New Jersey, 2007. pp. 17–25. DOI: 10.1002/9780470692448.ch2

[17] Vannan MA, Pedrizzetti G, Li P, Gurudevan S, Houle H, Main J, et al. Effect of cardiac resynchronization therapy on longitudinal and circumferential left ventricular mechanics by velocity vector imaging: description and initial clinical application of a novel method using high-frame rate B-mode echocardiographic images. Echocardiography. 2005;22:826–830. DOI: 10.1111/j.1540-8175.2005.00172.x

[18] Biswas M, Sudhakar S, Nanda NC, Buckberg G, Pradhan M, Roomi AU, Gorissen W, Houle H. Two- and three-dimensional speckle tracking echocardiography: clinical aplications and future directions. Echocardiography. 2013;30:88–105. DOI: 10.1111/echo.12079

[19] Voigt JU, Pedrizzetti G, Lysyansky P, Marwick TH, Houle H, Baumann R et al. Definitions for a common standard for 2D speckle tracking echocardiography: consensus document of the EACVI/ASE/industry task force to standardize deformation imaging. J Am Soc Echocardiogr. 2015;28(2):183–193. DOI: 10.1016/j.echo.2014.11.003

[20] Hurlburt HM, Aurigemma GP, Hill JC, Narayanan A, Gaasch WH, Vinch CS, et al. Direct ultrasound measurement of longitudinal, circumferential, and radial strain using 2-dimensional strain imaging in normal adults. Echocardiography. 2007;24:723–731. DOI: 10.1111/j.1540-8175.2007.00460.x

[21] Yingchoncharoen T, Agarwal S, Popovic ZB, Marwick TH. Normal ranges of left ventricular strain: a meta-analysis. J Am Soc Echocardiogr. 2013;26:185–191. DOI: 10.1016/j.echo.2012.10.008

[22] Nguyen JS, Lakkis NM, Bobek J, Goswami R, Dokainish H. Systolic and diastolic myocardial mechanics in patients with cardiac disease and preserved ejection fraction: impact of left ventricular filling pressure. J Am Soc Echocardiogr. 2010;23:1273–1280. DOI: 10.1016/j.echo.2010.09.008

[23] Amundsen BH, Helle-Valle T, Edvardsen T, Torp H, Crosby J, Lyseggen E, et al. Noninvasive myocardial strain measurement by speckle tracking echocardiography: validation against sonomicrometry and tagged magnetic resonance imaging. J Am Coll Cardiol. 2006;47:789–793. DOI: 10.1016/j.jacc.2005.10.040

[24] Cho GY, Chan J, Leano R, Strudwick M, Marwick TH. Comparison of two-dimensional speckle and tissue velocity based strain and validation with harmonic phase magnetic resonance imaging. Am J Cardiol. 2006;97:1661–1666. DOI: 10.1016/j.amjcard.2005.12.063

[25] Papademetris X, Sinusas AJ, Dione DP, Duncan JS. Estimation of 3D left ventricular deformation from echocardiography. Med Image Anal. 2001;5:17–28. DOI: 10.1016/S1361-8415(00)00022-0

[26] Elen A, Choi HF, Loeckx D, Gao H, Claus P, Suetens P, et al. Three-dimensional cardiac strain estimation using spatio-temporal elastic registration of ultrasound images: a feasibility study. IEEE Trans Med Imaging. 2008;27:1580–1591. DOI: 10.1109/TMI.2008.2004420

[27] Crosby J, Amundsen BH, Hergum T, Remme EW, Langeland S, Torp H. 3-D speckle tracking for assessment of regional left ventricular function. Ultrasound Med Biol. 2009;35:458–471. DOI: 10.1016/j.ultrasmedbio.2008.09.011

[28] Hayat D, Kloeckner M, Nahum J, Ecochard-Dugelay E, Dubois-Rande JL, Jean-Francois D, et al. Comparison of real-time three-dimensional speckle tracking to magnetic resonance imaging in patients with coronary heart disease. Am J Cardiol. 2012;109:180–186. DOI: 10.1016/j.amjcard.2011.08.030

[29] Abate E, Hoogslag GE, Antoni ML, Nucifora G, Delgado V, Holman ER, et al. Value of three-dimensional speckle-tracking longitudinal strain for predicting improvement of left ventricular function after acute myocardial infarction. Am J Cardiol. 2012;110:961–967. DOI: 10.1016/j.amjcard.2012.05.023

[30] Kleijn SA, Aly MF, Terwee CB, van Rossum AC, Kamp O. Three-dimensional speckle tracking echocardiography for automatic assessment of global and regional left ventricular function based on area strain. J Am Soc Echocardiogr. 2011;24:314–321. DOI: 10.1016/j.echo.2011.01.014

[31] Kleijn SA, Aly MF, Knol DL, Terwee CB, Jansma EP, Abd El-Hady YA, et al. A meta-analysis of left ventricular dyssynchrony assessment and prediction of response to cardiac resynchronization therapy by three-dimensional echocardiography. Eur Heart J Cardiovasc Imaging. 2012;13:763–775. DOI: 10.1093/ehjci/jes041

[32] Yodwut C, Weinert L, Klas B, Lang RM, Mor-Avi V. Effects of frame rate on three-dimensional speckle-tracking-based measurements of myocardial deformation. J Am Soc Echocardiogr. 2012;25:978–985. DOI: 10.1016/j.echo.2012.06.001

[33] Urbano-Moral JA, Patel AR, Maron MS, Arias-Godinez JA, Pandian NG. Three-dimensional speckle-tracking echocardiography: methodological aspects and clinical potential. Echocardiography. 2012;29:997–1010. DOI: 10.1111/j.1540-8175.2012.01773.x

[34] Urbano-Moral JA, Rowin EJ, Maron MS, Crean A, Pandian NG. Investigation of global and regional myocardial mechanics with 3-dimensional speckle tracking echocardiography and relations to hypertrophy and fibrosis in hypertrophic cardiomyopathy. Circ Cardiovasc Imaging. 2014;7:11–19. DOI: 10.1161/CIRCIMAGING.113.000842

[35] Perez de Isla L, Millan M, Lennie V, Quezada M, Guinea J, Macaya C, et al. Area strain: normal values for a new parameter in healthy people. Rev Esp Cardiol. 2011;64:1194–1197. DOI: 10.1016/j.recesp.2011.03.021

[36] Thomas JD, Badano LP. EACVI-ASE-industry initiative to standardize deformation imaging: a brief update from the co-chairs. Eur Heart J Cardiovasc Imaging. 2013;14:1039–1040. DOI: 10.1093/ehjci/jet184

[37] Voigt JU, Pedrizzetti G, Lysyansky P, Marwick TH, Houle H, Baumann R, et al. Definitions for a common standard for 2D speckle tracking echocardiography: consensus document of the EACVI/ASE/Industry Task Force to standardize deformation imaging. Eur Heart J Cardiovasc Imaging. 2015;16:1–11. DOI: 10.1093/ehjci/jeu184

[38] Heggemann F, Weiss C, Hamm K, Kaden J, Suselbeck T, Papavassiliu T, et al. Global and regional myocardial function quantification by two-dimensional strain in Takotsubo cardiomyopathy. Eur J Echocardiogr. 2009;10:760–764. DOI: 10.1093/ejechocard/jep062

[39] Shimoni S, Gendelman G, Ayzenberg O, Smirin N, Lysyansky P, Edri O, et al. Differential effects of coronary artery stenosis on myocardial function: the value of myocardial strain analysis for the detection of coronary artery disease. J Am Soc Echocardiogr. 2011;24:748–757. DOI: 10.1016/j.echo.2011.03.007

[40] Becker M, Hoffmann R, Kuhl HP, Grawe H, Katoh M, Kramann R, et al. Analysis of myocardial deformation based on ultrasonic pixel tracking to determine transmurality in chronic myocardial infarction. Eur Heart J. 006;27:2560–2566. DOI: 10.1093/eurheartj/ehl288

[41] Chan J, Hanekom L, Wong C, Leano R, Cho GY, Marwick TH. Differentiation of subendocardial and transmural infarction using two-dimensional strain rate imaging to assess short-axis and long-axis myocardial function. J Am Coll Cardiol. 2006;48:2026–2033. DOI: 10.1016/j.jacc.2006.07.050

[42] Tan YT, Wenzelburger F, Lee E, Heatlie G, Leyva F, Patel K, et al. The pathophysiology of heart failure with normal ejection fraction: exercise echocardiography reveals complex abnormalities of both systolic and diastolic ventricular function involving torsion, untwist, and longitudinal motion. J Am Coll Cardiol. 2009;54:36–46. DOI: 10.1016/j.jacc.2009.03.037

[43] Gorcsan J, 3rd, Tanabe M, Bleeker GB, Suffoletto MS, Thomas NC, Saba S, et al. Combined longitudinal and radial dyssynchrony predicts ventricular response after resynchronization therapy. J Am Coll Cardiol. 2007;50:1476–1483. DOI: 10.1016/j.jacc.2007.06.043

[44] Delgado V, van Bommel RJ, Bertini M, Borleffs CJ, Marsan NA, Arnold CT, et al. Relative merits of left ventricular dyssynchrony, left ventricular lead position, and myocardial scar to predict long-term survival of ischemic heart failure patients undergoing cardiac

resynchronization therapy. Circulation. 2011;123:70–78. DOI: 10.1161/CIRCULATIONAHA.110.945345

[45] Bellavia D, Abraham TP, Pellikka PA, Al-Zahrani GB, Dispenzieri A, Oh JK, et al. Detection of left ventricular systolic dysfunction in cardiac amyloidosis with strain rate echocardiography. J Am Soc Echocardiogr. 2007;20:1194–1202. DOI: 10.1016/j.echo.2007.02.025

[46] Delgado V, Tops LF, van Bommel RJ, van der Kley F, Marsan NA, Klautz RJ, et al. Strain analysis in patients with severe aortic stenosis and preserved left ventricular ejection fraction undergoing surgical valve replacement. Eur Heart J. 2009;30:3037–3047. DOI: 10.1093/eurheartj/ehp351

[47] De Isla LP, De Agustin A, Rodrigo JL, Almeria C, del Carmen Manzano M, Rodriguez E, et al. Chronic mitral regurgitation: a pilot study to assess preoperative left ventricular contractile function using speckle-tracking echocardiography. J Am Soc Echocardiogr. 2009;22:831–838. DOI: 10.1016/j.echo.2009.04.016

[48] Sengupta PP, Krishnamoorthy VK, Abhayaratna WP, Korinek J, Belohlavek M, Sundt TM, 3rd, et al. Disparate patterns of left ventricular mechanics differentiate constrictive pericarditis from restrictive cardiomyopathy. JACC Cardiovasc Imaging. 2008;1:29–38. DOI: 10.1016/j.jcmg.2007.10.006

[49] Kalam K, Otahal P, Marwick TH. Prognostic implications of global LV dysfunction: a systematic review and meta-analysis of global longitudinal strain and ejection fraction. Heart. 2014;100:1673–1680. DOI: 10.1136/heartjnl-2014-305538

[50] Bijnens B, Claus P, Weidemann F, Strotmann J, Sutherland GR. Investigating cardiac function using motion and deformation analysis in the setting of coronary artery disease. Circulation. 2007;116:2453–2464. DOI: 10.1161/CIRCULATIONAHA.106.684357

[51] Turschner O, D'Hooge J, Dommke C, Claus P, Verbeken E, De Scheerder I, et al. The sequential changes in myocardial thickness and thickening which occur during acute transmural infarction, infarct reperfusion and the resultant expression of reperfusion injury. Eur Heart J. 2004;25:794–803. DOI: 10.1016/j.ehj.2004.01.006

[52] Carlhall CJ, Lindstrom L, Wranne B, Nylander E. Atrioventricular plane displacement correlates closely to circulatory dimensions but not to ejection fraction in normal young subjects. Clin Physiol. 2001;21:621–628. DOI: 10.1046/j.1365-2281.2001.00356.x

[53] Zaky A, Nasser WK, Feigenbaum H. A study of mitral valve action recorded by reflected ultrasound and its application in the diagnosis of mitral stenosis. Circulation. 1968;37:789–799. DOI: 10.1161/01.CIR.37.5.789

[54] Roberson DA, Cui W. Tissue Doppler imaging measurement of left ventricular systolic function in children: mitral annular displacement index is superior to peak velocity. J Am Soc Echocardiogr. 2009;22:376–382. DOI: 10.1016/j.echo.2009.01.008

[55] Voigt JU, Exner B, Schmiedehausen K, Huchzermeyer C, Reulbach U, Nixdorff U, et al. Strain-rate imaging during dobutamine stress echocardiography provides objective evidence of inducible ischemia. Circulation. 2003;107:2120–2126. DOI: 10.1161/01.CIR.0000065249.69988.AA

[56] Weidemann F, Dommke C, Bijnens B, Claus P, D'Hooge J, Mertens P, et al. Defining the transmurality of a chronic myocardial infarction by ultrasonic strain-rate imaging: implications for identifying intramural viability: an experimental study. Circulation. 2003;107:883–888. DOI: 10.1161/01.CIR.0000050146.66577.4B

[57] Asanuma T, Uranishi A, Masuda K, Ishikura F, Beppu S, Nakatani S. Assessment of myocardial ischemic memory using persistence of post-systolic thickening after recovery from ischemia. JACC Cardiovasc Imaging. 2009;2:1253–1261. DOI: 10.1016/j.jcmg.2009.07.008

[58] Bragadeesh T, Jayaweera AR, Pascotto M, Micari A, Le DE, Kramer CM, et al. Post-ischaemic myocardial dysfunction (stunning) results from myofibrillar oedema. Heart. 2008;94:166–171. DOI: 10.1136/hrt.2006.102434

[59] Merli E, Sutherland GR, Bijnens B, Fischer A, Chaparro M, Karu T, et al. Usefulness of changes in left ventricular wall thickness to predict full or partial pressure reperfusion in ST-elevation acute myocardial infarction. Am J Cardiol. 2008;102:249–256. DOI: 10.1016/j.amjcard.2008.03.047

[60] Marciniak A, Claus P, Sutherland GR, Marciniak M, Karu T, Baltabaeva A, et al. Changes in systolic left ventricular function in isolated mitral regurgitation. A strain rate imaging study. Eur Heart J. 2007;28:2627–2636. DOI: 10.1093/eurheartj/ehm072

[61] Pandis D, Sengupta PP, Castillo JG, Caracciolo G, Fischer GW, Narula J, et al. Assessment of longitudinal myocardial mechanics in patients with degenerative mitral valve regurgitation predicts postoperative worsening of left ventricular systolic function. J Am Soc Echocardiogr. 2014;27:627–638. DOI: 10.1016/j.echo.2014.02.008

[62] Florescu M, Benea DC, Rimbas RC, Cerin G, Diena M, Lanzzillo G, et al. Myocardial systolic velocities and deformation assessed by speckle tracking for early detection of left ventricular dysfunction in asymptomatic patients with severe primary mitral regurgitation. Echocardiography. 2012;29:326–333. DOI: 10.1111/j.1540-8175.2011.01563.x

[63] Kumanohoso T, Otsuji Y, Yoshifuku S, Matsukida K, Koriyama C, Kisanuki A, et al. Mechanism of higher incidence of ischemic mitral regurgitation in patients with inferior myocardial infarction: quantitative analysis of left ventricular and mitral valve geometry in 103 patients with prior myocardial infarction. J Thorac Cardiovasc Surg. 2003;125:135–143. DOI: 10.1067/mva.2003.78

[64] Gustafsson U, Lindqvist P, Morner S, Waldenstrom A. Assessment of regional rotation patterns improves the understanding of the systolic and diastolic left ventricular

function: an echocardiographic speckle-tracking study in healthy individuals. Eur J Echocardiogr. 2009;10:56–61. DOI: 10.1093/ejechocard/jen141

[65] Zito C, Cusma-Piccione M, Oreto L, Tripepi S, Mohammed M, Di Bella G, et al. In patients with post-infarction left ventricular dysfunction, how does impaired basal rotation affect chronic ischemic mitral regurgitation? J Am Soc Echocardiogr. 2013;26:1118–1129. DOI: 10.1016/j.echo.2013.04.017

[66] Singh A, Steadman CD, McCann GP. Advances in the understanding of the pathophysiology and management of aortic stenosis: role of novel imaging techniques. Can J Cardiol. 2014;30:994–1003. DOI: 10.1016/j.cjca.2014.03.008

[67] Shah PK. Should severe aortic stenosis be operated on before symptom onset? Severe aortic stenosis should not be operated on before symptom onset. Circulation. 2012;126:118–125. DOI: 10.1161/CIRCULATIONAHA.111.079368

[68] Carabello BA. Should severe aortic stenosis be operated on before symptom onset? Aortic valve replacement should be operated on before symptom onset. Circulation. 2012;126:112–117. DOI: 0.1161/CIRCULATIONAHA.111.079350

[69] Carabello BA. The relationship of left ventricular geometry and hypertrophy to left ventricular function in valvular heart disease. J Heart Valve Dis. 1995;4 Suppl 2:S132–138; discussion S138–139. DOI: none

[70] Baltabaeva A, Marciniak M, Bijnens B, Moggridge J, He FJ, Antonios TF, et al. Regional left ventricular deformation and geometry analysis provides insights in myocardial remodelling in mild to moderate hypertension. Eur J Echocardiogr. 2008;9:501–508. DOI: 10.1016/j.euje.2007.08.004

[71] Yingchoncharoen T, Gibby C, Rodriguez LL, Grimm RA, Marwick TH. Association of myocardial deformation with outcome in asymptomatic aortic stenosis with normal ejection fraction. Circ Cardiovasc Imaging. 2012;5:719–725. DOI: 10.1161/CIRCIMAGING.112.977348

[72] Nishimura RA, Otto CM, Bonow RO, Carabello BA, Erwin JP, 3rd, Guyton RA, et al. 2014 AHA/ACC guideline for the management of patients with valvular heart disease: executive summary: a report of the American College of Cardiology/American Heart Association Task Force on practice guidelines. Circulation. 2014;129:2440–2492. DOI: 10.1161/CIR.0000000000000029

[73] Hawkins NM, Petrie MC, Burgess MI, McMurray JJ. Selecting patients for cardiac resynchronization therapy: the fallacy of echocardiographic dyssynchrony. J Am Coll Cardiol. 2009;53:1944–1959. DOI: 10.1016/j.jacc.2008.11.062

[74] Marciniak M, Bijnens B, Baltabaeva A, Marciniak A, Parsai C, Claus P, et al. Interventricular interaction as a possible mechanism for the presence of a biphasic systolic velocity profile in normal left ventricular free walls. Heart. 2008;94:1058–1064. DOI: 10.1136/hrt.2007.126938

[75] Suffoletto MS, Dohi K, Cannesson M, Saba S, Gorcsan J, 3rd. Novel speckle-tracking radial strain from routine black-and-white echocardiographic images to quantify dyssynchrony and predict response to cardiac resynchronization therapy. Circulation. 2006;113:960–968. DOI: 10.1161/CIRCULATIONAHA.105.571455

[76] Carasso S, Rakowski H, Witte KK, Smith P, Carasso D, Garceau P, et al. Left ventricular strain patterns in dilated cardiomyopathy predict response to cardiac resynchronization therapy: timing is not everything. J Am Soc Echocardiogr. 2009;22:242–250. DOI: 10.1016/j.echo.2008.12.003

[77] Russell K, Eriksen M, Aaberge L, Wilhelmsen N, Skulstad H, Remme EW, et al. A novel clinical method for quantification of regional left ventricular pressure-strain loop area: a non-invasive index of myocardial work. Eur Heart J. 2012;33:724–733. DOI: 10.1093/eurheartj/ehs016

[78] Russell K, Eriksen M, Aaberge L, Wilhelmsen N, Skulstad H, Gjesdal O, et al. Assessment of wasted myocardial work: a novel method to quantify energy loss due to uncoordinated left ventricular contractions. Am J Physiol Heart Circ Physiol. 2013;305:H996–1003. DOI: 10.1152/ajpheart.00191.2013

[79] Galderisi M. Diastolic dysfunction and diabetic cardiomyopathy: evaluation by Doppler echocardiography. J Am Coll Cardiol. 2006;48:1548–1551. DOI: 10.1016/j.jacc.2006.07.033

[80] Guo R, Wang K, Song W, Cong T, Shang ZJ, Sun YH, et al. Myocardial dysfunction in early diabetes patients with microalbuminuria: a 2-dimensional speckle tracking strain study. Cell Biochem Biophys. 2014;70:573–578. DOI: 10.1007/s12013-014-9958-8

[81] Shim CY, Park S, Choi EY, Kang SM, Cha BS, Ha JW, et al. Is albuminuria an indicator of myocardial dysfunction in diabetic patients without overt heart disease? A study with Doppler strain and strain rate imaging. Metabolism. 2008;57:448–452. DOI: 10.1016/j.metabol.2007.11.003

[82] Ernande L, Rietzschel ER, Bergerot C, De Buyzere ML, Schnell F, Groisne L, et al. Impaired myocardial radial function in asymptomatic patients with type 2 diabetes mellitus: a speckle-tracking imaging study. J Am Soc Echocardiogr. 2010;23:1266–1272. DOI: 10.1016/j.echo.2010.09.007

[83] Ernande L, Bergerot C, Rietzschel ER, De Buyzere ML, Thibault H, Pignonblanc PG, et al. Diastolic dysfunction in patients with type 2 diabetes mellitus: is it really the first marker of diabetic cardiomyopathy? J Am Soc Echocardiogr. 2011;24:1268–1275 e1261. DOI: 10.1016/j.echo.2011.07.017

[84] Karagoz A, Bezgin T, Kutluturk I, Kulahcioglu S, Tanboga IH, Guler A, et al. Subclinical left ventricular systolic dysfunction in diabetic patients and its association with retinopathy: a 2D speckle tracking echocardiography study. Herz. 2014. DOI: 10.1007/s00059-014-4138-6

[85] Hooning MJ, Botma A, Aleman BM, Baaijens MH, Bartelink H, Klijn JG, et al. Long-term risk of cardiovascular disease in 10-year survivors of breast cancer. J Natl Cancer Inst. 2007;99:365–375. DOI: 10.1093/jnci/djk064

[86] Doyle JJ, Neugut AI, Jacobson JS, Grann VR, Hershman DL. Chemotherapy and cardiotoxicity in older breast cancer patients: a population-based study. J Clin Oncol. 2005;23:8597–8605. DOI: 10.1200/JCO.2005.02.5841

[87] Lang RM, Bierig M, Devereux RB, Flachskampf FA, Foster E, Pellikka PA, et al. Recommendations for chamber quantification: a report from the American Society of Echocardiography's Guidelines and Standards Committee and the Chamber Quantification Writing Group, developed in conjunction with the European Association of Echocardiography, a branch of the European Society of Cardiology. J Am Soc Echocardiogr. 2005;18:1440–1463. DOI: 10.1016/j.echo.2005.10.005

[88] Thavendiranathan P, Grant AD, Negishi T, Plana JC, Popovic ZB, Marwick TH. Reproducibility of echocardiographic techniques for sequential assessment of left ventricular ejection fraction and volumes: application to patients undergoing cancer chemotherapy. J Am Coll Cardiol. 2013;61:77–84. DOI: 10.1016/j.jacc.2012.09.035

[89] Cardinale D, Colombo A, Lamantia G, Colombo N, Civelli M, De Giacomi G, et al. Anthracycline-induced cardiomyopathy: clinical relevance and response to pharmacologic therapy. J Am Coll Cardiol. 2010;55:213–220. DOI: 10.1016/j.jacc.2009.03.095

[90] Neilan TG, Jassal DS, Perez-Sanz TM, Raher MJ, Pradhan AD, Buys ES, et al. Tissue Doppler imaging predicts left ventricular dysfunction and mortality in a murine model of cardiac injury. Eur Heart J. 2006;27:1868–1875. DOI: 10.1093/eurheartj/ehl013

[91] Sawaya H, Sebag IA, Plana JC, Januzzi JL, Ky B, Cohen V, et al. Early detection and prediction of cardiotoxicity in chemotherapy-treated patients. Am J Cardiol. 2011;107:1375–1380. DOI: 10.1016/j.amjcard.2011.01.006

[92] Fallah-Rad N, Walker JR, Wassef A, Lytwyn M, Bohonis S, Fang T, et al. The utility of cardiac biomarkers, tissue velocity and strain imaging, and cardiac magnetic resonance imaging in predicting early left ventricular dysfunction in patients with human epidermal growth factor receptor II-positive breast cancer treated with adjuvant trastuzumab therapy. J Am Coll Cardiol. 2011;57:2263–2270. DOI: 10.1016/j.jacc.2010.11.063

[93] Poterucha JT, Kutty S, Lindquist RK, Li L, Eidem BW. Changes in left ventricular longitudinal strain with anthracycline chemotherapy in adolescents precede subsequent decreased left ventricular ejection fraction. J Am Soc Echocardiogr. 2012;25:733–740. DOI: 10.1016/j.echo.2012.04.007

[94] Sawaya H, Sebag IA, Plana JC, Januzzi JL, Ky B, Tan TC, et al. Assessment of echocardiography and biomarkers for the extended prediction of cardiotoxicity in patients treated with anthracyclines, taxanes, and trastuzumab. Circ Cardiovasc Imaging. 2012;5:596–603. DOI: 10.1161/CIRCIMAGING.112.973321

[95] Sirbu C, Herbots L, D'Hooge J, Claus P, Marciniak A, Langeland T, et al. Feasibility of strain and strain rate imaging for the assessment of regional left atrial deformation: a study in normal subjects. Eur J Echocardiogr. 2006;7:199–208. DOI: 10.1016/j.euje.2005.06.001

[96] Cameli M, Lisi M, Focardi M, Reccia R, Natali BM, Sparla S, et al. Left atrial deformation analysis by speckle tracking echocardiography for prediction of cardiovascular outcomes. Am J Cardiol. 2012;110:264–269. DOI: 10.1016/j.amjcard.2012.03.022

[97] Vianna-Pinton R, Moreno CA, Baxter CM, Lee KS, Tsang TS, Appleton CP. Two-dimensional speckle-tracking echocardiography of the left atrium: feasibility and regional contraction and relaxation differences in normal subjects. J Am Soc Echocardiogr. 2009;22:299–305. DOI: 10.1016/j.echo.2008.12.017

[98] Okamatsu K, Takeuchi M, Nakai H, Nishikage T, Salgo IS, Husson S, et al. Effects of aging on left atrial function assessed by two-dimensional speckle tracking echocardiography. J Am Soc Echocardiogr. 2009;22:70–75. DOI: 10.1016/j.echo.2008.11.006

[99] D'Hooge J, Heimdal A, Jamal F, Kukulski T, Bijnens B, Rademakers F, et al. Regional strain and strain rate measurements by cardiac ultrasound: principles, implementation and limitations. Eur J Echocardiogr. 2000;1:154–170. DOI: 10.1053/euje.2000.0031

[100] Meris A, Faletra F, Conca C, Klersy C, Regoli F, Klimusina J, et al. Timing and magnitude of regional right ventricular function: a speckle tracking-derived strain study of normal subjects and patients with right ventricular dysfunction. J Am Soc Echocardiogr. 2010;23:823–831. DOI: 10.1016/j.echo.2010.05.009

[101] Kleijn SA, Aly MF, Terwee CB, van Rossum AC, Kamp O. Reliability of left ventricular volumes and function measurements using three-dimensional speckle tracking echocardiography. Eur Heart J Cardiovasc Imaging. 2012;13:159–168. DOI: 10.1093/ejechocard/jer174

[102] Gayat E, Ahmad H, Weinert L, Lang RM, Mor-Avi V. Reproducibility and inter-vendor variability of left ventricular deformation measurements by three-dimensional speckle-tracking echocardiography. J Am Soc Echocardiogr. 2011;24:878–885. DOI: 10.1016/j.echo.2011.04.016

Chapter 6

Cardiac Imaging in Hypertrophic Cardiomyopathy

Dai-Yin Lu and Ming-Chong Hsiung

Additional information is available at the end of the chapter

http://dx.doi.org/10.5772/64364

Abstract

Hypertrophic cardiomyopathy (HCM) is a relatively common inherited cardiomyopathy, which is occasionally challenging to differentiate from hypertensive heart disease and athlete hearts on the basis of morphologic or functional abnormalities alone. Imaging studies provide solutions for most clinical needs, from diagnosis, anatomical and functional assessment, family screening, risk stratification, to monitoring of treatment response. Generally, transthoracic echocardiography is used as first-line imaging tool to establish the diagnosis. A multimodality imaging approach (cardiac magnetic resonance, cardiac computed tomography, and cardiac nuclear imaging) is also encouraged in the assessment of these patients. The choice of imaging tool should be based on a broad perspective and expert knowledge of what each technique has to offer, including its specific advantages and disadvantages. In this chapter, we discuss the utility and pitfalls of established imaging modalities and discuss the evolving role of novel echocardiographic imaging modalities.

Keywords: cardiac computed tomography, cardiovascular magnetic resonance, echocardiography, hypertrophic cardiomyopathy, nuclear imaging

1. Introduction

1.1. Definition and prevalence

Hypertrophic cardiomyopathy (HCM) is the most common inherited cardiac disease presented with exercise intolerance, heart failure, cardiac arrhythmias and sudden cardiac death [1]. Across different ethnicities, the prevalence is approximately 0.2% [2]. This estimated frequency in the general population appears to exceed the relatively low visit of HCM in cardiology practices, implying that the most affected individuals remain undiagnosed, probably in most cases without symptoms or shortened life expectancy [3]. The clinical diagnosis of HCM is based on the demonstration of asymmetric left ventricular hypertrophy (LVH) with maximal wall thickness ≥15 mm, in the absence of other cardiac or systemic cause that would produce such magnitude of hypertrophy.

1.2. Natural history and clinical course

The natural history is generally benign in vast majority of patients, with a life span close to general population [4]. However, hemodynamic-related symptoms secondary to dynamic left ventricular outflow tract (LVOT) obstruction as well as myopathy-related complications may happen. Although symptoms may occur at any age, they are more common between young adult and middle age. Development of symptoms at older age is generally associated with less severe forms of the disease.

Although HCM presents primarily with ventricular septal hypertrophy, a key recognizable feature has been dynamic LVOT obstruction and HCM has been regarded as a predominantly obstructive disease [5]. Left ventricular outflow tract (LVOT) obstruction may be noted at rest or during physiological exercise in 50–70% of the HCM patients [6]. LVOT obstruction at rest, defined as ≥30 mmHg, is a strong, independent predictor for progression of heart failure and death [7, 8]. Accordingly, current AHA/ACC/ESC guidelines classify HCM patients based on their LVOT gradients into obstructive (resting and provoked gradients ≥30 mmHg); latent obstructive (resting <30 and provoked ≥30 mmHg); non-obstructive (resting and provoked gradients <30 mmHg) [3, 4].

HCM also represents the most frequent cause of sudden cardiac death (SCD), one of the most serious complications, in young athletes in countries without systematic sport screening programs. Dynamic LVOT obstruction and disarrayed myocardial fiber impair diastolic function of left ventricle, followed by enlargement of left atrium and heart failure with preserved ejection fraction (EF). Atrial fibrillation (AF) is also a clinical presentation secondary to left atrial enlargement, which may later cause cardioembolic events and the following disability in the middle and older age groups.

2. The role of imaging in HCM

Multimodality imaging—echocardiography, cardiac magnetic resonance, cardiac computed tomography, and cardiac nuclear imaging—provide comprehensive information. Patients with HCM usually require long-term follow-up. It is suggested that transthoracic echocardiography be performed every 1–2 years and cardiac magnetic resonance at least once after the diagnosis is made, yet the strategy needs to be individualized (**Table 1**).

2.1. Role of echocardiography in evaluation of HCM (Table 2) [9]

2.1.1. Anatomical evaluation

HCM presents primarily with LVH, which progresses with time (**Figure 1**). The presentation is rare when in childhood, and the growth of LVH becomes more obvious during adolescence.

http://dx.doi.org/10.5772/64364

Other systemic causes of LVH (obesity, athlete heart, systemic hypertension, aortic stenosis, or infiltrative disease) should be ruled out first before the diagnosis is confirmed. The pattern of hypertrophy and LV volume can be analyzed by echocardiography. Ventricular volumes are generally normal or slightly lower, and the biplane Simpson's method has been applied to the measurement of LV volumes and EF [10]. Three-dimensional (3D) echocardiography has also been shown to provide more accurate means of quantification, [11] yet the references for HCM are limited.

	Indications	Strengths	Limitations
Echocardiography	• First line imaging tool in screening and follow-up	• Real time • Repeatable • Demonstrate dynamic change • Provide hemodynamic information	• Imaging quality depends on patient's acoustic window • Interpretation operator dependent
Cardiac magnetic resonance (CMR)	• Anatomic evaluation • Fibrosis assessment • Differential diagnosis	• Good spatial resolution • Fibrosis assessment	• No real-time information • Contrast needed • Not applicable for every patient (with metallic device or pacemaker)
Cardiac nuclear imaging (CNI)	• Perfusion assessment • Metabolism	• Information of microvascular disease	• Radiation • Low spatial resolution

Table 1. Imaging tools in HCM.

Screening	
LV	Presence of hypertrophy and its distribution; report should include measurements f LV dimensions and wall thickness (septal, posterior, and maximum)
	Ejection fraction
	Diastolic function (comments n LV relaxation and filling pressures)
	Dynamic obstruction at rest and with Valsalva maneuver; report should identify the site of obstruction and the gradient
MV	Mitral valve and papillary muscle evaluation, including the direction, mechanism, and severity of mitral regurgitation; if needed, TEE should be performed to satisfactorily answer these questions
RV	RV hypertrophy and whether RV dynamic obstruction is present
PA	Pulmonary artery systolic pressure
LA	LA volume indexed to body surface area
Guidance	TEE is recommended to guide surgical myectomy, and TTE or TEE for alcohol septal ablation

LA = left atrium; LV = left ventricle; MV = mitral valve; PA = pulmonary artery; RV = right ventricle; TEE = transesophageal echocardiography (Adapted with permission from Nagueh et al. [9]).

Table 2. Echocardiogrophic evaluations of patients with HCM.

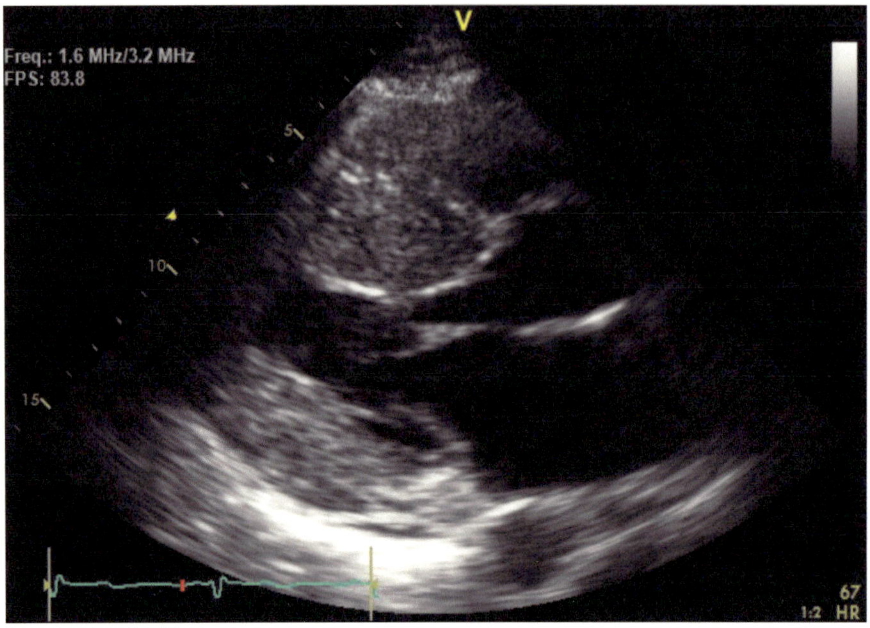

Figure 1. Left ventricular thickness, evaluated at septum and free wall level, is considered abnormal when ≥ 15 mm, and defined asymmetrical in presence of a septal to free wall thickness ratio between 1.3 and 1.5.

2.1.2. Hemodynamic evaluation

A key recognizable feature has been dynamic LVOT obstruction, and HCM has been regarded as a predominantly obstructive disease [5]. Patients with LVOT obstruction, defined by the presence of a peak gradient higher than 30 mmHg at rest or after provocative maneuvers (Valsalva, standing, and exercise) is a strong, independent predictor for progression of heart failure and death [7, 8] (**Figure 2**). Structural abnormalities of the mitral valve apparatus in HCM include hypertrophy of the papillary muscles, resulting in anterior displacement of papillary muscles, and mitral valve elongation [12, 13]. Systolic anterior motion (SAM) is defined as the systolic motion of the mitral leaflet, mainly anterior leaflet, or chordae into LVOT, resulting in outlet narrowing and flow disturbance. SAM also impairs the mitral leaflet coaptation, followed by regurgitation (**Figure 3**). The anterior leaflet motion is greater than that of the posterior leaflet during SAM and an interleaflet gap occurs, resulting in a typically posteriorly directed jet of mitral regurgitation. The anterior leaflet has a greater surface area and hence greater redundancy and mobility. If a concentric regurgitation jet is found in HCM patients, concomitant mitral valvulopathy should be carefully evaluated.

2.1.3. Assessment of LV systolic function

The ejection fraction of left ventricle in HCM patients is generally normal or even increased. However, patients with significant hypertrophy may have small LV end-diastolic volumes and the following lower stroke volumes despite a normal LVEF. LV systolic dysfunction is usually

http://dx.doi.org/10.5772/64364

defined as LVEF < 50%. When present, the prognosis is markedly worse. In addition to 2D imaging, Doppler echocardiography has been used to assess subclinical LV systolic dysfunction. Tissue Doppler imaging measures the velocity of myocardial motion. A lower systolic (Sa) or reduced early diastolic (Ea or e') velocities can occur before overt hypertrophy develops [14].

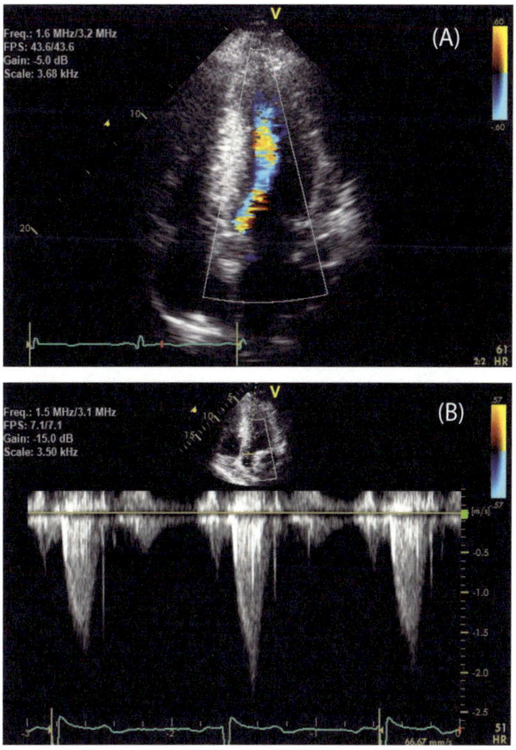

Figure 2. (A) Asymmetric septal hypertrophy may cause narrowing of the left ventricular outflow tract, resulting in turbulent flow. (B) Doppler analysis across the LVOT in dynamic obstructive HCM results in a characteristic signal with a late-peaking dagger-shaped appearance.

2.1.4. Assessment of LV diastolic function

Reduction in ventricular compliance and increased stiffness due to myocardial fibrosis coupled with a reduction of chamber volume and suction play a role in the pathophysiology of diastolic dysfunction in patients with HCM. LV and left atrial (LA) filling abnormalities have been reported in patients with HCM, irrespective of the presence and extent of LV hypertrophy. Tissue Doppler echocardiography indicates impaired myocardial relaxation regardless of symptoms or severity of LVOT obstruction [15]. Although tissue Doppler echocardiography has been successfully used to estimate filling pressures in a variety of cardiac disorders [16, 17], it is not as reliable in patients with hypertrophic cardiomyopathy as in patients with left ventricular systolic dysfunction [18]. In a study consisting of 35 patients, LV filling pressures can be estimated with reasonable accuracy in HCM patients by measuring mitral early diastolic inflow/flow propagation velocity or ratio of early diastolic mitral flow velocity to the early diastolic mitral septal annulus motion velocity (E/e′) [19]. Whereas a later report with symptomatic HCM patients concluded Doppler echocardiographic estimates of left ventricular filling pressure with the use of transmitral flow and mitral annular velocities correlated modestly with direct measurement of left atrial pressure [20]. Despite of this inconsistency in filling pressure estimation, tissue Doppler imaging remains a useful tool for risk stratification of patients with HCM [21]. A higher septal E/e′ predicts patients with HCM who are at risk of sustained ventricular tachycardia (VT), implantable cardioverter defibrillator (ICD) discharge, cardiac arrest or sudden cardiac death [22, 23].

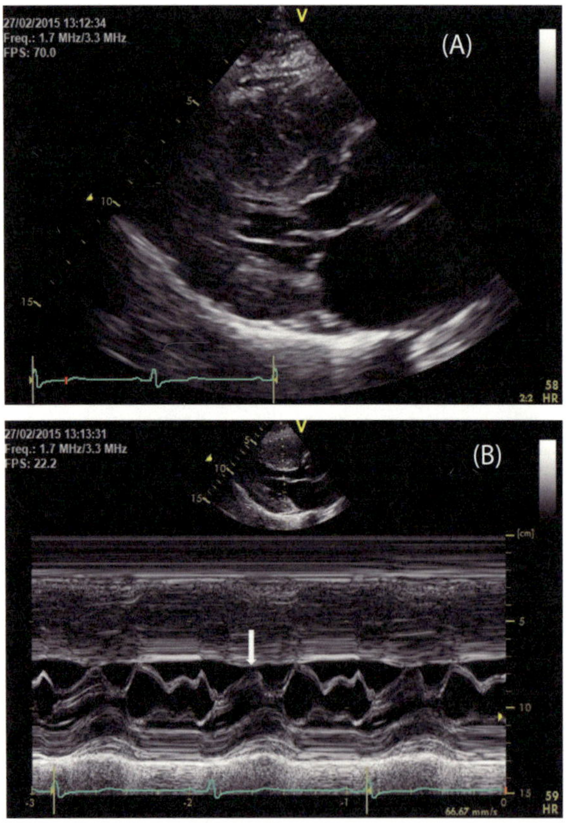

Figure 3. Systolic anterior motion (SAM) of anterior mitral leaflet at mid to late systolic phase (A) parasternal long axis view, 2D; (B) parasternal long axis view, M-mode.

LA volume is mainly secondary to diastolic dysfunction, mitral regurgitation and atrial myopathy. LA enlargement is generally assessed by 2D or M-mode linear dimensions. However, it is important to recognize that linear dimensions, particularly anteroposterior measurements of the LA, may not measure true LA size, as LA remodeling frequently happens asymmetrically [24]. Increased LA volume is an independent indicator of functional capacity [25] and an LA volume index of >34 ml/m² has been shown to be predictive of a more severe LVH, diastolic dysfunction, and adverse cardiovascular outcomes [26].

2.2. Role of deformation imaging in HCM

2.2.1. TDI-derived strain

Although tissue Doppler velocity was considered as a technique for evaluation of regional myocardial performance, the utility is limited in distinguishing myocardial contractility from passive motion. Such restriction later leads to the development of strain imaging. Strain is a measure of tissue deformation and is defined as the change in length normalized to the original length. The rate at which this change occurs is called strain rate (SR). In contrast to tissue Doppler velocity, which examines myocardial motion relative to the transducer, strain measures myocardial motion relative to the adjacent myocardium [27]. When the left ventricle contracts, the myocardium shortens in longitudinal and circumferential direction (negative value in strain) and thickens in the radial direction (positive value in strain) (**Figure 4**) [28]. Strain rate (SR) represents the local rate of myocardial deformation (**Figure 5**) [29]. Weidemann et al. (30) firstly described the use of TDI-derived strain for the evaluation of HCM in a case report of a child with non-obstructive HCM. Tissue Doppler velocities were found to be normal in all the septal segments interrogated. However, systolic longitudinal strain SR was significantly decreased in the mid septal region with no significant changes in the basal regions when compared with healthy children [30]. Later reports also confirmed similar findings in adults with HCM [31, 32].

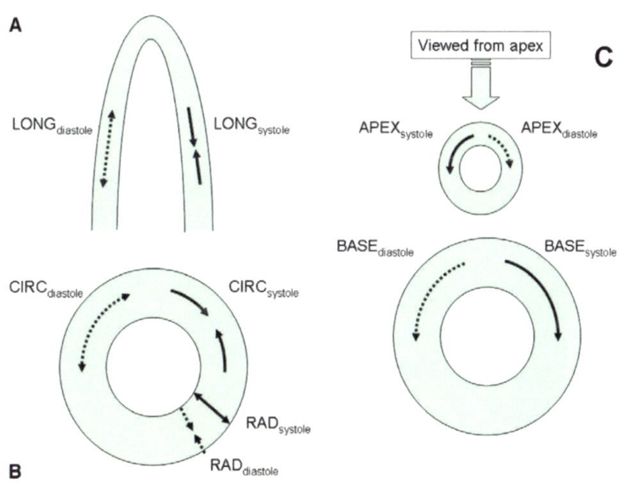

Figure 4. Graphic representation of the principal myocardial deformations: longitudinal (A), radial and circumferential (B), and torsion (C). The direction of deformation in systole is shown as solid lines and that in diastole is shown as dashed lines. LONG indicates longitudinal; RAD, radial; and CIRC, circumferential. (Reprinted with permission from Abraham et al. [28]).

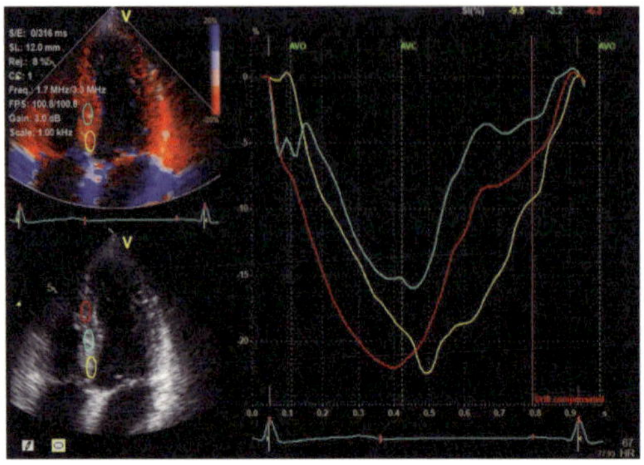

Figure 5. Strain analysis from tissue Doppler imaging from three representative regions of interest (ROIs) in LV septal wall.

2.2.2. 2D strain or speckle tracking imaging

The interaction of ultrasound with the myocardium produces unique acoustic patterns, also known as "speckles." These speckles can be tracked over time and speckle displacement can be used to calculate the tissue velocity and strain [33]. This method is not based on the Doppler principle and relatively angle independent [34]. Deformation is calculated with frame-by-frame speckle displacement, yielding angle independent parameters of myocardial contraction, and gives longitudinal, transverse strain and strain rate in long-axis images (**Figure 6**). Similarly, radial and circumferential strain or strain rate may be analyzed by the short-axis images. In a study for patients with familial non-obstructive HCM, average longitudinal was reduced in affected individuals compared with healthy controls, despite apparently normal systolic function. In addition, no significant difference in the values obtained by TDI versus 2D strain echocardiography was observed [35]. A recent study of patients with HCM and preserved systolic function demonstrated attenuated longitudinal strain, increased circumferential strain, and normal overall systolic LV twist or torsion [36].

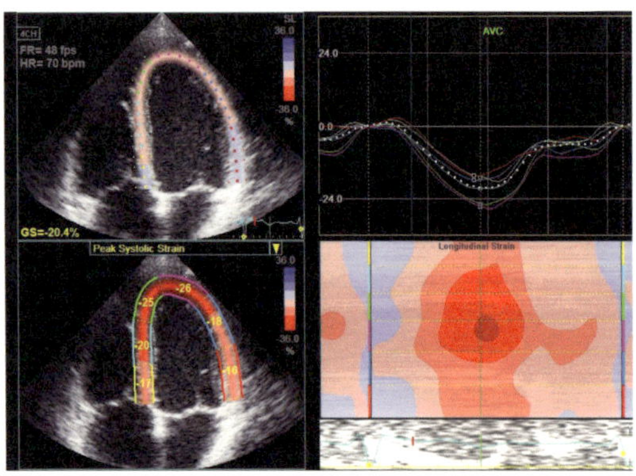

Figure 6. Strain analysis from two-dimensional speckle tracking from apical four chamber view.

2.3. Application of interventional echocardiography in HCM

2.3.1. Alcohol septal ablation (ASA)

2D echo is useful in search of suitable patients for ASA. During the procedure under transthoracic echocardiographic guidance, injection of echo contrast into a septal perforator branch of the left anterior descending artery helps determine whether the selected branch to occlude supplies the appropriate myocardium where SAM contacts interventricular septum (**Figure 7**) [37]. For patients with suboptimal transthoracic echo window, transesophageal echo imaging may be another option.

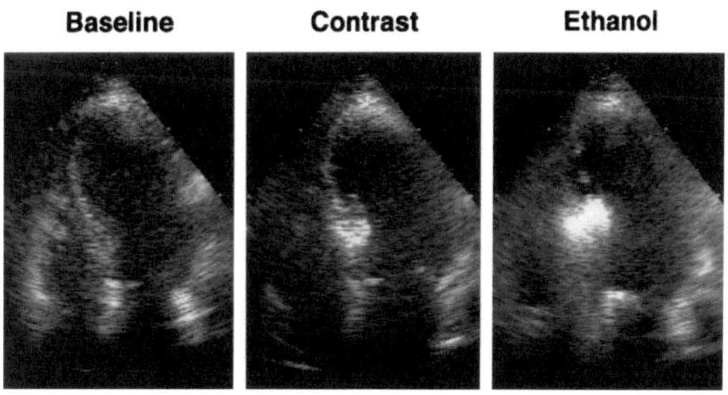

Figure 7. Myocardial contrast echocardiography of the hypertrophied septum after injection of sonicated albumin (Contrast) and ethanol (Reprinted wth permission from Nagueh et al. [37]).

2.3.2. Surgical myectomy and mitral surgery

It is important to have a real-time imaging analysis in the peri-procedural assessment of HCM patients undergoing myectomy, with or without mitral surgery. Intraoperative Transesophageal echocardiography (TEE) plays a key role in surgery, assessing mechanisms of LVOTO, mechanism of MR, extension of myocardial region that need to be removed and other possible intra-operative complications.

2.4. Other imaging modality

*2.4.1. Cardiac magnetic resonance (**Table 3**) [38]*

2.4.1.1. Anatomical evaluation

Cardiac magnetic resonance (CMR) should be considered in the initial evaluation of all patients with HCM when clinic resources are available [4]. It provides comprehensive evaluation of both the ventricle, including assessment of wall thickness [39–41] and the chamber volumes, with high quality of spatial and temporal resolution (**Figure 8**) [38]. CMR may be more sensitive than echocardiography in detecting LVH [40]. The extension of LVH can be defined using CMR as focal (1–2 hypertrophic segments), intermediate (3–7 segments), and diffuse (8–16 hypertrophic segments). CMR can also give more precise measurement in maximal diastolic wall thickness [42].

Left ventricle volumes, mass and ejection fraction
Location, type, distribution of hypertrophy, maximal wall thickness and diastolic wall thickness to volume ratio
Degree of asymmetry
LVOT or mid-cavity obstruction
LGE: presence or absence; pattern and extension
Evidence of MR
Description of mitral valve apparatus (leaflets, chordae, papillary muscles) and its relation to obstruction or MR

LGE = late gadolinium enhancement; LVOT = left ventricular outlet tract; MR = mitral regurgitation. (Adapted with permission from Cardim et al. [38].)

Table 3. CMR evaluations of patients with HCM.

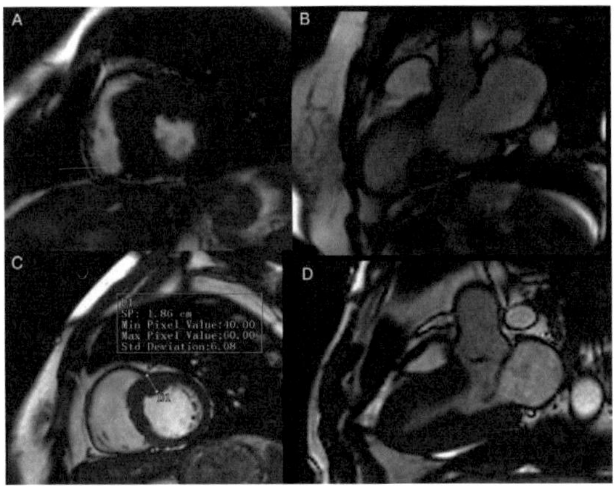

Figure 8. Cardiac MR in HCM patients. Cine CMR-SSFP in different HCM patients. (A) Basal short-axis view, asymmetric LVH with lateral wall sparing. (B) Three-chamber view, mid-ventricular hypertrophy of the medial segments of the posterior wall and anterior interventricular septum. (C) short-axis view, LVH localized in the anteroseptal wall (18 mm), undetected by echocardiography. (D) Three-chamber view, systolic phase. (Reprinted with permission from Cardim et al. [38]).

2.4.1.2. *Tissue characterization*

CMR is the most important technique in tissue characterization. The principle of late gadolinium enhancement (LGE) in CMR is based on those tissues, with an expanded extracellular space that provides a larger distribution volume for the conventional CMR contrast agents, which occupy extravascular and extracellular space. Within 30 minutes, differences between the tissue with normal and expanded extracellular volumes are large and LGE imaging is acquired (**Figure 9**) [43]. Current LGE protocols provide a very high spatial resolution (≤1 mm) and also provide a very high contrast to noise ratio, allowing to delineate small amounts of myocardial fibrosis. In HCM patients, there is frequent [44] and progressive [45] fibrosis. Two major patterns of LGE distribution are demonstrated: Intramural LGE was seen within the hypertrophied segments, which are thought to be reflective of replacement fibrosis [46]. RV insertion points LGE corresponds to interstitial fibrosis and myocyte disarray [47].

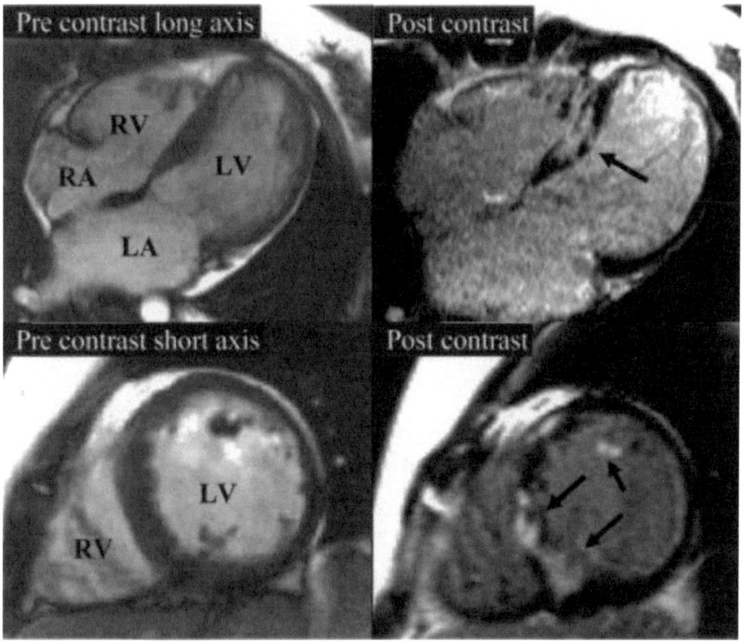

Figure 9. Pre- and post-contrast CMR images demonstrating enhancement. The pre-contrast images are the diastolic frames of fast imaging with steady-state precession cine loops. In the post-contrast images, normal myocardium appears dark. There is a large area of septal enhancement, with additional papillary muscle enhancement and subendocardial enhancement of the lateral wall. The total extent of enhancement was 25% of the left ventricular mass. (Reprinted with permission from Moon et al. [43]).

2.4.2. Cardiac nuclear imaging

Single photon-emission computed tomography (SPECT) myocardial perfusion imaging with Thallium-201 and Tc-99 m labelled tracers often demonstrate reversible (suggestive of ischemia) and fixed defects (scar), even when there is no obvious epicardial coronary artery disease [48]. The positive predictive value for SPECT study in HCM is relatively low for epicardial coronary artery disease compared to a high negative predictive value. Ischemic and scarring have been demonstrated a predictor of worse outcome, including adverse remodeling, systolic dysfunction and sudden cardiac death [49]. In obstructive HCM patients, improvement of perfusion may be observed when the obstruction is relieved after myectomy (**Figure 10**) [38, 50].

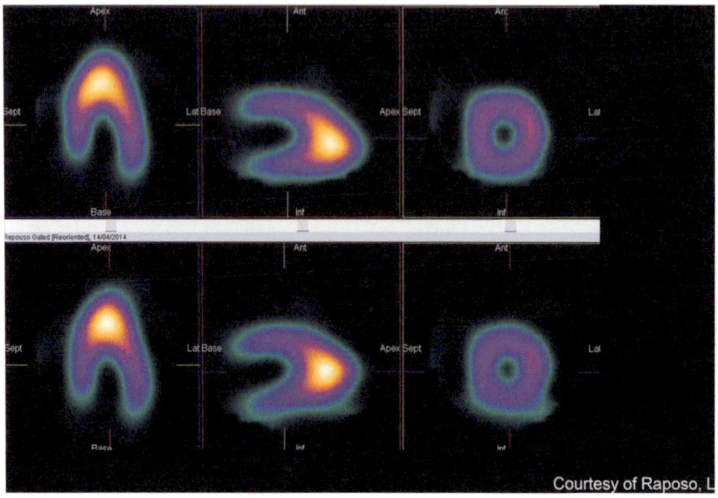

Figure 10. Functional imaging of ischemia with single photon-emission computed tomography (SPECT) with Tc-99m-Sestamibi in a 34-year-old male patient with HCM with history of chest pain in the absence of epicardial coronary artery disease). Stress (upper row) and rest (lower row). A fixed, non-reversible defect (scar) in the basal segments of the LV was found, with a non-coronary artery distribution. The apical perfusion is normal. However, this pattern may be a false perfusion defect due to increased hypertrophic mid-ventricular and apical uptake of the radiotracer. (Reprinted with permission from Cardim et al. [38]).

Using N-13-labelled ammonia and O-15-labelled water, proton emission tomography (PET) imaging detects absolute myocardial blood flow in patients with HCM. In contrast to SPECT, PET allows the direct quantification of myocardial blood flow (**Figure 11**) [38]. PET imaging

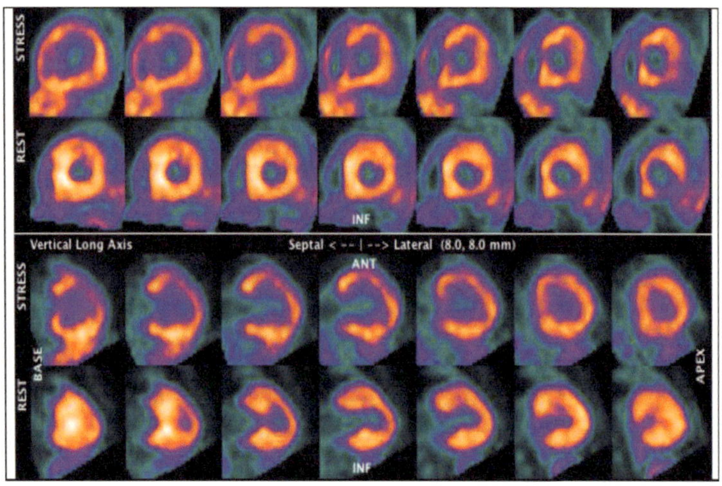

Figure 11. Functional imaging of ischemia with nuclear proton emission tomography (PET). Stress dipyridamole (upper row) and rest (lower row) $^{13}NH_3$ perfusion images in an 14-year-old girl diagnosed with HCM with interventricular septum (IVS) 29 mm. Stress: LV dilation and subendocardial hypoperfusion (IVS and antero-lateral wall). Rest: increased IVS $^{13}NH_3$ uptake is seen, indicative of IVS hypertrophy. (Reprinted with permission from Cardim et al. [38]).

is the most reliable noninvasive quantitative method for assessing myocardial ischemia in HCM [51].

3. Summary

Echocardiography remains the first-line imaging tool in the assessment of HCM patients, while the role of cardiac MR and nuclear imaging is getting more and more important, providing specific clinical information, which echocardiography is unable to give. The assessment of fibrosis, tissue characterization, and myocardial function, represents imaging future priorities of HCM imaging.

Author details

Dai-Yin Lu[1,2] and Ming-Chong Hsiung[3*]

*Address all correspondence to: hsiungmc@gmail.com

1 Division of Cardiology, Department of Medicine, Taipei Veterans General Hospital, Taipei, Taiwan

2 Department of Medicine, National Yang-Ming University, Taipei, Taiwan

3 Division of Cardiology, Heart Center, Chen-Hsin General Hospital, Taipei, Taiwan

References

[1] Maron BJ, Ommen SR, Semsarian C, Spirito P, Olivotto I, Maron MS. Hypertrophic cardiomyopathy: present and future, with translation into contemporary cardiovascular medicine. Journal of the American College of Cardiology. 2014;64(1):83–99.

[2] Maron BJ, McKenna WJ, Danielson GK, Kappenberger LJ, Kuhn HJ, Seidman CE, et al. American College of Cardiology/European Society of Cardiology clinical expert consensus document on hypertrophic cardiomyopathy. A report of the American College of Cardiology Foundation Task Force on Clinical Expert Consensus Documents and the European Society of Cardiology Committee for Practice Guidelines. Journal of the American College of Cardiology. 2003;42(9):1687–713.

[3] Gersh BJ, Maron BJ, Bonow RO, Dearani JA, Fifer MA, Link MS, et al. 2011 ACCF/AHA Guideline for the Diagnosis and Treatment of Hypertrophic Cardiomyopathy: a report of the American College of Cardiology Foundation/American Heart Association Task Force on Practice Guidelines. Developed in collaboration with the American Associa-

tion for Thoracic Surgery, American Society of Echocardiography, American Society of Nuclear Cardiology, Heart Failure Society of America, Heart Rhythm Society, Society for Cardiovascular Angiography and Interventions, and Society of Thoracic Surgeons. Journal of the American College of Cardiology. 2011;58(25):e212–60.

[4] Elliott PM, Anastasakis A, Borger MA, Borggrefe M, Cecchi F, et al. 2014 ESC Guidelines on diagnosis and management of hypertrophic cardiomyopathy: the Task Force for the Diagnosis and Management of Hypertrophic Cardiomyopathy of the European Society of Cardiology (ESC). European Heart Journal. 2014;35(39):2733–79.

[5] Maron BJ, Maron MS, Wigle ED, Braunwald E. The 50-year history, controversy, and clinical implications of left ventricular outflow tract obstruction in hypertrophic cardiomyopathy from idiopathic hypertrophic subaortic stenosis to hypertrophic cardiomyopathy: from idiopathic hypertrophic subaortic stenosis to hypertrophic cardiomyopathy. Journal of the American College of Cardiology. 2009;54(3):191–200.

[6] Maron MS, Olivotto I, Zenovich AG, Link MS, Pandian NG, Kuvin JT, et al. Hypertrophic cardiomyopathy is predominantly a disease of left ventricular outflow tract obstruction. Circulation. 2006;114(21):2232–9.

[7] Maron MS, Olivotto I, Betocchi S, Casey SA, Lesser JR, Losi MA, et al. Effect of left ventricular outflow tract obstruction on clinical outcome in hypertrophic cardiomyopathy. The New England Journal of Medicine. 2003;348(4):295–303.

[8] Elliott PM, Gimeno JR, Tome MT, Shah J, Ward D, Thaman R, et al. Left ventricular outflow tract obstruction and sudden death risk in patients with hypertrophic cardiomyopathy. European Heart Journal. 2006;27(16):1933–41.

[9] Nagueh SF, Bierig SM, Budoff MJ, Desai M, Dilsizian V, Eidem B, et al. American Society of Echocardiography clinical recommendations for multimodality cardiovascular imaging of patients with hypertrophic cardiomyopathy: Endorsed by the American Society of Nuclear Cardiology, Society for Cardiovascular Magnetic Resonance, and Society of Cardiovascular Computed Tomography. Journal of the American Society of Echocardiography: Official Publication of the American Society of Echocardiography. 2011;24(5):473–98.

[10] Lang RM, Bierig M, Devereux RB, Flachskampf FA, Foster E, Pellikka PA, et al. Recommendations for chamber quantification: a report from the American Society of Echocardiography's Guidelines and Standards Committee and the Chamber Quantification Writing Group, developed in conjunction with the European Association of Echocardiography, a branch of the European Society of Cardiology. Journal of the American Society of Echocardiography: Official Publication of the American Society of Echocardiography. 2005;18(12):1440–63.

[11] Caselli S, Pelliccia A, Maron M, Santini D, Puccio D, Marcantonio A, et al. Differentiation of hypertrophic cardiomyopathy from other forms of left ventricular hypertrophy

http://dx.doi.org/10.5772/64364

by means of three-dimensional echocardiography. The American Journal of Cardiology. 2008;102(5):616–20.

[12] Grigg LE, Wigle ED, Williams WG, Daniel LB, Rakowski H. Transesophageal Doppler echocardiography in obstructive hypertrophic cardiomyopathy: clarification of pathophysiology and importance in intraoperative decision making. Journal of the American College of Cardiology. 1992;20(1):42–52.

[13] Klues HG, Maron BJ, Dollar AL, Roberts WC. Diversity of structural mitral valve alterations in hypertrophic cardiomyopathy. Circulation. 1992;85(5):1651–60.

[14] Nagueh SF, Bachinski LL, Meyer D, Hill R, Zoghbi WA, Tam JW, et al. Tissue Doppler imaging consistently detects myocardial abnormalities in patients with hypertrophic cardiomyopathy and provides a novel means for an early diagnosis before and independently of hypertrophy. Circulation. 2001;104(2):128–30.

[15] Maron BJ, Spirito P, Green KJ, Wesley YE, Bonow RO, Arce J. Noninvasive assessment of left ventricular diastolic function by pulsed Doppler echocardiography in patients with hypertrophic cardiomyopathy. Journal of the American College of Cardiology. 1987;10(4):733–42.

[16] Nagueh SF, Middleton KJ, Kopelen HA, Zoghbi WA, Quinones MA. Doppler tissue imaging: a noninvasive technique for evaluation of left ventricular relaxation and estimation of filling pressures. Journal of the American College of Cardiology. 1997;30(6):1527–33.

[17] Yamamoto K, Nishimura RA, Chaliki HP, Appleton CP, Holmes DR, Jr., Redfield MM. Determination of left ventricular filling pressure by Doppler echocardiography in patients with coronary artery disease: critical role of left ventricular systolic function. Journal of the American College of Cardiology. 1997;30(7):1819–26.

[18] Nishimura RA, Appleton CP, Redfield MM, Ilstrup DM, Holmes DR, Jr., Tajik AJ. Noninvasive doppler echocardiographic evaluation of left ventricular filling pressures in patients with cardiomyopathies: a simultaneous Doppler echocardiographic and cardiac catheterization study. Journal of the American College of Cardiology. 1996;28(5):1226–33.

[19] Nagueh SF, Lakkis NM, Middleton KJ, Spencer WH, 3rd, Zoghbi WA, Quinones MA. Doppler estimation of left ventricular filling pressures in patients with hypertrophic cardiomyopathy. Circulation. 1999;99(2):254–61.

[20] Geske JB, Sorajja P, Nishimura RA, Ommen SR. Evaluation of left ventricular filling pressures by Doppler echocardiography in patients with hypertrophic cardiomyopathy: correlation with direct left atrial pressure measurement at cardiac catheterization. Circulation. 2007;116(23):2702–8.

[21] Kitaoka H, Kubo T, Okawa M, Takenaka N, Sakamoto C, Baba Y, et al. Tissue doppler imaging and plasma BNP levels to assess the prognosis in patients with hypertrophic

cardiomyopathy. Journal of the American Society of Echocardiography: Official Publication of the American Society of Echocardiography. 2011;24(9):1020–5.

[22] Efthimiadis GK, Giannakoulas G, Parcharidou DG, Karvounis HI, Mochlas ST, Styliadis IH, et al. Clinical significance of tissue Doppler imaging in patients with hypertrophic cardiomyopathy. Circulation Journal: Official Journal of the Japanese Circulation Society. 2007;71(6):897–903.

[23] Kitaoka H, Kubo T, Hayashi K, Yamasaki N, Matsumura Y, Furuno T, et al. Tissue Doppler imaging and prognosis in asymptomatic or mildly symptomatic patients with hypertrophic cardiomyopathy. European Heart Journal Cardiovascular Imaging. 2013;14(6):544–9.

[24] Lester SJ, Ryan EW, Schiller NB, Foster E. Best method in clinical practice and in research studies to determine left atrial size. The American Journal of Cardiology. 1999;84(7): 829–32.

[25] Sachdev V, Shizukuda Y, Brenneman CL, Birdsall CW, Waclawiw MA, Arai AE, et al. Left atrial volumetric remodeling is predictive of functional capacity in nonobstructive hypertrophic cardiomyopathy. American Heart Journal. 2005;149(4):730–6.

[26] Yang H, Woo A, Monakier D, Jamorski M, Fedwick K, Wigle ED, et al. Enlarged left atrial volume in hypertrophic cardiomyopathy: a marker for disease severity. Journal of the American Society of Echocardiography: Official Publication of the American Society of Echocardiography. 2005;18(10):1074–82.

[27] Marwick TH. Measurement of strain and strain rate by echocardiography: ready for prime time? Journal of the American College of Cardiology. 2006;47(7):1313–27.

[28] Abraham TP, Dimaano VL, Liang HY. Role of tissue Doppler and strain echocardiography in current clinical practice. Circulation. 2007;116(22):2597–609.

[29] Gilman G, Khandheria BK, Hagen ME, Abraham TP, Seward JB, Belohlavek M. Strain rate and strain: a step-by-step approach to image and data acquisition. Journal of the American Society of Echocardiography: Official Publication of the American Society of Echocardiography. 2004;17(9):1011–20.

[30] Weidemann F, Mertens L, Gewillig M, Sutherland GR. Quantitation of localized abnormal deformation in asymmetric nonobstructive hypertrophic cardiomyopathy: a velocity, strain rate, and strain Doppler myocardial imaging study. Pediatric Cardiology. 2001;22(6):534–7.

[31] Yang H, Sun JP, Lever HM, Popovic ZB, Drinko JK, Greenberg NL, et al. Use of strain imaging in detecting segmental dysfunction in patients with hypertrophic cardiomyopathy. Journal of the American Society of Echocardiography: Official Publication of the American Society of Echocardiography. 2003;16(3):233–9.

[32] Sengupta PP, Mehta V, Arora R, Mohan JC, Khandheria BK. Quantification of regional nonuniformity and paradoxical intramural mechanics in hypertrophic cardiomyop-

athy by high frame rate ultrasound myocardial strain mapping. Journal of the American Society of Echocardiography: Official Publication of the American Society of Echocardiography. 2005;18(7):737–42.

[33] Leitman M, Lysyansky P, Sidenko S, Shir V, Peleg E, Binenbaum M, et al. Two-dimensional strain-a novel software for real-time quantitative echocardiographic assessment of myocardial function. Journal of the American Society of Echocardiography: Official Publication of the American Society of Echocardiography. 2004;17(10):1021–9.

[34] Amundsen BH, Helle-Valle T, Edvardsen T, Torp H, Crosby J, Lyseggen E, et al. Noninvasive myocardial strain measurement by speckle tracking echocardiography: validation against sonomicrometry and tagged magnetic resonance imaging. Journal of the American College of Cardiology. 2006;47(4):789–93.

[35] Serri K, Reant P, Lafitte M, Berhouet M, Le Bouffos V, Roudaut R, et al. Global and regional myocardial function quantification by two-dimensional strain: application in hypertrophic cardiomyopathy. Journal of the American College of Cardiology. 2006;47(6):1175–81.

[36] Carasso S, Yang H, Woo A, Vannan MA, Jamorski M, Wigle ED, et al. Systolic myocardial mechanics in hypertrophic cardiomyopathy: novel concepts and implications for clinical status. Journal of the American Society of Echocardiography: Official Publication of the American Society of Echocardiography. 2008;21(6):675–83.

[37] Nagueh SF, Lakkis NM, He ZX, Middleton KJ, Killip D, Zoghbi WA, et al. Role of myocardial contrast echocardiography during nonsurgical septal reduction therapy for hypertrophic obstructive cardiomyopathy. Journal of the American College of Cardiology. 1998;32(1):225–9.

[38] Cardim N, Galderisi M, Edvardsen T, Plein S, Popescu BA, D'Andrea A, et al. Role of multimodality cardiac imaging in the management of patients with hypertrophic cardiomyopathy: an expert consensus of the European Association of Cardiovascular Imaging Endorsed by the Saudi Heart Association. European Heart Journal Cardiovascular Imaging. 2015;16(3):280.

[39] Maron MS, Appelbaum E, Harrigan CJ, Buros J, Gibson CM, Hanna C, et al. Clinical profile and significance of delayed enhancement in hypertrophic cardiomyopathy. Circulation Heart Failure. 2008;1(3):184–91.

[40] Rickers C, Wilke NM, Jerosch-Herold M, Casey SA, Panse P, Panse N, et al. Utility of cardiac magnetic resonance imaging in the diagnosis of hypertrophic cardiomyopathy. Circulation. 2005;112(6):855–61.

[41] Maron BJ, Haas TS, Lesser JR. Images in cardiovascular medicine. Diagnostic utility of cardiac magnetic resonance imaging in monozygotic twins with hypertrophic cardiomyopathy and identical pattern of left ventricular hypertrophy. Circulation. 2007;115(24):e627-8.

[42] Moon JC, Fisher NG, McKenna WJ, Pennell DJ. Detection of apical hypertrophic cardiomyopathy by cardiovascular magnetic resonance in patients with non-diagnostic echocardiography. Heart. 2004;90(6):645–9.

[43] Moon JC, McKenna WJ, McCrohon JA, Elliott PM, Smith GC, Pennell DJ. Toward clinical risk assessment in hypertrophic cardiomyopathy with gadolinium cardiovascular magnetic resonance. Journal of the American College of Cardiology. 2003;41(9): 1561–7.

[44] Petersen SE, Jerosch-Herold M, Hudsmith LE, Robson MD, Francis JM, Doll HA, et al. Evidence for microvascular dysfunction in hypertrophic cardiomyopathy: new insights from multiparametric magnetic resonance imaging. Circulation. 2007;115(18):2418–25.

[45] Todiere G, Aquaro GD, Piaggi P, Formisano F, Barison A, Masci PG, et al. Progression of myocardial fibrosis assessed with cardiac magnetic resonance in hypertrophic cardiomyopathy. Journal of the American College of Cardiology. 2012;60(10):922–9.

[46] Moravsky G, Ofek E, Rakowski H, Butany J, Williams L, Ralph-Edwards A, et al. Myocardial fibrosis in hypertrophic cardiomyopathy: accurate reflection of histopathological findings by CMR. JACC Cardiovascular Imaging. 2013;6(5):587–96.

[47] Moon JC, Reed E, Sheppard MN, Elkington AG, Ho SY, Burke M, et al. The histologic basis of late gadolinium enhancement cardiovascular magnetic resonance in hypertrophic cardiomyopathy. Journal of the American College of Cardiology. 2004;43(12):2260–4.

[48] O'Gara PT, Bonow RO, Maron BJ, Damske BA, Van Lingen A, Bacharach SL, et al. Myocardial perfusion abnormalities in patients with hypertrophic cardiomyopathy: assessment with thallium-201 emission computed tomography. Circulation. 1987;76(6): 1214–23.

[49] Dilsizian V, Bonow RO, Epstein SE, Fananapazir L. Myocardial ischemia detected by thallium scintigraphy is frequently related to cardiac arrest and syncope in young patients with hypertrophic cardiomyopathy. Journal of the American College of Cardiology. 1993;22(3):796–804.

[50] Cannon RO, 3rd, Dilsizian V, O'Gara PT, Udelson JE, Tucker E, Panza JA, et al. Impact of surgical relief of outflow obstruction on thallium perfusion abnormalities in hypertrophic cardiomyopathy. Circulation. 1992;85(3):1039–45.

[51] Maron MS, Olivotto I, Maron BJ, Prasad SK, Cecchi F, Udelson JE, et al. The case for myocardial ischemia in hypertrophic cardiomyopathy. Journal of the American College of Cardiology. 2009;54(9):866–75.

Chapter 7

Noninvasive Measurement of Pulmonary Capillary Wedge Pressure by Speckle Tracking Echocardiography

Masanori Kawasaki

Additional information is available at the end of the chapter

http://dx.doi.org/10.5772/64864

Abstract

The severity of left-sided heart failure can be evaluated by pulmonary capillary wedge pressure (PCWP) because PCWP reflects left ventricular (LV) filling pressure. Owing to developments in echocardiographic technology, speckle tracking echocardiography (STE) has allowed automatic construction of time-left atrial (LA) volume (LAV) curves. Thus, we developed a novel index based on a combination of LAV and LA function that would estimate PCWP using STE. The following regression equation described the relationship between PCWP that was obtained by right-heart catheterization and active LAEF/minimum LAV index (volume was indexed to body surface area: LAVI) in the patients with sinus rhythm: PCWP = 10.8–12.4 [$\log_{10}$ (active LAEF/minimum LAVI)] (r = −0.86, p <0.001) (measurements from the apical 4-chamber view). We defined this index [$\log_{10}$ (active LAEF/minimum LAVI)] as the kinetics-tracking index (KT index). The PCWP estimated by the KT index (ePCWP) had a strong correlation with PCWP obtained by right-heart catheterization (r = 0.92, p <0.001). The ePCWP measured by STE could be a useful parameter to improve clinical outcomes in patients with heart failure.

Keywords: speckle tracking echocardiography, heart failure, pulmonary capillary wedge pressure

1. Noninvasive assessment of PCWP

1.1. Introduction

Regardless of the presence of abnormal left ventricular (LV) systolic fraction, chronic heart failure (HF) causes cardiac disease or cardiac death. The physiological cause in patients with

HF with preserved ejection fraction (HFPEF) is a diastolic dysfunction [1]. Evaluation of left atrial (LA) pressure is a useful parameter for the diagnosis and treatment of HF. However, measurement of pulmonary capillary wedge pressure (PCWP) or LV filling pressure is an invasive method, and there have been few noninvasive indices that can precisely estimate PCWP or LV filling pressure. Therefore, the establishment of a noninvasive parameter to easily and accurately predict PCWP is important for the clinical diagnosis of HF.

LA volume (LAV) has been thought to reflect elevated LV filling pressure and serves as a parameter to evaluate prognosis of cardiac disease [2–4]. LV filling pressure and LV diastolic function can be estimated by the regional tissue velocity of the mitral annulus measured during early filling (e′) or the ratio of peak early transmitral flow velocity (E) to regional tissue velocity of the mitral annulus measured during early filling (E/e′) [5–8]. However, these parameters do not necessarily reflect the conditions of myocardial expansion during mid and late diastole [8].

Speckle tracking echocardiography (STE) has allowed the automatic construction of time-left atrial (LA) volume curves due to developments in echocardiographic technology [9]. STE has also permitted the evaluation of phasic LA function and volume [10, 11]. LA function and volume are directly influenced by LV diastolic function. Therefore, the combined parameter of LA function and volume would be useful to estimate PCWP. A novel index based on the combination of LA function and volume evaluated by the time-LA volume curve using STE would be more accurate to evaluate PCWP than conventional parameters such as E/e′ and LAV.

1.2. Methods

1.2.1. Subjects and study protocol

The study group consisted of a training study and a testing study. Patients in normal sinus rhythm (NSR), patients with chronic atrial fibrillation (AF) and patients with moderate-to-severe mitral valve regurgitation (MR), who were referred for clinically-indicated right-heart catheterization, were evaluated. In the training study, we measured LAV and LA emptying function (LAEF) in patients in sinus rhythm without chronic AF or moderate-to-severe MR to derive a novel index that gave the best estimate of PCWP. Four parameters based on various combinations of active or total LAEF and minimum or maximum LAV were used to estimate PCWP. In the testing study, we evaluated the reliability and accuracy of the novel index in patients in sinus rhythm, patients with chronic AF and patients with moderate-to-severe MR. Volume was indexed to body surface area (LAV index: LAVI). Transthoracic echocardiography was performed in the left lateral decubitus position by two experienced sonographers just before right-heart catheterization (within 1 hour). As recommended by the American Society of Echocardiography, measurements of phasic LAV were made from the apical 2- and 4-chamber views [12].

1.2.2. Echocardiographic studies and invasive measurements of PCWP

Total LAEF (reservoir function), active LAEF (booster pump function) and passive LAEF (conduit function) were measured to estimate phasic LA function (**Figure 1**). Total, active and

http://dx.doi.org/10.5772/64864

passive LAEF were defined as (maximum LAV – minimum LAV)/maximum LAV × 100%, (pre-atrial contraction LAV – minimum LAV)/pre-atrial contraction LAV × 100% and (maximum LAV – pre-atrial contraction LAV)/maximum LAV × 100%, respectively. The measurements of LAV and LA function were averaged from three consecutive beats. The reliability of the quantification of phasic LAV and LA function by STE has been established in previous studies [10, 11].

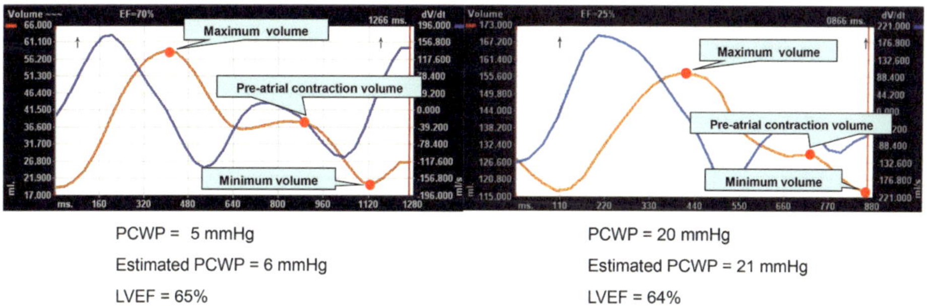

Figure 1. Representative time-left atrial volume curves in two patients. The patient on the left had a PCWP measured by right-heart catheterization of 5 mmHg, whereas the one on the right had a PCWP of 20 mmHg. Red lines are the time-left atrial volume curves, and blue lines are the dV/dt curves. PCWP: pulmonary capillary wedge pressure; LVEF: left ventricular ejection fraction.

A pulmonary artery balloon-occlusion catheter was connected to a fluid-filled transducer that was balanced before the study with the transducer located at the mid-axillary line. By the use of fluoroscopy, the wedge position was verified and the mean PCWP was measured.

1.3. Results

1.3.1. Association between PCWP and echocardiographic parameters in the training and testing studies

From the combination of LV function and volume, the following four parameters were calculated in the training study to predict PCWP:

1. Total LAEF/minimum LAVI

2. Total LAEF/maximum LAVI

3. Active LAEF/minimum LAVI

4. Active LAEF/maximum LAVI.

In the training study, all of these indices were found to be logarithmically correlated with PCWP obtained by right-heart catheterization (**Figure 2**). Therefore, we used the logarithm of these parameters in linear regression analyses. E/e′ and the logarithm of these four indices along with phasic LAVI and phasic LA function were linearly correlated with PCWP measured by right-heart catheterization (**Figure 3**). The logarithm of active LAEF/minimum LAVI had the strongest correlation with PCWP obtained by right-heart catheterization among all of the echocardiographic parameters (**Figure 3**). We defined this novel index [$\log_{10}$ (active LAEF/ minimum LAVI)] as the kinetics-tracking index (KT index).

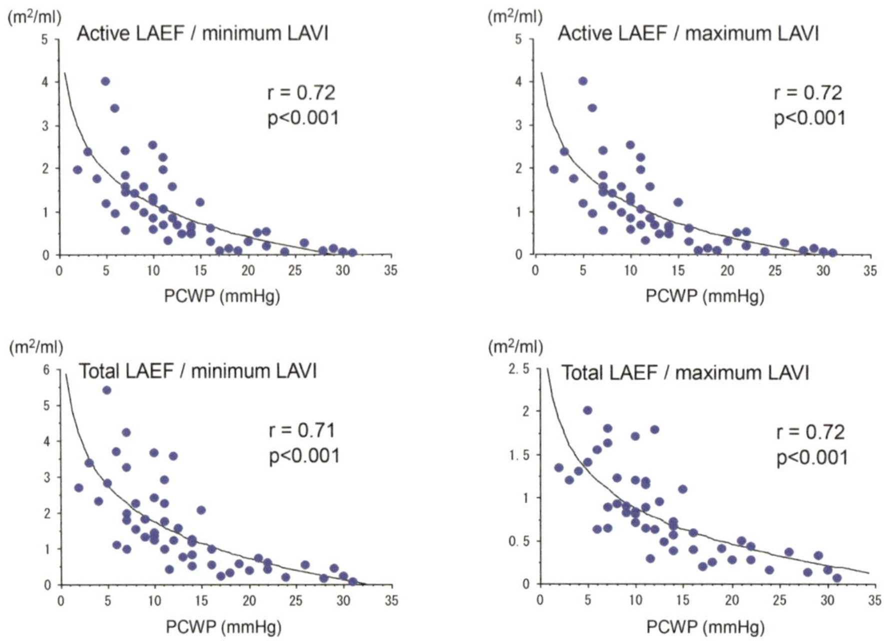

Figure 2. Relationship between pulmonary capillary wedge pressure measured by right-heart catheterization and the combined parameters of left atrial function and volume in the training study (n=50). The logarithm of each index was used in linear regression analysis. PCWP: pulmonary capillary wedge pressure; LAEF: left atrial emptying function; LAVI: left atrial volume index.

The following regression equation described the relationship between PCWP and active LAEF/ minimum LAVI in patients with sinus rhythm:

PCWP = 10.8–12.4 [$\log_{10}$ (active LAEF/minimum LAVI)] ($r = -0.86$, $p < 0.001$) (measurements from the apical four-chamber view);

PCWP = 11.5–12.1 [$\log_{10}$ (active LAEF/minimum LAVI)] ($r = -0.87$, $p < 0.001$) (measurements from the apical two- and four-chamber view).

In patients with chronic AF, total LAEF was substituted for active LAEF because pre-atrial contraction LAV was not present during AF. Only the KT index was found to be an independent predictor of PCWP among the various echocardiographic parameters by multiple regression analysis.

There was a strong correlation between the PCWP estimated by the KT index and PCWP obtained by right-heart catheterization ($r = 0.92$, $p < 0.001$). **Figure 4** showed the relationship between PCWP estimated by the KT index and PCWP obtained by right-heart catheterization in the testing study.

http://dx.doi.org/10.5772/64864

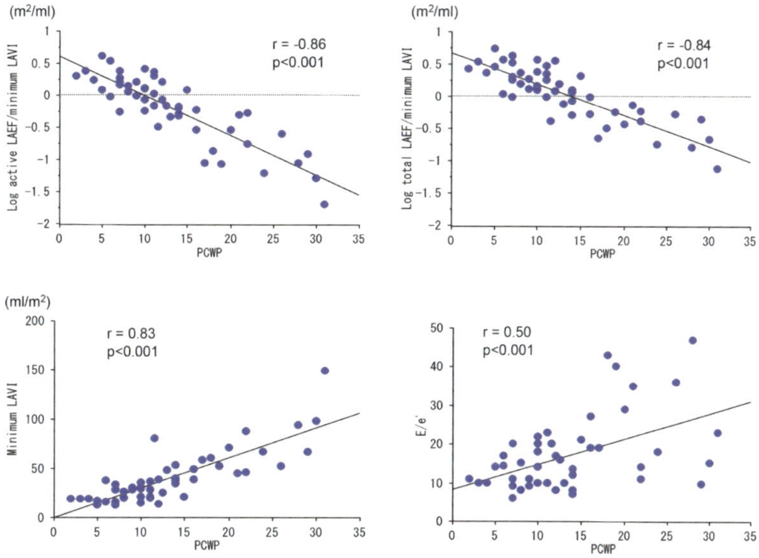

Figure 3. Relationship between pulmonary capillary wedge pressure measured by right-heart catheterization and echocardiographic parameters in the training study (n=50). PCWP: pulmonary capillary wedge pressure; LAEF: left atrial emptying function; LAVI: left atrial volume index. Note that the KT index was better than LAV alone and E/e′ for estimation of PCWP.

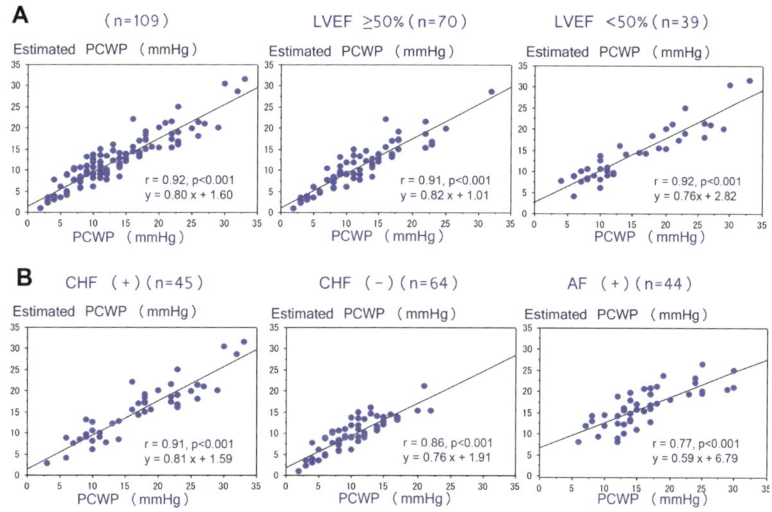

Figure 4. (**A**) Relationship between pulmonary capillary wedge pressure measured by right-heart catheterization and estimated by the KT index in patients in the testing study and in the subgroups with left ventricular ejection fraction (LVEF) ≥50% and LVEF <50%. The relationships were evaluated by simple linear regression analysis. (**B**) Relationship between pulmonary capillary wedge pressure measured by right-heart catheterization and estimated by the KT index in patients in the testing study, in the subgroups with (CHF+) or without (CHF−) symptoms of congestive heart failure and in the subgroup with chronic atrial fibrillation (AF+). The relationships were evaluated by simple linear regression analysis.

1.4 Discussion

1.4.1. Establishment of the KT index

A previous experimental study reported that the LA pressure-volume relationship consists of two loops arranged in a horizontal figure-of-eight pattern that incorporates both the active (A loop) and passive (V loop) components of LA function [13]. Dernellis et al. [14] reported that there was a linear correlation between minimum LAVI and LA pressure in subjects with normal atrial function, patients with acute myocardial infarction and patients with chronic HF. LA volume increases in proportion to the deterioration of LV diastolic function [15, 16]. Therefore, we employed LAV as the denominator in the KT index to evaluate PCWP. Likewise, active LAEF decreases in proportion to the deterioration of LV diastolic function [17]. Therefore, we employed active LAEF as the numerator in the KT index to evaluate PCWP. Moreover, the logarithmic correlation between LV filling pressure and LA distensibility [(max LAVI – min LAVI)/min LAVI] that is similar to the total LAEF [(max LAVI –min LAVI)/max LAVI] is reported [16]. Therefore, we determined the logarithmic association between ePCWP and LA function. Based on our equation, the KT index decreased in proportion to the increase of PCWP.

In the patients with chronic AF, we calculated the regression equation using the data in the testing study and obtained the following regression equation: PCWP (measured by catheterization) = 10.5–12.5 KT index ($r = 0.76$). Intriguingly, PCWP obtained by the KT index in patients with chronic AF had good agreement with PCWP obtained by right-heart catheterization, even using the same regression equation as in patients in NSR. A possible explanation that the ratio of pre-AC LAVI to min LAVI (1.191) (similar ratio to active LAEF) in patients in NSR was similar to the ratio of max LAVI to min LAVI (1.213) (similar ratio to total LAEF) in the patients with chronic AF.

1.4.2. Diagnostic accuracy of KT index and E/e′ for the prediction of PCWP

It was reported that e′ represents regional tissue velocity and e′ reflects LV relaxation and has a good correlation with PCWP [7, 18]. However, e′ is associated not only with active relaxation but also with lengthening load and elastic recoil of left ventricle [19]. Thus, e′ does not directly reflect intrinsic LV relaxation. The E wave is also associated with loading conditions (afterload and preload) [20, 21]. Therefore, E/e′ does not directly reflect atrial active function that is associated with LV stiffness or the condition of diastasis that occurs during mid and late diastole. Therefore, E/e′ is an index that evaluates only early diastole. In the present study, there was a significant but moderate correlation between E/e′ and PCWP obtained by right-heart catheterization ($r = 0.50$), as well as in a previous study ($r = 0.47$) [17]. Several parameters (LAEF [17] and isovolumetric myocardial acceleration obtained by tissue Doppler imaging [22]) were reported to predict LV filling pressure or PCWP. However, the correlation coefficient ($r = -0.63$ and $r = 0.74$) between LV filling pressure and PCWP was less than that in the present study ($r = -0.87$). In addition, the prediction by isovolumetric myocardial acceleration was limited to patients with left ventricular ejection fraction (LVEF) <55% and E/e′ <8 or >15 [22]. In healthy subjects or in patients with acute decompensated HF, the correlation between E/e′

and LV filling pressure was not significant [23, 24]. We proposed a combination of minimum LAVI and active LAEF (KT index) that evaluates LA features throughout diastole to estimate LV filling pressure to overcome the limitations of E/e′.

2. Impacts of gender and healthy aging on PCWP

2.1. Introduction

Measurement of intracardiac pressure such as PCWP or LV filling pressure is useful for the stratification of LV diastolic dysfunction that can lead to HF due to hypertension and aging [25, 26]. However, measurement of PCWP or LV filling pressure is an invasive method, and there have been few noninvasive indices that can precisely estimate PCWP or LV filling pressure. The KT index was a more accurate and useful predictor of PCWP than E/e′ [27].

There have been no previous reports that evaluated PCWP in healthy subjects in a relatively large population because there has been no noninvasive method to measure PCWP in healthy subjects. Therefore, the aim of the present study was to evaluate the impact of gender and healthy aging without hypertension on ePCWP and other echocardiographic parameters.

2.2. Methods

2.2.1. Subjects and study protocol

Healthy subjects, who were free of cardiovascular or other systemic disease and not taking any medications, were included in the study. All the subjects had to have normal findings based on a physical checkup once every year or school physical checkup once every 3 years. We included subjects who were more than 40 years old with a normal electrocardiogram (ECG), but with chest discomfort or pain and shown to be free from cardiovascular disease evaluated by multidetector computed tomography, myocardial scintigraphy or left heart catheterization. We also included subjects more than 40 years old with a normal ECG, but with chest discomfort or pain and shown to be free from cardiovascular disease evaluated by exercise stress ECG. Although we included subjects who had a normal chest x-ray and echocardiographic findings according to the recommendations of the American Society of Echocardiography [12], we also included patients who had trivial valvular regurgitation and those with abnormal values of diastolic function parameters such as E/A and E/e′. Measurements of echocardiography were made according to the criteria of the American Society of Echocardiography [12]. Doppler measurements of mitral inflow E-wave and A-wave velocity were obtained, and tissue Doppler measurements of mitral e′ wave velocity were made at the septal annulus. Total, passive, active LAEF and KT index were also measured.

2.3. Results

2.3.1. Impacts of healthy aging and gender on echocardiographic parameters

The LVEF was not significantly different among the eight age groups of both males and females. The minimum, maximum and pre-atrial contraction LAVI significantly increased with advancing age, resulting in a deterioration of passive and total LAEF. E/e′ and E/A (indicators of LV diastolic function) with advancing age. However, ePCWP was maintained due to compensation by an increase in active LAEF. As shown in **Figure 5**, maximum and minimum LAVI in octogenarians were greater than those in subjects in their thirties, forties and fifties in both males and females.

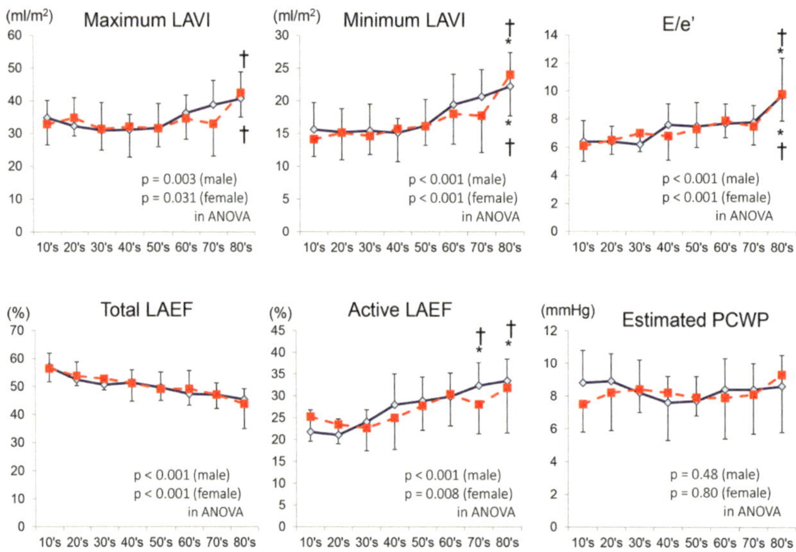

Figure 5. Left atrial volume and function in each decade. Solid blue line: male; broken red line: female. LAVI: left atrial volume index, LAEF: left atrial emptying function, PCWP: pulmonary capillary wedge pressure, ANOVA: one-way analysis of variance. *$p<0.05$ vs. twenties; †$p<0.05$ vs. thirties, forties and fifties;

2.3.2. Relationship between age and LV diastolic dysfunction

The relationships between age and the echocardiographic parameters that indicated LV diastolic dysfunction are shown in **Figure 6**. As age increased, the echocardiographic parameters, such as E/A and E/e′ (indicators of LV diastolic function) deteriorated to the same extent in males and females (slope of E/A: −0.021 in females and −0.021 in males) (slope of E/e′: 0.039 in females and 0.041 in males). However, there was no significant relationship between age and ePCWP. This suggested that ePCWP was maintained around 8 mmHg due to compensation by an increase in active LAEF in subjects without cardiovascular disease. Contrary, the compensation for LV diastolic dysfunction by an increase in active LAEF was more efficient in males than in females (slope=0.11) (slope=0.18, p=0.060 vs. females).

http://dx.doi.org/10.5772/64864

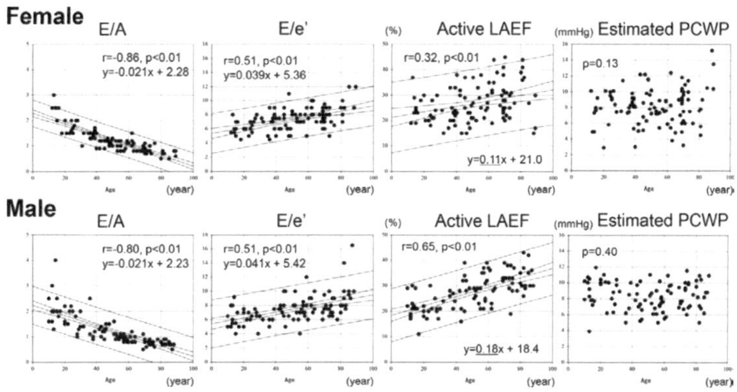

Figure 6. Relationships between age and the echocardiographic parameters. LAEF: left atrial emptying function, PCWP: pulmonary capillary wedge pressure. Center line indicates regression line. Inner lines indicate 95% confidence interval of the regression line. Outer lines indicate 95% confidence interval of the raw data.

2.4. Discussion

2.4.1. The clinical value of estimated PCWP in healthy subjects

HF affects many conditions of LV fluid volume and pressure status. The noninvasive measurement of PCWP in healthy subjects as well as patients with HF is useful for the quantitative stratification of intravascular fluid pressure and volume status to predict prognosis of HF. However, there have been few studies that evaluated PCWP in healthy subjects in a relatively large population because the measurement of PCWP requires an invasive method such as right-heart catheterization. PCWP in healthy subjects was maintained regardless of deterioration of LV diastolic function due to compensation by an increase in active LAEF in the present study. A previous study demonstrated that LV diastolic dysfunction, evaluated by E/A and E/e′, deteriorated with advancing age in healthy subjects [28]. However, that report did not evaluate PCWP. Another study also demonstrated echocardiographic parameters using three-dimensional echocardiography in healthy subjects [29]. That study focused only on volumetric parameters in the left atrium. However, the present study focused on ePCWP and LA function as well as LAV and demonstrated that the deterioration of LV diastolic function due to aging was compensated by LA function; thus, PCWP was maintained.

2.4.2. Estimated PCWP in healthy subjects

A few studies that elucidated PCWP in the healthy subjects in small populations have been performed. In a previous study, PCWP was evaluated by right-heart catheterization in 70 healthy volunteers. The PCWP in these healthy volunteers was around 12 mmHg and did not differ among seniors (50% men, 70 ± 3 years old), late middle age (48% men, 57 ± 4 years old), early middle age (32% men, 42 ± 5 years old) and young (57% men, 28 ± 4 years old) [30], whereas E/A deteriorated from 1.9 to 0.8. PCWP measured by right-heart catheterization (12 mmHg) was slightly higher than that in the present study (8 mmHg), whereas this finding that did not differ with advancing age reinforced the present results. This discrepancy of PCWP (12 and 8 mmHg) may be due to the fact that evaluation of PCWP measured by right-heart catheterization was performed by an invasive method that imposed a physical burden on the healthy volunteers, whereas ePCWP measurement by STE did not impose a physical burden on the healthy subjects. Previous study reported PCWP that was measured by right-heart catheterization in 50 healthy, elderly, nonsedentary volunteers who had a normal echocardiographic and ECG findings and was free of pulmonary, cardiovascular, systemic disease, shortness of breath and chest pain. The PCWP in these subjects was around 9 mmHg (65 ± 10 years old, 74% men) [31]. This value was similar to ePCWP in the present study.

2.4.3. *Atrial function of males and females*

The maximum LAVI in octogenarians was greater than the values in subjects in their thirties, forties and fifties regardless of gender, whereas deterioration of passive LAEF developed almost two decades earlier in both males and females. These results were the same as the results of a previous study [32]. In the present study, however, there was compensation by an increase of active LAEF only in male septuagenarians and octogenarians. Another intriguing finding in the present study was that as age increases, the echocardiographic parameters that reflect LV diastolic dysfunction deteriorated to the same extent in both males and females. However, compensation for deterioration of LV diastolic function by an increase in active LAEF was more pronounced in males (slope = 0.18) than females (slope = 0.11). In males, there was a stronger correlation between E/A and active LAEF, and between E/e′ and active LAEF than in females. The slopes of these two regression lines indicate that the strength of the compensation for deterioration of LV diastolic function was also lesser in females than males. Compensation by an increase in active LAEF was less prominent in females than males. The Framingham Heart Study demonstrated that the prevalence of congestive HF in septuagenarians was higher in males than females [33]. However, the prevalence of congestive HF in octogenarians was lower in males than in females. The 11-year follow-up study reported that female gender was associated with new onset of HFPEF, whereas male gender was associated with new onset of HFPEF, after adjusting for age [34]. In the present study, compensation for deterioration of LV diastolic function by an increase in active LAEF was more increased only in male octogenarians than female octogenarians. This may explain why HFPEF occurs more frequently in females than in males.

2.4.4. *Clinical implications*

The potential clinical application of the present methods and findings is broad. Noninvasive measurement of ePCWP is useful for the evaluation for intravascular fluid volume and pressure status to identify the onset of HF. Stratification of the risk of HF in patients as well as healthy subjects using PCWP is important for understanding when and why HF develops. The ePCWP that is measured by KT index also may be applicable for the determination of appropriate dry weight during dialysis and prediction of the onset of AF.

Author details

Masanori Kawasaki

Address all correspondence to: masanori@ya2.so-net.ne.jp

Department of Cardiology, Gifu University Graduate School of Medicine, Gifu, Japan

References

[1] Zile MR, Baicu CF, Gaasch WH. Diastolic heart failure - abnormalities in active relaxation and passive stiffness of the left ventricle. N Engl J Med 2004;350:1953–1959.

[2] Lee JS, Shim CY, Wi J, Joung B, Ha JW, Lee MH, Pak HN. Left ventricular diastolic function is closely associated with mechanical function of the left atrium in patients with paroxysmal atrial fibrillation. Circ J 2013;77:697–704.

[3] Appleton CP, Galloway JM, Gonzalez MS, Gaballa M, Basnight MA. Estimation of left ventricular filling pressures using two-dimensional and Doppler echocardiography in adult patients with cardiac disease: additional value of analyzing left atrial size, left atrial ejection fraction and the difference in duration of pulmonary venous and mitral flow velocity at atrial contraction. J Am Coll Cardiol 1993;2:1972–1982.

[4] Douglas PS. The left atrium: a biomarker of chronic diastolic dysfunction and cardiovascular disease risk. J Am Coll Cardiol 2003;42:1206–1207.

[5] Kato T, Noda A, Izawa H, Nishizawa T, Somura F, Yamada A, Nagata K, Iwase M, Nakao A, Yokota M. Myocardial velocity gradient as a noninvasively determined index of left ventricular diastolic dysfunction in patients with hypertrophic cardiomyopathy. J Am Coll Cardiol 2003;42:278–285.

[6] Nagueh SF, Middleton KJ, Kopelen HA, Zoghbi WA, Quinones MA. Doppler tissue imaging: a noninvasive technique for evaluation of left ventricular relaxation and estimation of filling pressures. J Am Coll Cardiol 1997;30:1527–1533

[7] Nagueh SF, Mikati I, Kopelen HA, Middleton KJ, Quinones MA, Zoghbi WA. Doppler estimation of left ventricular filling pressure in sinus tachycardia: a new application of tissue Doppler imaging. Circulation 1998;98:1644–1650.

[8] Maurer MS, Spevack D, Burkhoff D, Kronzon I. Diastolic dysfunction: can it be diagnosed by Doppler echocardiography? J Am Coll Cardiol 2004;44:1543–1549.

[9] Onishi N, Kawasaki M, Tanaka R, Sato H, Saeki M, Nagaya M, Sato N, Minatoguchi S, Watanabe T, Ono K, Arai M, Noda T, Amano K, Goto K, Watanabe S, Minatoguchi S. Comparison between left atrial features in well-controlled hypertensive patients and

normal subjects assessed by three-dimensional speckle tracking echocardiography. J Cardiol 2014;63:291–295.

[10] Ogawa K, Hozumi T, Sugioka K, Iwata S, Otsuka R, Takagi Y, Yoshitani H, Yoshiyama M, Yoshikawa J. Automated assessment of left atrial function from time-left atrial volume curves using a novel speckle tracking imaging method. J Am Soc Echocardiogr 2009;22:63–69.

[11] Hirose T, Kawasaki M, Tanaka R, Ono K, Watanabe T, Iwama M, Noda T, Watanabe S, Takemura G, Minatoguchi S. Left atrial function assessed by speckle tracking echocardiography as a predictor of new-onset non-valvular atrial fibrillation: results from a prospective study in 580 adults. Eur Heart J Cardiovasc Img 2012;13:243–250.

[12] Lang RM, Bierig M, Devereux RB, Flachskampf FA, Foster E, Pellikka PA, Picard MH, Roman MJ, Seward J, Shanewise JS, Solomon SD, Spencer KT, Sutton MS, Stewart WJ; Chamber Quantification Writing Group; American Society of Echocardiography's Guidelines and Standards Committee; European Association of Echocardiography. Recommendations for chamber quantification: a report from the American Society of Echocardiography's Guidelines and Standards Committee and the Chamber Quantification Writing Group, developed in conjunction with the European Association of Echocardiography, a branch of the European Society of Cardiology. J Am Soc Echocardiogr. 2005;18:1440–1463.

[13] Pagel PS, Kehl F, Gare M, Hettrick DA, Kersten JR, Warltier DC. Mechanical function of the left atrium: new insights based on analysis of pressure-volume relations and Doppler echocardiography. Anesthesiology 2003;98:975–994.

[14] Dernellis JM, Stefanadis CI, Zacharoulis AA, Toutouzas PK. Left atrial mechanical adaptation to long-standing hemodynamic loads based on pressure-volume relation. Am J Cardiol 1998;81:1138–1143.

[15] Pritchett AM, Mahoney DW, Jacobsen SJ, Rodeheffer RJ, Karon BL, Redfield MM. Diastolic dysfunction and left atrial volume: A population-based study. J Am Coll Cardiol 2005;45:87–92.

[16] Hsiao SH, Huang WC, Lin KL, Chiou KR, Kuo FY, Lin SK, Cheng CC. Left atrial distensibility and left ventricular filling pressure in acute versus chronic severe mitral regurgitation. Am J Cardiol 2010;105:709–715.

[17] Hsiao SH, Chiou KR, Lin KL, Lin SK, Huang WC, Kuo FY, Cheng CC, Liu CP. Left atrial distensibility and E/e′ for estimating left ventricular filling pressure in patients with stable angina. A comparative echocardiography and catheterization study. Circ J. 2011;75:1942–1950.

[18] Ommen SR, Nishimura RA, Appleton CP, Miller FA, Oh JK, Redfield MM, Tajik AJ. Clinical utility of Doppler echocardiography and tissue Doppler imaging in the estimation of left ventricular filling pressure: a comparative simultaneous Doppler catheterization study. Circulation 2000;102:1788–1794.

[19] Tschope C, Paulus WJ. Doppler echocardiography yields dubious estimates of left ventricular diastolic pressure. Circulation 2009;120:810–820.

[20] Stoddard MF, Pearson AC, Kern MJ, Ratcliff J, Mrosek DG, Labovitz AJ. Influence of alteration in preload on the pattern of left ventricular diastolic filling as assessed by Doppler echocardiography in humans. Circulation 1989;79:1226–1236.

[21] Nishimura RA, Abel MD, Hatle LK, Tajik AJ. Relation of pulmonary vein to mitral flow velocities by transesophageal Doppler echocardiography: effect of different loading conditions. Circulation 1990;81:1488–1497.

[22] Salem Omar AM, Tanaka H, Matsumoto K, Tatsumi K, Miyoshi T, Hiraishi M, Tsuji T, Kaneko A, Ryo K, Fukuda Y, Kawai H, Hirata K. Tissue Doppler imaging-derived myocardial acceleration during isovolumetric contraction predicts pulmonary capillary wedge pressure in patients with reduced ejection fraction. Circ J 2012;76:1399–1408.

[23] Mullens W, Borowski AG, Curtin RJ, Thomas JD, Tang WH. Tissue Doppler imaging in the estimation of intracardiac filling pressure in decompensated patients with advanced systolic heart failure. Circulation 2009;119:62–70.

[24] Firstenberg MS, Levine BD, Garcia MJ, Greenberg NL, Cardon L, Morehead AJ, Zuckerman J, Thomas JD. Relationship of echocardiographic indices to pulmonary capillary wedge pressures in healthy volunteers. J Am Coll Cardiol 2000;36:1664–1669.

[25] Baicu CF, Zile MR, Aurigemma GP, Gaasch WH. Left ventricular systolic performance, function, and contractility in patients with diastolic heart failure. Circulation 2005;111:2306–2312.

[26] Saeki M, Sato N, Kawasaki M, Tanaka R, Nagaya M, Watanabe T, Ono K, Noda T, Zile MR, Minatoguchi S. Left ventricular layer function in hypertension assessed by myocardial strain rate using novel one-beat real-time three-dimensional speckle tracking echocardiography with high volume rates. Hypertens Res. 2015;38:551–559. doi: 10.1038/ 21 hr.2015.47.

[27] Kawasaki M, Tanaka R, Ono K, Minatoguchi S, Watanabe T, Iwama M, Hirose T, Arai M, Noda T, Watanabe S, Zile MR, Minatoguchi S. A novel ultrasound predictor of pulmonary capillary wedge pressure assessed by the combination of left atrial volume and function: A speckle tracking echocardiography study. J Cardiol 2015;66:253–262.

[28] Daimon M, Watanabe H, Abe Y, Hirata K, Hozumi T, Ishii K, Ito H, Iwakura K, Izumi C, Matsuzaki M, Minagoe S, Abe H, Murata K, Nakatani S, Negishi K, Yoshida K, Tanabe K, Tanaka N, Tokai K, Yoshikawa J; JAMP Study Investigators. Normal values of echocardiographic parameters in relation to age in a healthy Japanese population: the JAMP study. Circ J. 2008;72:1859–1866.

[29] Fukuda S, Watanabe H, Daimon M, Abe Y, Hirashiki A, Hirata K, Ito H, Iwai-Takano M, Iwakura K, Izumi C, Hidaka T, Yuasa T, Murata K, Nakatani S, Negishi K, Nishigami K, Nishikage T, Ota T, Hayashida A, Sakata K, Tanaka N, Yamada S, Yamamoto K,

Yoshikawa J. Normal values of real-time 3-dimensional echocardiographic parameters in a healthy Japanese population: the JAMP-3D Study. Circ J 2012;76:1177–1181.

[30] Carrick-Ranson G, Hastings JL, Bhella PS, Shibata S, Fujimoto N, Palmer MD, Boyd K, Levine BD. Effect of healthy aging on left ventricular relaxation and diastolic suction. Am J Physiol Heart Circ Physiol 2012;303:H315-H322.

[31] Guron CW, Persson A, Wikh R, Caidahl K. Can the left ventricular early diastolic tissue-to-blood time interval be used to identify a normal pulmonary capillary wedge pressure? Eur J Echocardiogr 2007;8:94–101.

[32] Boyd AC, Schiller NB, Leung D, Ross DL, Thomas L. Atrial dilation and altered function are mediated by age and diastolic function but not before the eighth decade. JACC Cardiovasc Imaging 2011;4:234–242.

[33] Pitt B. Part II: New insights into the epidemiology and pathophysiology of heart failure. J Am Coll Cardiol 1993;22:6A-13A.

[34] Brouwers FP, de Boer RA, van der Harst P, Voors AA, Gansevoort RT, Bakker SJ, Hillege HL, van Veldhuisen DJ, van Gilst WH. Incidence and epidemiology of new onset heart failure with preserved vs. reduced ejection fraction in a community-based cohort: 11-year follow-up of PREVEND. Eur Heart J. 2013;34:1424–1431.

Chapter 8

The Role of Echocardiography in the Management of Patients Undergoing a Ventricular Assist Device Implantation and/or Transplantation

Tomoko Kato, Takashi Nishimura, Shunei Kyo,
Kenji Kuwaki, Hiroyuki Dada and Atsushi Amano

Additional information is available at the end of the chapter

http://dx.doi.org/10.5772/65095

Abstract

Heart transplantation (HTx) is a curative treatment for patients with advanced heart failure (HF); however, since transplant opportunities are severely limited due to donor shortage, the left ventricular assist device (LVAD) has become a standard therapy for patients awaiting HTx. The role of echocardiography as a primary imaging modality to monitor the allograft function in transplant recipients as well as to optimize LVAD settings in LVAD recipients has been expanding. The purpose of this review is to highlight the clinical role of echocardiography in the management of patients undergoing LVAD implantation and/or HTx. In particular, we overview (1) how to detect LVAD malfunction and device-associated complication in LVAD recipients and (2) echocardiographic assessments of cardiac allograft rejection in transplant recipients.

Keywords: heart failure, transplant, rejection, ventricular assist device, echocardiography

1. Introduction

Heart transplantation (HTx) provides considerable survival benefits for patients with end-stage heart failure, but it is available for only a small fraction of such patients all over the world due to donor shortage [1]. Therefore, many heart transplant candidates require long-term support by a left ventricular assist device (LVAD) while they await transplantation [1, 2]. More recently, mechanical circulatory support has evolved into a standard therapy for patients with advanced heart failure, not only as a bridge to cardiac transplantation but also as a destination therapy or a bridge to myocardial recovery [3].

Echocardiography is a primary imaging modality in the assessment of cardiac structure and function in patients with advanced HF. In addition, echocardiography can be performed at the patient's bedside, and results are immediately available. In this review, we highlight the effectiveness of echocardiography in the management of patients undergoing LVAD implantation and/or HTx.

2. Echocardiography in LVAD recipients

A growing number of heart transplant candidates require long-term support by an LVAD while they await cardiac transplantation. Further, LVAD therapy has become a standard therapy for patients with advanced HF, not only as a bridge to cardiac transplantation but also as a destination therapy or a bridge to myocardial recovery. Here, we focused on the usefulness of echocardiography in patients undergoing LVAD implantation.

2.1. Preoperative assessment

It is important to assess the LVAD eligibility and rule out any contraindications against LVAD surgery prior to an operation. Several structural issues that can be surgically corrected at the time of LVAD implantation should be carefully evaluated prior to the LVAD surgery. The presence of clots, especially at the apex, should be carefully assessed because it will increase the risk of inflow cannula obstructions and/or perioperative stroke. Intracardiac shunts, including patent foramen ovale, should also be carefully assessed before and during surgery. Intracardiac shunts must be closed at the time of LVAD surgery. Further, coexisting valvular heart disease should be assessed prior to the LVAD procedure. Concomitant valvular surgery can be performed at the time of LVAD implantation; however, although such an additional approach can provide possible benefits, data regarding its long-term effect are limited, and the indications are still controversial. Another important issue to be carefully evaluated preoperatively includes right ventricular (RV) function because right ventricular failure (RVF) after LVAD placement is associated with increased morbidity and mortality.

2.1.1. Preoperative valvular assessment

Regarding tricuspid regurgitation (TR), several previous papers have revealed that tricuspid annular dilatation is highly associated with post-LVAD right ventricular failure [4]. Kukucka M et al. reviewed 122 patients without significant TR at the time of VAD implant and found that a tricuspid annulus diameter >43 mm was an independent predictor of survival after LVAD (**Figure 1**). On the other hand, whether the TR should be surgically managed at the time of LVAD surgery is controversial. Dunlay et al. performed a literature search of randomized controlled trials and observational studies (including 3249 patients) that compared the outcome of concomitant tricuspid valve surgery at the time of LVAD with that of LVAD alone [5]. They found that the addition of valvular surgery at the time of the LVAD procedure prolonged cardiopulmonary bypass times by an average of 31 minutes, but no differences were found between the groups for acute renal failure, early mortality, or the need for a right ventricular assist device. Having said that, a recent paper from Columbia University suggested that concomitant tricuspid valve procedures at the time of LVAD surgery can be performed safely and protect against worsening tricuspid regurgitation during the first two years of support [6]. In either case, the severity of TR and annular size need to be assessed preoperatively. Surgeons should also bear in mind that preexisting severe TR, especially with annular size >43 mm, is at higher risk of adverse events after surgery.

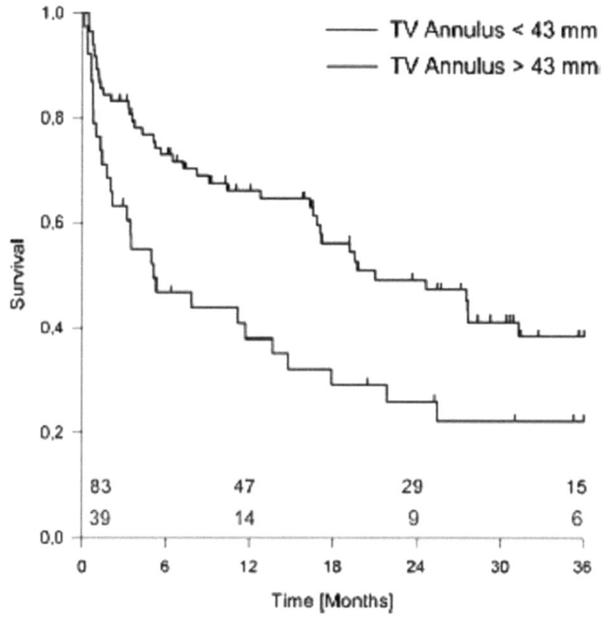

Figure 1. The impact on tricuspid valve annulus dilation on post-LVAD survival (quoted from Ref. [4]). Kaplan-Meier survival curves of patients with tricuspid valve (TV) annulus diameter <43 mm (blue) and >43 mm (red). Censored patients are represented by vertical marks. Numbers of patients at risk at 0, 12, 24, and 36 months of follow-up are presented above the x-axis (log-rank test, p = 0.007).

Aortic insufficiency (AI) occurs in up to 50% of patients within 1 year after continuous flow LVAD implantation. Although de novo AI can be commonly seen postoperatively, the presence of more than mild AI as well as any structural abnormality, as detected by transthoracic echocardiography (TTE), should be reported to the LVAD surgery team. In cases with poor TTE images, the results derived from intraoperative transesophageal echocardiography (TEE) should be carefully discussed. The valvular morphology, valvular calcification, possible fusion, and myxomatous changes should also be reported to the surgeons. The recently published comprehensive review of AI post-LVAD by Cowger et al. suggested the importance of intraoperative TEE to detect unmasked AI [7]. During the initiation of continuous flow LVAD support, as LV filling pressures drop with early unloading, the gradient between the aortic root and the LV increases, potentially exposing significant AI that was previously unrecognized. Because AI severity can be associated with an increase in pump speeds, we can quantitatively assess AI severity at different pump speeds to consider the necessity of concomitant aortic valve surgery in an operating room. This review summarized the risk and benefits of aortic valve surgery at the time of LVAD (**Table 1**).

Strategy	Pros	Cons
Partial closure with a single central stitch (Park's stitch)	• Simple and effective when the leaflet tissue has adequate tensile strength to hold sutures • Permit blood ejection through the aortic valve	• Questionable durability • Risk of progression to aortic stenosis • Need for AVR in the event of myocardial recovery leading to LVAD explant
Modified Park's stitch—additional pledgeted mattress suture between the central stitch and each commissure	• Relatively simple and can be effective, even if leaflets are thin • Permits blood ejection through the aortic valve but could be reduced compared to single central stitch	• Questionable durability • Risk of progression to aortic stenosis • Need for AVR in the event of myocardial recovery leading to LVAD explant
Complete closure of the ventriculo-aortic juncture with a circular patch	• Simple with relatively fast repair time • Long-term durability	• No blood ejection through the aortic valve • Risk of thrombus formation • Risk of death in the case of pump stoppage or failure
Replacement of incompetent aortic valve with bioprosthetic valve	• Maintenance of valve opening in the postoperative period • Testing for cardiac recovery • Tolerance to exercise	• Increase CPB and cross-clamp time • Risk of leaflet fusion • Risk of valvular and subvalvular thrombus formation due to fresh suture lines combined with decreased flow across the new valve

Table 1. Pros and cons of surgical management strategies of the native aortic valve (quoted from Ref. [7]).

Mitral valve insufficiency has fewer effects on postoperative outcome compared with aortic and tricuspid valve insufficiency. Indeed, a significant number of patients who had severe mitral regurgitation due to annulus dilatation and tethered pupillary muscle preoperatively showed a remarkable decrease in mitral regurgitation flow under LVAD support [8]. Although mitral valve surgery at the time of LVAD implant to correct severe mitral regurgitation does not affect postoperative mortality or cause other adverse events, the procedure can be considered in cases undergoing an LVAD procedure as a bridge to recovery. In addition, concomitant mitral valve repair can decrease pulmonary vascular resistance [9]. Kitada et al. investigated preoperative echocardiographic features associated with persistent mitral regurgitation after LVAD implantation (**Figure 2**) [10]. They found that the posterior displacement of the coapta-

http://dx.doi.org/10.5772/65095

tion point of a mitral leaflet (30 vs. 24 mm), papillary muscle distance (49 vs. 43 mm), and tethering area (353 vs. 299 mm²) before surgery were greater in patients who had persistent moderate to severe mitral regurgitation post-LVAD than those in patients who did not have significant MR postoperatively. A multivariate analysis showed that the posterior displacement was the only independent predictor for persistent MR.

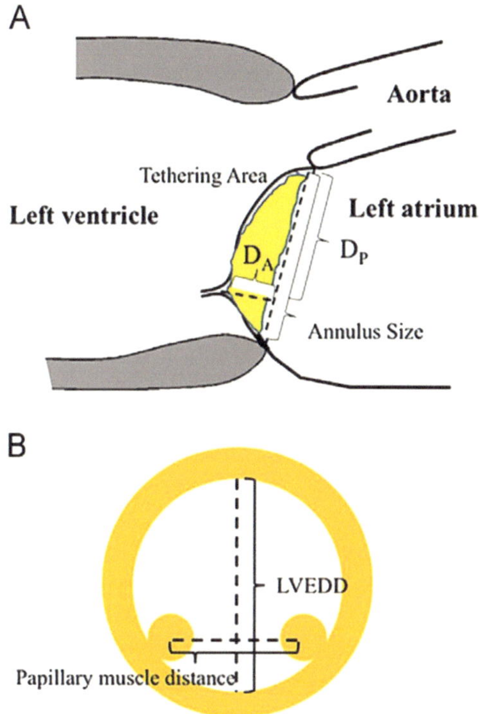

Figure 2. The measurements of echocardiographic parameters to quantify the mitral leaflet configurations in 2D echocardiography (quoted from Ref. [10]). DA, apical displacement; DP, posterior displacement; LVEDD, left ventricular end diastolic dimension.

2.1.2. Preoperative and perioperative right ventricular assessment

Right ventricular failure (RVF) remains a major cause of morbidity and mortality following LVAD surgery. The incidence of RVF post-LVAD is 10–30% despite the recent improvements in device technology and postoperative patient management. Under LVAD support, right ventricular (RV) preload increases as a result of increased circulatory volume, whereas RV afterload is expected to decrease, secondary to improvement in pulmonary vascular resistance [11]. A sepal wall shift induced by LVAD alters the RV structure, which may worsen RV contractile and relaxation abnormalities. Therefore, when considering RV systolic and diastolic reserve before and also after surgery, it is important to identify which patients may need RV-specific mechanical and medical support post-LVAD [12].

Study	Patients	RVF definition and rate	Multivariable predictors	Echocardiographic RV parameters considered
Michigan RV failure risk score (2008)[a]	197 LVADs 28 CF-LVAD 94% BTT	Need for RVAD/ inotropes RVF rate: 35%	Preoperative vasopressors (4 pts) AST ≥80 IU/L (2 pts) Bilirubin ≥2.0 mg/dL (2.5 pts) Creatinine ≥2.3 mg/dL (3 pts)	RV systolic function (visual semiquantitative) TR (visual semiquantitative)
Penn RVAD risk score[b] (2008)	266 LVADs 6 CF-LVAD BTT vs. DT not reported	Need for RVAD RVF rate: 37%	Cardiac index ≤2.2 L/min/m^2 RVSWI ≤0.25 mm Hg × L/m^2 Severe RV dysfunction Creatinine ≥1.9 mg/dL Prior cardiac surgery Systolic BP ≤96 mm Hg	RV systolic function (visual semiquantitative)
Utah RV risk score[c] (2010)	175 LVADs 25 CF-LVAD 58% BTT, 42% DT	Need for RVAD/ inotropes/ inhaled NO RVF rate: 44%	DT indication (3.5 pts) IABP (4 pts) PVR (1–4 pts) Inotrope dependency (2.5 pts) Obesity (2 pts) ACEI or ARB use (−2.5 pts) β-blocker use (2 pts)	Right atrial area
Kormos[d] (2010)	484 LVADs All CF-LVAD BTT 100%	Need for RVAD/ inotropes RVF rate: 20.2%	CVP/PCWP >0.63 (OR, 2.3) Need for preoperative ventilator support (OR, 5.5)BUN >39 mg/dL (OR, 2.1)	None
Pittsburgh Decision Tree[e] (2012)	183 LVADs 40 CF-LVAD BTT vs. DT not reported	Need for RVAD RVF rate: 15%	Age, heart rate, transpulmonary gradient; right atrial pressure; INR, white blood cell count, ALT, number of inotropic agents	None
CRITT[f] (2013)	167 LVADs, all CF-LVAD 51 BiVADsBTT vs. DT not reported	Need for BiVAD RVF rate: 23%	CVP >15 mm Hg (C) Severe RV dysfunction (R) Preoperative intubation (I) Severe TR (T) Heart rate >100 (tachycardia [T])	RV systolic function (visual semiquantitative) Severe TR (visual semiquantitative)

ACEI, angiotensin-converting enzyme inhibitor; ALT, alanine aminotransferase; ARB, angiotensin receptor blocker; AST, aspartate aminotransferase; BiVAD, biventricular assist device; BP, blood pressure; BTT, bridge to transplantation; BUN, blood urea nitrogen; CF, continuous flow; CRITT, central venous pressure-RV dysfunction-preoperative intubation-severe tricuspid regurgitation-tachycardia; CVP, central venous pressure; DT, destination therapy; IABP; intra-aortic balloon pump; INR, international normalized ratio; ITT, intention to treat; LVAD, left ventricular assist device; NO, nitric oxide; OR, odds ratio; PCWP, pulmonary capillary wedge pressure; PVR, pulmonary vascular resistance; RV, right ventricle; RVAD, right ventricular assist device; RVF, right ventricular failure; RVSWI, right ventricular stroke work index; and TR, tricuspid regurgitation.

The data were obtained from the following papers: (a) Matthews JC, et al. J Am Coll Cardiol. 2008;51:2163–2172; (b) Fitzpatrick JR III, et al. J Heart Lung Transplant. 2008;27:1286–1292; (c) Drakos SG, et al. Am J Cardiol. 2010;105:1030–1035; (d) Kormos RL, et al; HeartMate II Clinical Investigators. J Thorac Cardiovasc Surg. 2010;139:1316–1324; (e) Wang Y, et al. J Heart Lung Transplant. 2012;31:140–149; (f) Atluri P, et al. Ann Thorac Surg. 2013;96:857–863.

Table 2. Clinical risk prediction scores for right ventricular failure in left ventricular assist device recipients (quoted from Ref. [13]).

http://dx.doi.org/10.5772/65095

Table 2 summarizes the clinical risk prediction scores that have been cited in the recently published review literature [13]. In addition to these risk scores, serial echocardiographic assessments are helpful in evaluating RV functional reserve prior to surgery. Previously reported echocardiographic parameters associated with the risk for developing RVF after LVAD implantation have included tricuspid annular dilation (>43 mm) [4], tricuspid annular motion (8 vs. 15 mm) [14], and RV-to-LV end-diastolic diameter ratio (>0.72) [15]. However, it is sometimes technically difficult to obtain ideal RV images that allow quantitative assessments of patients with advanced heart failure, particularly if the patients are severely congested, intubated, and/or have a markedly enlarged left ventricle (LV) that obscures the right ventricle (RV) [16]. Kato et al. focused only on left-sided 2D echo parameters that can predict RVF post-LVAD. They showed that patients with relatively small LV size, preserved LV contraction, and a dilated left atrium were at higher risk for RVF after LVAD surgery (**Figure 3**) [16]. In addition to the conventional echo parameters, Grant et al. reported that the incremental role of RV strain to predict RVF [17]. More recently, Kato et al. reported that serial echocardiograms using tissue Doppler imaging (TDI) and speckle tracking echocardiography (STE) before and soon after (within 72 hours) LVAD surgery may aid in identifying the need to initiate targeted RVF-specific therapy [12]. In this study, RV stiffness (as reflected by TDI-derived E/E′) and decreased RV contractility (as reflected by TDI-derived S′ and RV longitudinal strain) before and soon after LVAD surgery were found to be useful parameters to include in the perioperative management of LVAD patients (**Figure 4**).

(A) LV-Echo-for-RVF Score Point based on 2D left-sided echocardiography

Points	0	1	2
LVEDd (mm)	>78	78-70	<70
LVEF (%)	< 19	19-33	>33
LAD/LVEDd	< 0.63	0.63-0.68	> 0.68

Sum of the points

(B) Sensitivity and specificity of LV-Echo-for RVF score for post-LVAD RVF

LV-Echo-for-RVF Score	≥1	≥2	≥3	≥4	≥5
Sensitivity (%)	100	97.1	88.6	71.4	42.9
Specificity (%)	14.5	32.9	47.4	67.1	80.3

(C)

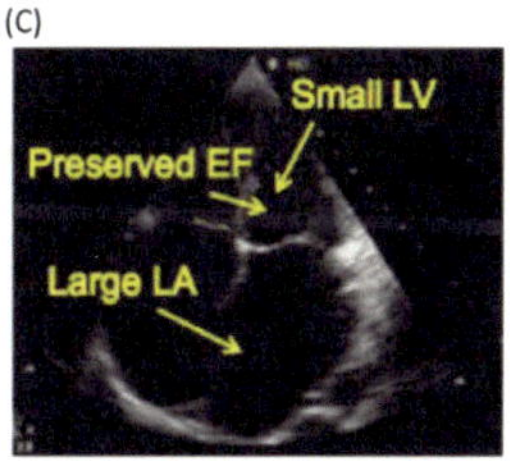

(D)

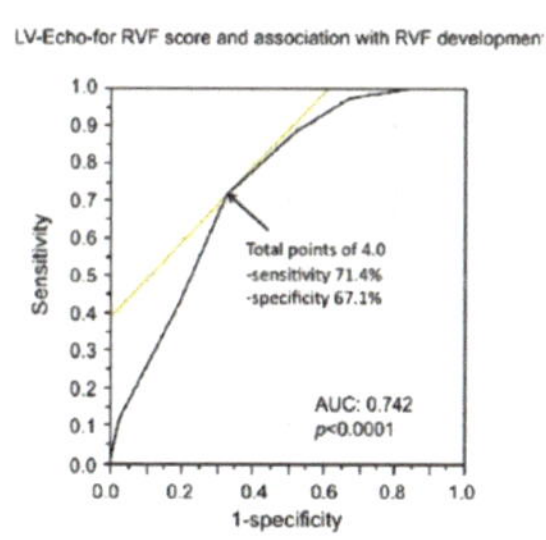

Figure 3. Left ventricular echocardiographic right ventricular failure score (LV-for-Echo-RVF) based on two-dimensional echocardiographic left-sided heart parameters (quoted from Ref. [16]). (A) Points associated with value of each variable. (B) Sensitivity and specificity of sum of points associated with right ventricular failure development after left ventricular assist device placement. (C) Representative 2D echo images in patients developing RVF post-LVAD. (D) Receiver operating characteristics curve for LV echocardiographic RVF score. AUC, area under the curve.

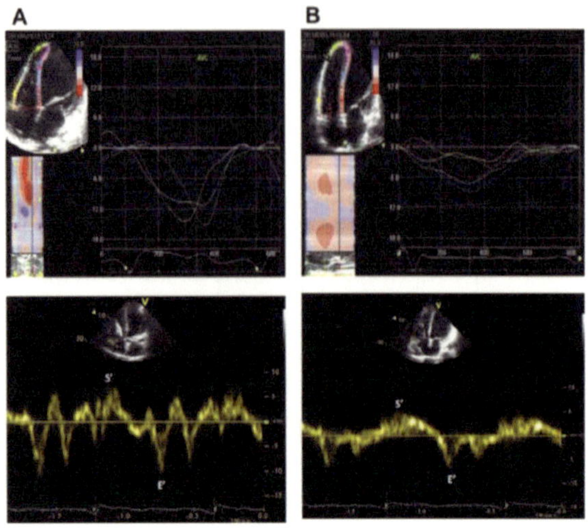

Figure 4. Representative global RV longitudinal strain and TDI obtained before surgery from a patient without RVF after LVAD and from a patient with RVF after LVAD (quoted from Ref. [18]). (A) The right ventricular (RV) global longitudinal strain; tissue Doppler image (TDI)-derived S′ and E′ for patient A was −14.3%, 7.8 cm/s and −10.8 cm/s, respectively. (B) These parameters were −6.2%, 4.6 cm/s and −5.3 cm/s, respectively. LVAD, left ventricular assist device; RVF, right ventricular failure.

2.2. Perioperative assessment

Other than the speed adjustment to avoid RV failure due to excessive RV preload by LVAD support, several important points should be evaluated by intraoperative TEE. First, de-airing of the heart chamber should be confirmed. Careful observation of trapped air at the site of anastomosis sites and around the LVAD inflow/outflow cannula is required [18]. Second, adjusting LV speed to maintain appropriate LV unloading without a septal shift under TEE guidance is required. The positioning of the inflow cannula at the apex should be monitored by TEE as well. Third, as mentioned above, the existence of valvular diseases and intracardiac shunts, which can be corrected simultaneously at the time of LVAD implantation, should be communicated to the surgeons. Finally, pericardial effusion and its amount should also be carefully observed by TEE. Cardiac tamponade can occur relatively often because patients under LVAD support require sufficient anticoagulation soon after surgery to prevent clot formation at the cannula and inside the device.

2.3. Postoperative assessment

Table 3 illustrates the checklist that will help sonographers/echocardiologists to perform an LVAD echo. In general, we can simply summarize the purposes of echo in LVAD recipients as follows: (1) to carefully monitor device malfunction, (2) to adjust appropriate LVAD setting/speed (appropriate peripheral perfusion and RV preload), and (3) to evaluate myocardial recovery and to seek optimal timing for LVAD weaning.

The points to be evaluated by TEE on a periodic basis are as follows: the location and thrombus at the inflow cannula; LV cavity diameters; septal position; RV function; valvular regurgitation, especially about the aortic valve opening/intervals and regurgitation.

View	Points to be checked
Parasternal views	• LV dimensions (ensure they are taken on axis) • AV opening (long acquisitions, use long and short axis, and M-mode) • Mitral regurgitation (tethering is the hallmark of functional regurgitation, and the degree may change according to LVAD rpm) • Consider evaluating cardiac output through RV out flow
Apical views	• Evaluate LV and RV function • Evaluate inlet cannula flow (position and suctioning) • Rule out thrombus in LV, RV, LA, and RA (use contrast as needed) • Evaluate aortic regurgitation
Image the inlet cannula	• Use multiple views including nonstandard • Rule out thrombus or other cause of obstruction (use contrast as needed) • Positioning (against LV wall)

Table 3. Echo LVAD checklist.

2.3.1. General postoperative assessment in LVAD recipients

Recommendations for device speed adjustment include the target measures of mean arterial pressure above 65 mmHg, maintaining the position of interventricular septum and shape, and intermittent aortic valve opening, under the condition of no more than mild mitral regurgitation to ensure appropriate unloading of the LV. Optimization of speed settings is extremely important to prevent several of the key complications associated with chronic LVAD support. The importance of ensuring the middle septal position for optimal RV function has been well established [19, 20].

Serially monitoring the timing and its interval of aortic valve opening in all LVAD recipients are necessary. Also, adjusting the LVAD speed to maintain the aortic valve opening is important to prevent the development of aortic valve regurgitation. At least 10 cardiac cycles should be recorded to evaluate the aortic valve opening. Because the interval of aortic valve opening, LV diameter, and grade of MR entirely depend on the degree of LV unloading, the LVAD setting together with the echo report needs to be recorded (**Figure 5**). Aortic regurgitation is sometimes seen with atypical timing (**Figure 6**) or continuously, both during the diastolic and systolic phases [21].

Cardiac output using RV outflow-derived Doppler estimation can be calculated as follows: cardiac output = stroke volume × heart rate, stroke volume = $\pi \times (\text{RV outflow diameter}/2)^2 \times$

time velocity integral at RV outflow. In patients who have at least an intermittent aortic valve opening, RV cardiac output minus LV outflow-derived cardiac output is equivalent to the estimated pump flow.

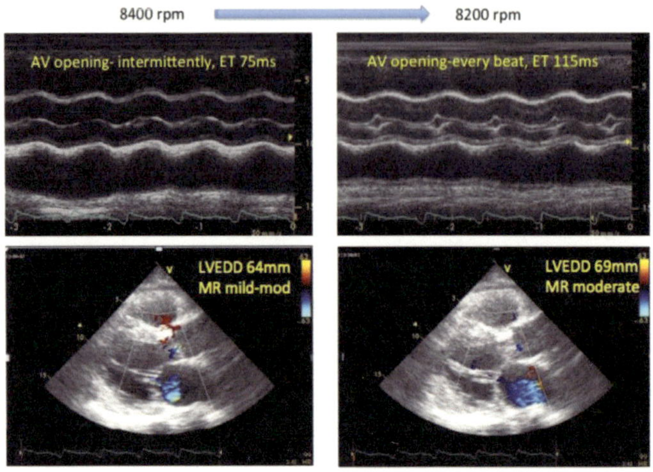

Figure 5. Representative images in a LVAD recipient with different LVAD speeds. This patient received HeartMate II (Thoratec Corp) implantation. Under 8400 rpm, the aortic valve opened intermittently, and the ejection time was only 75 ms. When we set the speed down to 8200, the aortic valve opened every beat, but due to less unloading, the LV diameter increased and the amount of mitral regurgitation also increased.

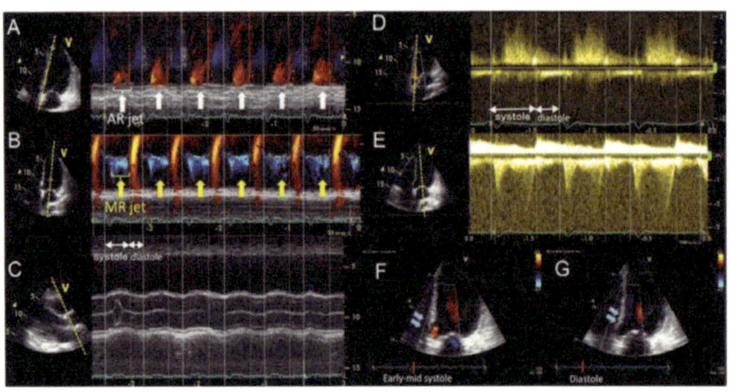

Figure 6. Aortic regurgitation during systolic phase accompanied by mitral regurgitation in patients with a continuous-flow left ventricular assist device (quoted from Ref. [22]). Echo images obtained from a patient undergoing LVAD implantation who showed systolic-phase aortic regurgitation (AR). The timing of the regurgitation jet started at the mid-systolic phase and ended at the early diastolic phase (A). The AR occurred slightly after the onset of mitral regurgitation (MR) (B), and both MR and AR timings were consistent with the systolic phase. No remarkable AR jet was documented during the diastolic phase. The AV was mostly closed throughout the cycles, which opens once every 8–10 beats (C). The mean pressure gradients of the trans-AV and trans-mitral valve based on the continuous wave Doppler measurements of AR (D) and MR flow (E) were 3.7 and 24.3 mmHg, respectively. The morphology of AV annulus changes through the cycles irrespective of the AV opening, with the AV annulus abnormally distorted and dilated during early mid-systole (F), whereas the septum wall as well as the AV annulus edge slightly pushed toward the LV during diastole (G).

Serial assessments of pulmonary artery pressure by Doppler-derived TR pressure gradients are also important. In general, LVAD support can successfully unload LV, which results in the correction of pulmonary hypertension due to left-sided heart failure. However, some patients have showed residual pulmonary vascular resistance post-LVAD; therefore, echo-guided optimal medical therapy, including the necessity of pulmonary dilators such as PDE5 inhibitors (sildenafil®, etc.), is required.

2.3.2. Detection of LVAD malfunction

The careful observation of the inflow cannula is critically important. By using multiple views, including nonstandard ones, the thrombus or other causes of obstruction should be ruled out. The direction of the inflow cannula should also be reported. The direction may sometimes change after the surgery and direct toward the lateral wall, which may cause suctioning or inadequate LVAD support. Contrast echocardiography can provide additional information. Detecting the outflow cannula obstruction by echocardiography is difficult, but practitioners should try to find a good echo window and investigate any abnormality, including kinking (**Figure 7**) [22, 23].

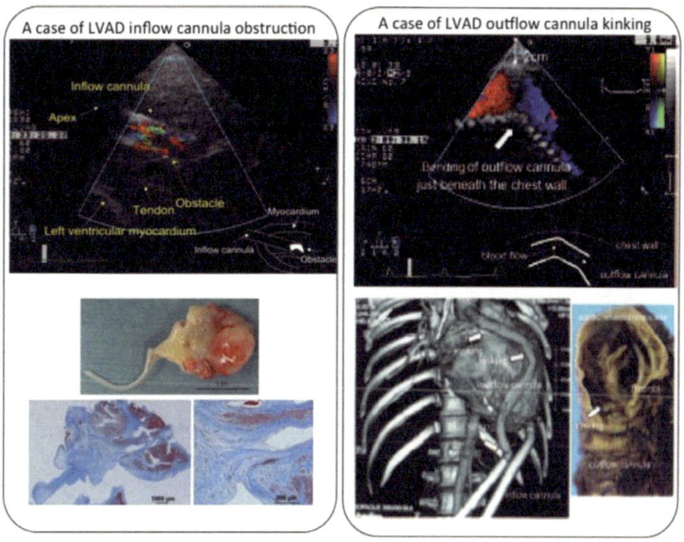

Figure 7. Cases of LVAD malfunction detected by echocardiography (quoted from Refs. [23, 24]). Left: A 29-year-old male developed low output syndrome 5 months after LVAD implantation. Echocardiography revealed pendulating obstacles at the inflow cannula of the LVAD. The obstacle was removed surgically, which histologically turned out to be myocardium with fibrous tissue and thrombi. Right: A 53-year-old man undergoing LVAD implantation developed low output syndrome. Echocardiography indicated distortion of the outflow cannula of the LVAD. A 3D CT also showed the kinking of the cannula. The autopsy revealed thrombus at the kinking site.

The protocol for a ramp study was established by Uriel N [20]. It is useful in optimizing LVAD settings and in diagnosing device malfunctions. Ramp test echocardiography can be performed at the time of discharge for speed optimization and/or if device malfunction is suspected (**Figure 8**) [24]. The patient's left ventricular size, the frequency of the aortic valve opening, valvular insufficiency, blood pressure, and continuous flow-LVAD parameters should be recorded according to the increments of the device speed. Serial assessments of ramp tests are also helpful to detect LVAD clots [24].

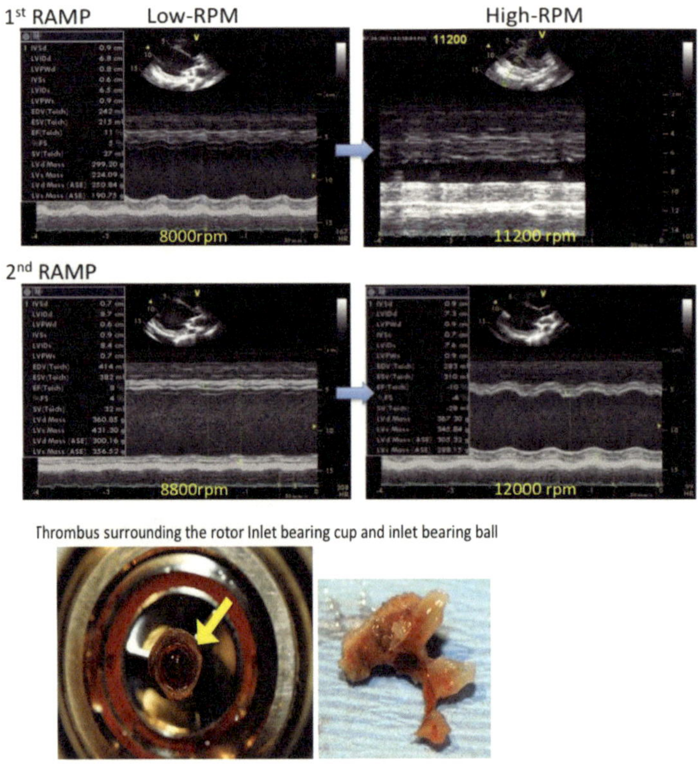

Figure 8. A representative case with device thrombosis was detected by a ramp echocardiography device (quoted from Ref. [24]). A case of a 29-year-old woman undergoing HeartMate II LVAD implantation; serial ramp studies were used to diagnose intradevice thrombus after device implantation. The first ramp study on postoperative day (POD) 26 revealed an adequate reduction in ventricular size according to the increase in LVAD. The patient was discharged home and received routine anticoagulation maintenance therapy. However, a second ramp test was performed on POD 56 due to increased lactase dehydrogenase and brain natriuretic peptide levels and showed a marked increase in the LV chamber size without an adequate response to the LVAD speed changes. Given the suspicion for partial pump thrombosis, the patient was immediately hospitalized and received intravenous heparin infusion. The patient eventually underwent cardiac transplant successfully, and the partial clot was found inside of the pump (lower panel).

2.3.3. *Assessment of native cardiac function*

It is important to assess native LV function, especially in patients receiving LVAD as a bridge to recovery. We cannot assess LV function without turning off the LVAD because it drastically affects preload and afterload; therefore, we need to reduce the LVAD speed under adequate anticoagulation during weaning test echocardiography. Strain assessment has been reported

http://dx.doi.org/10.5772/65095

to be more sensitive in evaluating the myocardial systolic and diastolic reserve, and 2D speckle tracing echocardiography for the assessment of myocardial recovery in LVAD recipients may be useful [25].

3. Echocardiography in transplant recipients

3.1. Donor heart evaluation

Evaluating a donor heart as accurately as possible at the time of procurement provides essential information to a recipient team leading the delicate posttransplant management of the heart [26]. If an organ procurement team has a cardiologist or sonographer who knows which patient is going to receive the heart, the team can gather detailed information by bedside echocardiography on the donor in light of the potential recipient's conditions at the organ procurement.

Measuring the heart size of the donor from bedside echocardiography at the time of organ procurement can provide useful information for judging the appropriateness of proceeding with the heart transplant in the case of a donor-recipient size mismatch. The wall thickness of the donor heart may also be useful information for optimizing the medical therapy after transplantation, as well as for deciding whether or not to use the organ. Information regarding the presence or absence of a septal defect would be of help to surgeons planning the additional procedure of septal closure at the time of transplantation. Information about the coronary flow in the left anterior descending artery of the donor heart, especially in cases with coronary risk factors, is useful for judging the availability of the heart, as well as for considering issues related to posttransplant medical management. Finally, information about preexisting localized wall motion abnormalities from bedside echocardiography is useful for speculating on the possibility of rejection or other reasons for wall motion abnormality after transplant surgery.

According to such information, the team can make a final decision whether or not to harvest the heart. For example, the donor heart may be relatively small for the potential recipient. If a donor heart with a lower limit of normal systolic function shows decreased coronary flow and localized right heart wall motion abnormality, the heart should be declined in cases where the potential recipients have moderately high pulmonary vascular resistance. Such recipients need to receive a donor heart with good right ventricular function.

3.2. A noninvasive rejection diagnosis

Advances in immunosuppressive therapy have resulted in a marked decrease in the incidence of acute allograft rejection in heart transplant recipients; however, acute rejection still remains an important determinant factor for long-term morbidity and mortality. Acute rejection can result in not only the immediate risk of graft loss or heart failure but also of subsequent allograft vasculopathy [27]. Therefore, early diagnosis of rejection and consequent timely treatment are crucial for the early and long-term care in heart transplant recipients. Detection of allograft rejection based on the findings derived from endomyocardial biopsy (EMB) is still a gold standard; however, EMB is invasive, cost and time consuming, and may have a possibility of sampling error and interobserver variability. Although many noninvasive modalities, including radionuclide imaging, MRI, and gene expression profiling, have been investigated for their potential to detect rejection, none of them have been found to be sufficient for replacing EMB. Echocardiography has been routinely used in the management of cardiac transplant recipients. Indeed, it is an easily applicable, repeatable, and powerful noninvasive tool in the management of posttransplant recipients [28].

Variables	Characteristics and pitfalls
LVEF ↓ LV %FS ↓	• Occurs in the late phase of the rejection process • Mild/moderate rejection cannot be detected
LV wall thickness ↑ LV mass ↑	• May be related to inflammatory cell infiltration • Myocardial edema/preoperative ischemia also cause increase in LV wall thickness; so difficult to interpret during early postoperative periods
Mitral E/A ratio ↑ Mitral DcT ↓ IVRT ↓	• Abnormal filling pattern/restrictive physiology is associated with rejection • Relatively pre/after-load dependent • Doppler angle dependent • Heart rate dependent (not appropriate for patients with tachycardia)
TEI Index* (MPI) ↑	• Can evaluate global ventricular performance (both systolic and diastolic) • Derived from Doppler-derived time intervals • HR independent
Pericardial effusion↑	• May be related to the inflammatory process of rejection, but can have many causes, especially during the early postoperative phase

A, late diastolic mitral inflow velocity; DcT, deceleration time; E, early diastolic mitral inflow velocity; EF, ejection fraction; FS, fractional shortening; LV, left ventricle, left ventricular; IVRT, isovolumic relaxation time; IMP, myocardial performance index. *MPI = (isovolumic contraction time – IVRT)/ejection time.

Table 4. Conventional echocardiographic variables associated with rejections (quoted from Ref. [29]).

3.2.1. Conventional echocardiography

Table 4 summarizes the conventional echocardiographic parameters associated with acute cellular rejection [28]. Conventional echocardiography soon after the surgery can provide information about global systolic and diastolic functions, wall motion abnormality, and the hemodynamics of the transplanted hearts. Any apparent abnormal findings such as remarkable systolic and/or diastolic impairment may acute or hyperacute rejection, including antibody-mediated rejection, although primary graft failure, donor-related graft dysfunction, and any perioperative accidents should also be considered. The ability of conventional echo parameters to detect rejection is still limited to severe clinically detectable rejection. However,

http://dx.doi.org/10.5772/65095

the findings are still useful for assessing responsiveness to treatment. In general, patients with rejection develop restrictive physiology accompanied by various degrees of systolic dysfunction. Valantine HA et al. reported that a 15% decrease in mitral deceleration time or isovolumic relaxation time (IVRT) is associated with biopsy proven rejection [29]. More recently, Sun et al. reported that a combination of IVRT less than 90 ms, a mitral E/A ratio more than 1.7, and other clinical parameters is independently associated with rejection [30]. However, because transplant recipients usually have higher resting heart rates than the nontransplant population due to denervation, their mitral E and A waves can be fused. Indeed, it is difficult to obtain clear Doppler waves from transplant recipients. They frequently have extended adhesion of the transplanted heart to the chest cavity, which hinders the acquisition of an appropriate Doppler angle. The TEI index or myocardial performance index (MPI), which is a parameter of a Doppler-derived combination of systolic and diastolic time intervals, is a useful parameter in patients with E-A fusion and high heart rate; therefore, the MPI has the potential to detect rejection more accurately than traditional Doppler indices [31]. Representative conventional 2D echo images associated with and without rejection are shown in **Figure 9**.

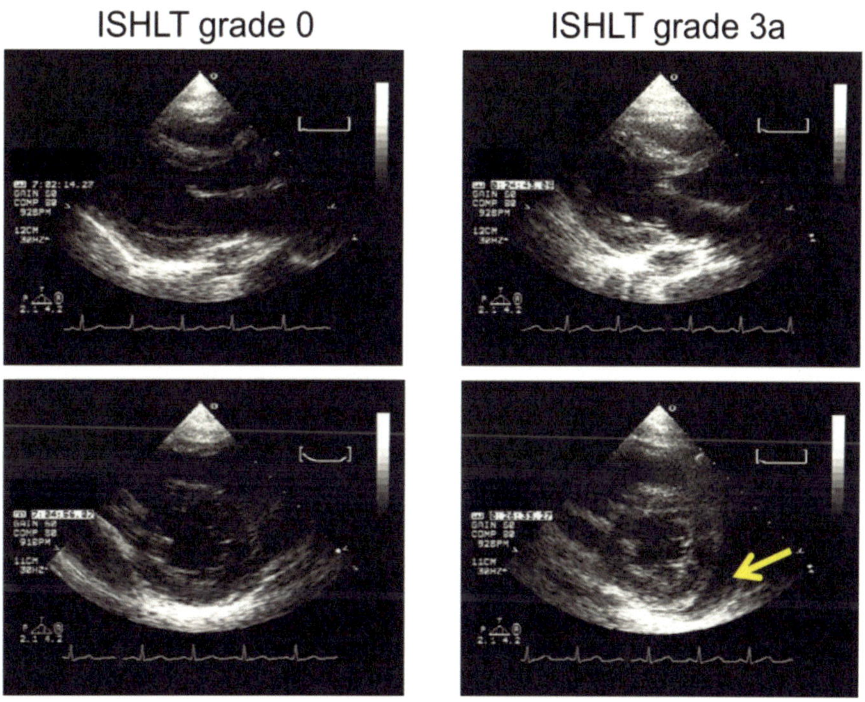

Figure 9. Representative 2D echocardiography in a patient with and without cellular rejection. Representative conventional 2D echocardiograms obtained from a 26-year-old female transplant recipient at the time when her EMB showed conventional ISHLT grade 0 (left) and ISHLT grade 3a rejection (right). The posterior wall thickness of LV and the LV mass index without rejection (left) were 9 mm and 88 g/m^2, respectively. The same parameters associated with rejection (right) were 13 mm and 112 g/m^2. The arrow in the right lower panel indicates a pericardial effusion. EMB, endomyocardial biopsies; ISHLT, International Society for Heart and Lung Transplantation; LV, left ventricular and left ventricle.

Variables	Characteristics and pitfalls
TDI derived E′ ↓ A′ ↓ E/E′ ↑	• Reflecting increased LV filling pressure/relaxation abnormalities • Angle dependent
TDI-derived longitudinal systolic strain ↓ TDI-derived radial systolic strain ↓	• Reflecting both systolic and diastolic abnormalities • Possibility of reflecting heterogeneous myocardial abnormalities • Ability to detect subclinical rejection • Angle dependent • Frame rate limitations
TDI-derived diastolic strain rate ↓	• Reflecting relaxation abnormalities • Ability to detect subclinical rejection • Angle dependent • Frame rate limitations
2D-STE-derived LV torsion ↓	• Reflecting relaxation abnormalities • Ability to detect subclinical rejection • Angle independent • Values can be calculated offline using stored 2D images
2D-STE-derived global radial systolic strain ↓	• Reflecting both systolic and diastolic abnormalities • Possibility of reflecting heterogeneous myocardial abnormalities • Ability to detect subclinical rejection • Angle independent • Values can be calculated offline using stored 2D images
2D-STE-derived systolic and diastolic global strain rate ↓	• May be more sensitive for the early detection of rejection than systolic and early diastolic global strains • Angle independent • Values can be calculated offline using stored 2D images

A′, late diastolic mitral annular velocity, E′, early diastolic mitral annular tissue velocity. * LV torsion = (apical end-systolic rotation) – (basal end-systolic rotation).

Table 5. Tissue-Doppler imaging and 2D-speckle-tracking echocardiography-derived variables associated with rejections (quoted from Ref. [29]).

3.2.2. Tissue Doppler imaging and speckle tracking echocardiography

Tissue Doppler imaging (TDI) enables the measurements of systolic and diastolic velocities within the myocardium. Several studies have evaluated the usefulness of TDI-derived mitral annular velocities to detect allograft rejection, which are summarized in **Table 5** [28]. Strain rate analysis has a potential to detect even mild rejection. Kato TS et al. reported that the attenuation of LV longitudinal strain and the diastolic strain rate derived from TDI were associated with conventional ISHLT (International Society for Heart and Lung Transplantation) grade 1b or higher rejection without hemodynamic alterations (**Figure 10**) [32]. Marciniak et al. found significantly lower LV longitudinal and radial peak systolic strain and strain rate values in patients with conventional ISHLT grade 1b or higher rejection. TDI-derived strain and strain rate potentially reflect abnormalities [33].

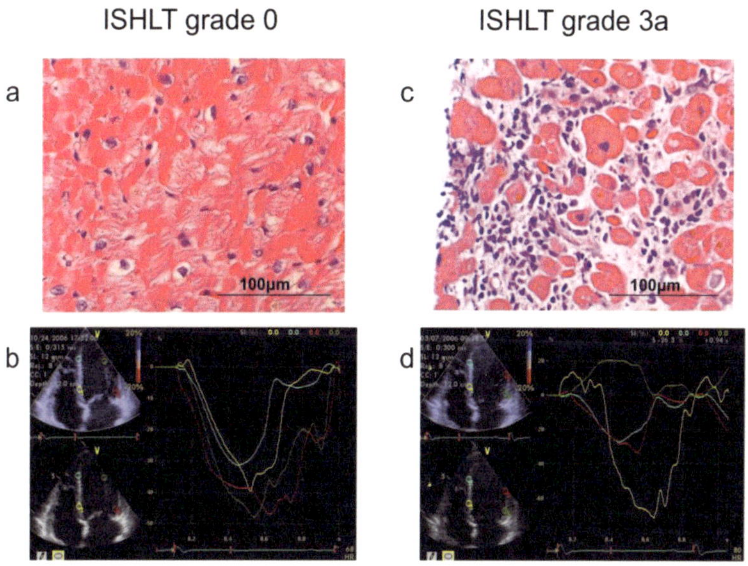

Figure 10. Representative TDI-derived strain analysis in a patient with and without rejection (quoted from Ref. [33]). Representative pathological findings for EMB specimens (a, b) and strain analysis (c, d) of HTx with ISHLT grade 0 (a, c) or 3a (b, d) rejection. Sections in (a) and (b) were stained with hematoxylin-eosin; scale bars, 100 mm. EMB, endomyocardial biopsies; HTx, heart transplant recipients; ISHLT, International Society for Heart and Lung Transplantation.

Two-dimensional speckle-tracking echocardiography (2D-STE) was developed as an angle-independent echocardiographic modality to evaluate cardiac mechanical function. The 2D-STE-derived parameters associated with rejection are also shown in **Table 5** [28]. The association between LV torsional deformation and rejection in transplant recipients has been reported since the 1980s. Sato et al. reported that 2D-STE-derived LV torsion values are decreased in patients with rejection, and the serial assessments of an intra-patients comparison showed that a cut-off value of a 25% reduction of LV torsion from the baseline is associated with ISHLT grade 2 or higher rejection, which returns to the baseline after adequate rejection treatment (**Figure 11**) [34]. LV global strains are also calculated using 2D-STE in an angle-independent manner. Sera F et al. reported that 2D-STE-derived LV global longitudinal strain was associated with treatment-requiring rejection [35] (**Figure 12**). In addition to its major advantage of angle independency, 2D-STE has other advantages over TDI, such as spatial resolution, translational artifacts, the sensitivity to signal noise, the time needed for data acquisition, and the necessity of employing expert readers. Three-dimensional (3D) STEs are useful echocardiographic modalities to assess various strain and rotation parameters more accurately than 2D-STE by tracking the same speckle throughout the cardiac cycle. However, it will take several years for the validation studies of 3D-STE to be performed to verify the value of rejection-detecting tools in heart transplant recipients.

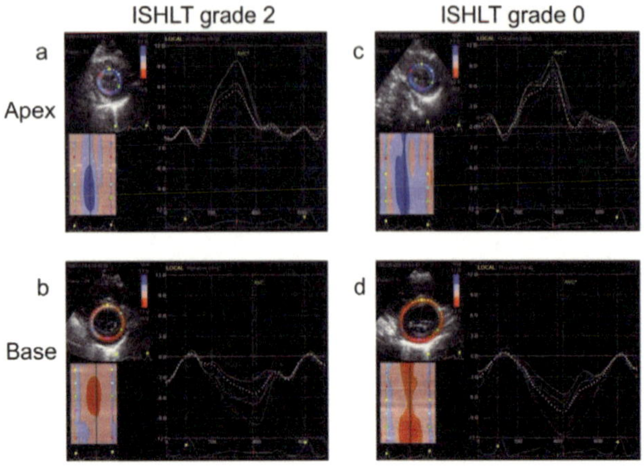

Figure 11. Representative 2D speckle-tracking echocardiogram and analysis of torsion in a patient with and without rejection. (quoted from Ref. [35]). Representative 2D-STE imaging with rotation curves obtained from the same recipient (a 32-year-old man) at LV short-axis views of the apex (a, c) and the base (b, d). Each color of the deformational curve represents one segment of the LV, and the dashed white curve depicts the mean rotation of six segments. The LV-tor, defined as the difference between apical basal end-systolic rotation when the patient had ISHLT grade 2 rejection, was 10.9 degrees (a, b). The LV torsion accompanied with ISHLT grade 0 after rejection treatment was 15.6 degrees (c, d). The % change of LV torsion in this patient at the time of rejection was approximately 30% decreased from his baseline. ISHLT, International Society for Heart and Lung Transplantation; LV, left ventricular; 2D-STE, 2D speckle-tracking echocardiography; EMB, endomyocardial biopsies; HTx, heart transplant recipients.

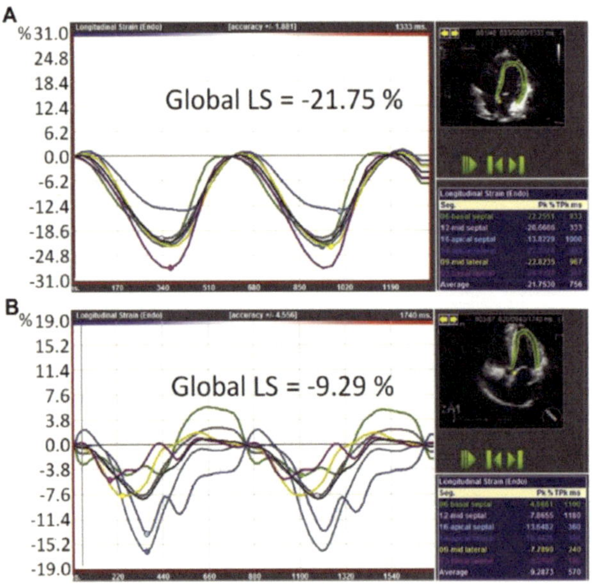

Figure 12. Representative 2D speckle tracking echocardiogram and analysis of global longitudinal strain in a patient with and without rejection (quoted from Ref. [36]). LS curves obtained from a patient without rejection (grade 0) (A) and another patient with grade 3a rejection (B). LS, longitudinal strain.

http://dx.doi.org/10.5772/65095

3.2.3. Transplant vasculopathy and echocardiography

Echocardiography is a helpful and an ideal noninvasive tool to detect transplant vasculopathy or chronic rejection as well. Dobutamine or/and exercise stress echocardiography has been used to detect allograft vasculopathy, especially for pediatric patients or those with renal insufficiency [36]. Decreases in strain and strain rates at rest and with dobutamine stress are also useful to detect significant transplant vasculopathy. Contrast echocardiography is another useful method.

Author details

Tomoko Kato[1,2*], Takashi Nishimura[1,2], Shunei Kyo[1,2], Kenji Kuwaki[1,2], Hiroyuki Dada[1,2] and Atsushi Amano[1,2]

*Address all correspondence to: rinnko@sannet.ne.jp

1 Juntendo University School of Medicine, Heart Center, Tokyo, Japan

2 Tokyo Metropolitan Geriatric Hospital, Institute of Gerontology, Tokyo, Japan

References

[1] Lund LH, Edwards LB, Kucheryavaya AY, Benden C, Dipchand AI, et al. The Registry of the International Society for Heart and Lung Transplantation: Thirty-second Official Adult Heart Transplantation Report – 2015; Focus Theme: Early Graft Failure. J Heart Lung Transplant 2015; 34:1244–1254.

[2] Kirklin JK, Naftel DC, Pagani FD, Kormos RL, Stevenson LW, et al. Seventh INTERMACS annual report: 15,000 patients and counting. J Heart Lung Transplant 2015; 34:1495–1504.

[3] Jorde UP, Kushwaha SS, Tatooles AJ, Naka Y, Bhat G, et al; HeartMate II Clinical Investigators. Results of the destination therapy post-food and drug administration approval study with a continuous flow left ventricular assist device: a prospective study using the INTERMACS registry (Interagency Registry for Mechanically Assisted Circulatory Support). J Am Coll Cardiol. 2014; 63:1751–1757.

[4] Kukucka M, Stepanenko A, Potapov E, Krabatsch T, Kuppe H, Habazettl H. Impact of tricuspid valve annulus dilation on mid-term survival after implantation of a left ventricular assist device. J Heart Lung Transplant 2012;31:967–971.

[5] Dunlay SM, Deo SV, Park SJ. Impact of tricuspid valve surgery at the time of left ventricular assist device insertion on postoperative outcomes. ASAIO J 2015; 61:15–20.

[6] Han J, Takeda K, Takayama H, Kurlansky PA, Mauro CM, et al. Durability and clinical impact of tricuspid valve procedures in patients receiving a continuous-flow left ventricular assist device. J Thorac Cardiovasc Surg 2016;151:520–527.

[7] Cowger J, Rao V, Massey T, Sun B, May-Newman K, et al. Comprehensive review and suggested strategies for the detection and management of aortic insufficiency in patients with a continuous-flow left ventricular assist device. J Heart Lung Transplant 2015;34:149–157. doi: 10.1016/j.healun.2014.09.045. Epub 2014 Oct 24.

[8] Stulak JM, Tchantchaleishvili V, Haglund NA, Davis ME, Schirger JA, et al. Uncorrected pre-operative mitral valve regurgitation is not associated with adverse outcomes after continuous-flow left ventricular assist device implantation. J Heart Lung Transplant 2015;34:718–723.

[9] Taghavi S, Hamad E, Wilson L, Clark R, Jayarajan SN, et al. Mitral valve repair at the time of continuous-flow left ventricular assist device implantation confers meaningful decrement in pulmonary vascular resistance. ASAIO J 2013;59:469–473.

[10] Kitada S, Kato TS, Thomas SS, Conwell SD, Russo C, et al. Pre-operative echocardiographic features associated with persistent mitral regurgitation after left ventricular assist device implantation. J Heart Lung Transplant 2013;32:897–904.

[11] Mikus E, Stepanenko A, Krabatsch T, Loforte A, Dandel M, et al. Reversibility of fixed pulmonary hypertension in left ventricular assist device support recipients. Eur J Cardiothorac Surg. 2011;40:971–977.

[12] Kato TS, Jiang J, Schulze PC, Jorde U, Uriel N, et al. Serial echocardiography using tissue Doppler and speckle tracking imaging to monitor right ventricular failure before and after left ventricular assist device surgery. JACC Heart Fail 2013;1:216–222.

[13] Hayek S, Sims DB, Markham DW, Butler J, Kalogeropoulos AP. Assessment of right ventricular function in left ventricular assist device candidates. Circ Cardiovasc Imaging 2014;7:379–389.

[14] Puwanant S, Hamilton KK, Klodell CT, Hill JA, Schofield RS, et al. Tricuspid annular motion as a predictor of severe right ventricular failure after left ventricular assist device implantation. J Heart Lung Transplant 2008;27:1102–1107.

[15] Kukucka M, Stepanenko A, Potapov E, Krabatsch T, Redlin M, et al. Right-to-left ventricular end-diastolic diameter ratio and prediction of right ventricular failure with continuous-flow left ventricular assist devices. J Heart Lung Transplant 2011;30:64–69.

[16] Kato TS, Farr M, Schulze PC, Maurer M, Shahzad K, et al. Usefulness of 2-dimensional echocardiographic parameters of the left side of the heart to predict right ventricular failure after left ventricular assist device implantation. Am J Cardiol 2012;109:246–251.

[17] Grant AD, Smedira NG, Starling RC, Marwick TH. Independent and incremental role of quantitative right ventricular evaluation for the prediction of right ventricular failure after left ventricular assist device implantation. J Am Coll Cardiol 2012;60:521–528.

[18] Ammar KA, Umland MM, Kramer C, Sulemanjee N, Jan MF, et al. The ABCs of left ventricular assist device echocardiography: a systematic approach. Eur Heart J Cardiovasc Imaging 2012;13:885–899.

[19] Topilsky Y, Hasin T, Oh JK, Borgeson DD, Boilson BA, et al. Echocardiographic variables after left ventricular assist device implantation associated with adverse outcome. Circ Cardiovasc Imaging 2011;4:648–661.

[20] Uriel N, Morrison KA, Garan AR, Kato TS, Yuzefpolskaya M, et al. Development of a novel echocardiography ramp test for speed optimization and diagnosis of device thrombosis in continuous-flow left ventricular assist devices: the Columbia ramp study. J Am Coll Cardiol 2012;60:1764–1775.

[21] Kato TS, Maurer MS, Sera F, Homma S, Mancini D. Aortic regurgitation during systolic-phase accompanied by mitral regurgitation in patients with continuous-flow left ventricular assist device. Eur Heart J Cardiovasc Imaging 2013;14:1022.

[22] Kato TS, Oda N, Hashimoto S, Ikeda Y, Ishibashi-Ueda H, Komamura K. Assist device malfunction due to kinking of cannula between heart and chest wall. Asian Cardiovasc Thorac Ann 2010;18:598.

[23] Oda N, Kato TS, Niwaya K, Komamura K. Unusual cause of left ventricular assist device failure: pendulating mass in the cavity. Eur J Cardiothorac Surg 2007;32:533.

[24] Kato TS, Colombo PC, Nahumi N, Kitada S, Takayama H, et al. Value of serial echo-guided ramp studies in a patient with suspicion of device thrombosis after left ventricular assist device implantation. Echocardiography 2014;31:E5–E9.

[25] Gupta DK, Skali H, Rivero J, Campbell P, Griffin L, et al. Assessment of myocardial viability and left ventricular function in patients supported by a left ventricular assist device. J Heart Lung Transplant 2014;33:372–381.

[26] Hashimoto S, Kato TS, Komamura K, Hanatani A, Niwaya K, et al. Utility of echocardiographic evaluation of donor hearts upon the organ procurement for heart transplantation. J Cardiol 2011;57:215–222.

[27] Raichlin E, Edwards BS, Kremers WK, Clavell AL, Rodeheffer RJ, et al. Acute cellular rejection and the subsequent development of allograft vasculopathy after cardiac transplantation. J Heart Lung Transplant 2009;28:320–327.

[28] Kato TS, Homma S, Mancini D. Novel echocardiographic strategies for rejection diagnosis. Curr Opin Organ Transplant 2013;18:573–580.

[29] Valantine HA, Yeoh TK, Gibbons R, McCarthy P, Stinson EB, et al. Sensitivity and specificity of diastolic indices for rejection surveillance: temporal correlation with endomyocardial biopsy. J Heart Lung Transplant 1991;10:757–765.

[30] Sun JP, Abdalla IA, Asher CR, Greenberg NL, Popović ZB, et al. Non-invasive evaluation of orthotopic heart transplant rejection by echocardiography. J Heart Lung Transplant 2005;24:160–165.

[31] Leonard GT Jr, Fricker FJ, Pruett D, Harker K, Williams B, Schowengerdt KO Jr. Increased myocardial performance index correlates with biopsy-proven rejection in pediatric heart transplant recipients. J Heart Lung Transplant 2006;25:61–66.

[32] Kato TS, Oda N, Hashimura K, Hashimura K, Hashimoto S, et al. Strain rate imaging would predict subclinical acute rejection in heart transplant recipients. Eur J Cardiothorac Surg 2010;37:1104–1110.

[33] Marciniak A, Eroglu E, Marciniak M, Sirbu C, Herbots L, et al. The potential clinical role of ultrasonic strain and strain rate imaging in diagnosing acute rejection after heart transplantation. Eur J Echocardiogr 2007;8:213–221.

[34] Sato T, Kato TS, Komamura K, Hashimoto S, Shishido T, et al. Utility of left ventricular systolic torsion derived from 2-dimensional speckle-tracking echocardiography in monitoring acute cellular rejection in heart transplant recipients. J Heart Lung Transplant 2011;30:536–543.

[35] Sera F, Kato TS, Farr M, Russo C, Jin Z, et al. Left ventricular longitudinal strain by speckle-tracking echocardiography is associated with treatment-requiring cardiac allograft rejection. J Card Fail 2014;20:359–364.

[36] Dedieu N, Greil G, Wong J, Fenton M, Burch M, Hussain T. Diagnosis and management of coronary allograft vasculopathy in children and adolescents. World J Transplant 2014;24(4):276–293.

Chapter 9

Assessment of Right Ventricle by Echocardiogram

Gunjan Choudhary, Arushi A. Malik,
Dwight Stapleton and Pratap C. Reddy

Additional information is available at the end of the chapter

http://dx.doi.org/10.5772/64781

Abstract

Assessment of right ventricular (RV) function is important to ascertain clinical outcome in patients with symptoms of right ventricular failure manifested as lower extremity swelling and abdominal congestion. RV function is not routinely assessed and reported in clinical practice. Unlike the bullet-shaped left ventricle (LV), RV has a complex geometry with a triangular shape. RV is further divided into the inlet, trabecular apex, and infundibulum or conus. RV evaluation involves quantifying afterload and preload, assessing the mechanism and severity of tricuspid regurgitation (TR), and quantitative evaluation of RV performance. For quantification of RV size and function, we can use intravenous contrast for endocardial tracing of RV border to measure RV dimensions, tricuspid annular plane systolic excursion (TAPSE), fractional area change (FAC), Doppler index of myocardial performance (Tei index or myocardial performance index), pulsed wave or color Doppler tissue imaging systolic velocity [s'], or strain imaging. For qualitative evaluation of RV, the RV size is compared to the LV size in parasternal, short axis, and subcostal projections.

Keywords: right ventricle, functional evaluation, right heart hemodynamics, echocardiography, clinical significance

1. Introduction

Historically, the importance of right ventricle (RV) has been underestimated and overlooked in clinical practice and literature. Usually, left ventricle (LV) function is most commonly reported and signified. Only in recent years, the importance of assessment of RV size and function in clinical management and treatment of cardiopulmonary disorders has been recognized [1]. RV dysfunction is associated with adverse clinical outcome [2–8] in patients with LV dysfunction, acute myocardial infarction, pulmonary embolism, pulmonary arterial hypertension, and congenital heart disease [9–11]. Hence, this has generated interest in the evaluation of RV function. RV dysfunction could be secondary to pressure or volume overload; from primary right heart disease or secondary to left heart diseases such as cardiomyopathy or valvular heart disease [12, 13] (**Tables 1** and **2**). RV dysfunction may affect by way of interventricular septal motion (ventricular interdependence) and by affecting LV preload.

RV cardiomyopathy
Arrhythmogenic right ventricular cardiomyopathy (ARVC)
Dilated cardiomyopathy
Endomyocardial fibrosis
Cirrhotic cardiomyopathy
Eosinophilic myocarditis
Peripartum cardiomyopathy
Uhl's anomaly
Sepsis
Viral myocarditis
Coronary artery disease

Table 1. Causes of RV contractile dysfunction.

RV pressure overload
All groups of pulmonary hypertension
Massive pulmonary embolism
ARDS
Eisenmenger syndrome
RV outflow obstruction
Pulmonic valve stenosis
Infundibular stenosis
(Tetralogy of Fallot, hypertrophic cardiomyopathy)
Mechanical ventilation
Hypoventilation
RV volume overload
Left to right shunt
Atrial septal defect
Anomalous pulmonary venous drainage
Pulmonary regurgitation
Tricuspid regurgitation
Primary
Infective endocarditis
Carcinoid syndrome
Rheumatic heart disease
Ebstein's anomaly
Secondary to tricuspid annular dilation from RV Dilation

Table 2. Causes of right ventricular overload.

http://dx.doi.org/10.5772/64781

Of all the noninvasive imaging modalities, echocardiography remains a mainstay in the evaluation of RV. Moreover, with advances in echocardiography the pathophysiology of RV has been better understood. In this chapter, we aim to review various methods to assess RV anatomy, function, and hemodynamics using two-dimensional (2D) echocardiography, color Doppler echocardiography, tissue Doppler imaging (TDI), three-dimensional (3D) echocardiography, and strain imaging echocardiography [12]. To identify RV pathology, guidelines have been published by the American Society of Echocardiography (ASE) on parameters and normal reference values (**Table 5**).

2. Location and anatomy of RV

The RV in the normal heart is the most anteriorly situated cardiac chamber located immediately behind the sternum and anterior to LV. It forms the majority of the anterior as well as the inferior border of the cardiac silhouette. Due to this unique anatomical location, assessment of RV size and function by transthoracic echocardiogram (TTE) may appear easy but assessment of RV function is challenging given the odd geometry of the crescent-shaped RV that wraps around conical LV. Furthermore, heavily trabeculated myocardium also limits the delineation of RV endocardial surface.

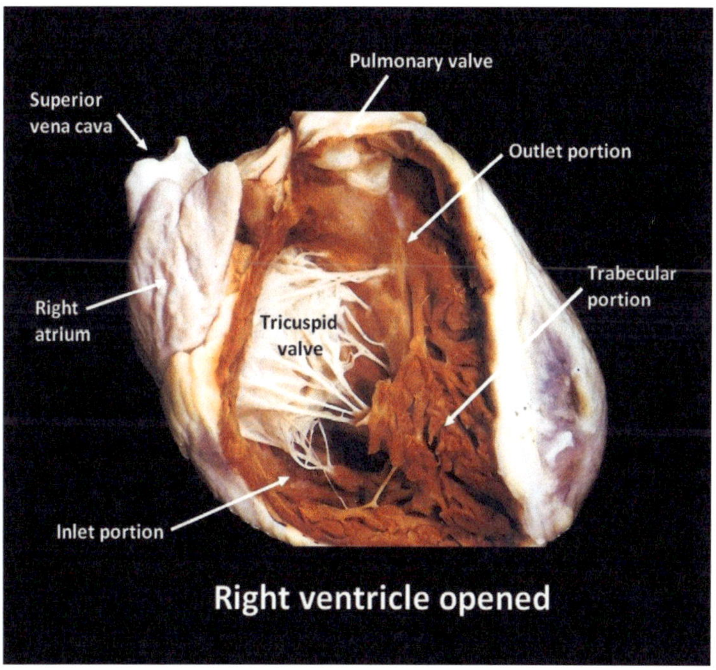

Figure 1. RV anatomy and myocardial fibers. The RV structure: illustrates the inlet, trabecular, and outlet components.

Unlike the LV that is ellipsoid or conical, the RV is crescent shaped or pyramidal, and its cavity has three components [14]: **Figure 1**

1. The muscular inlet comprising of the tricuspid valve, chordae tendineae, and three papillary muscles, which originate in ventricular wall and attach to anterior, posterior, and septal leaflets of the tricuspid valve via chordae tendineae.
2. Immobile apex with heavy, coarse trabeculations; two thick intracavitary muscle bands, the crista supraventricularis [15], and the moderator band attached to the right ventricular outflow tract (RVOT) extending from the interventricular septum (IVS) to the anterior RV wall. The apical part of the RV is heavily trabeculated and virtually an immobile part of the ventricle.
3. Smooth funnel-shaped myocardial outflow tract called infundibulum [14].

The RV is formed by free (anterior and posterior) wall and interventricular septum. Blood supply to the RV is by right coronary artery (equal in systole and diastole except in pressure overload and hypertrophy). The moderator band is supplied by the left anterior descending artery. The tricuspid valve has three papillary muscles and three cusps (anterior, posterior, and septal). The tricuspid valve is 2 mm more apical to the mitral valve. It is very important to be able to differentiate left ventricle from right ventricle based on morphology seen on an echocardiogram (**Table 3**).

Right ventricle is characterized by:
• More *apical position* of the tricuspid valve as compared to the mitral valve
• Presence of a moderator band
• Presence of more than three papillary muscles
• Three leaflets of the tricuspid valve with *septal* papillary attachments
• Presence of trabeculations (trabeculations can also be seen in the left ventricle in case of pathological noncompaction of the left ventricle)

Table 3. Morphological differences between the right ventricle from the left ventricle.

2.1. Musculature of ventricular wall

The RV has one-sixth the muscle mass of LV as it pumps against approximately one-sixth the resistance the LV encounters. However, the RV pumps equal cardiac output as LV. The RV ejection fraction (EF) is lower as RV end-diastolic volume is slightly larger than that of the left ventricle. Appropriately, the RV is adaptable as a volume pump but is likely to fail when subjected to acute pressure overload. The muscular wall of the RV excluding trabeculations is

http://dx.doi.org/10.5772/64781

3–5 mm thick [16]. RV is relatively thin walled having superficial subepicardial circumferential myofibers parallel to the atrioventricular groove that encircles the subpulmonary infundibulum and deeper subendocardial longitudinal myofibers. Unlike the relatively thick-walled LV, the RV lacks the third layer of spiral/oblique myofibers. Longitudinal fibers contract to result in inward/radial thickening. The septal motion is considered to contribute to both LV and RV function [17, 18] and is a major determinant of overall RV performance [17–19].

2.2. RV area

The RV area is measured in the apical four-chamber window at end-diastole by planimetry of the RV cavity. Delineation of the RV endocardium is challenging and should exclude trabeculations or moderator band; however, one should include the apex of the RV to avoid erroneous estimation. The normal reference limit for RV end-diastolic area is ≤24 cm^2 in men and ≤20 cm^2 in women [14].

2.3. RV wall thickness

The RV wall thickness can be measured by M-mode or 2D echocardiography from either the left parasternal window or subcostal window at the level of the tip of the anterior tricuspid leaflet. RV hypertrophy is seen in infiltrative and hypertrophic cardiomyopathy, whereas RV wall thinning is seen in Uhl anomaly and arrhythmogenic RV cardiomyopathy. When measuring the RV wall thickness, it is essential to exclude RV trabeculations, papillary muscle, thickened pericardium, and epicardial fat. The normal cutoff is 0.5 cm from either parasternal long axis (PLAX) or subcostal windows.

2.4. RV linear dimensions

RV size can be measured from the apical four-chamber view at end-diastole wherein RV should appear almost two-thirds of the size of LV on qualitative assessment. The RV is enlarged in acute pressure and volume overload. The absence of standard reference points in RV imaging serves as a limitation in using transthoracic echocardiogram. The RV may appear viable in size when RV imaging is done through various cut planes depending on the probe rotation [20]. In the four-chamber view, the focus should be on the right ventricular chamber "RV Focused view" for better imaging of the RV lateral wall and to maximize the RV size. One should adjust the transducer to attain maximal plane to avert underestimation and to avoid overestimation by positioning the transducer over the cardiac apex with the plane through the left ventricle in the center of the cavity. The basal diameter is the maximal short-axis dimension in the basal, one-third of the right ventricle. The mid-cavity diameter is measured at the level of the LV papillary muscles in mid-third of the RV, and the longitudinal dimension is measured from the plane of the tricuspid annulus to the RV apex. ASE guidelines for the right heart assessment recommend measurement of the following dimensions: RV basal-apical four-chamber view, RV wall thickness (subcostal long axis view), proximal RVOT PSAX (parasternal short axis) view at the great vessels level, and distal RVOT PLAX view (**Figure 2**).

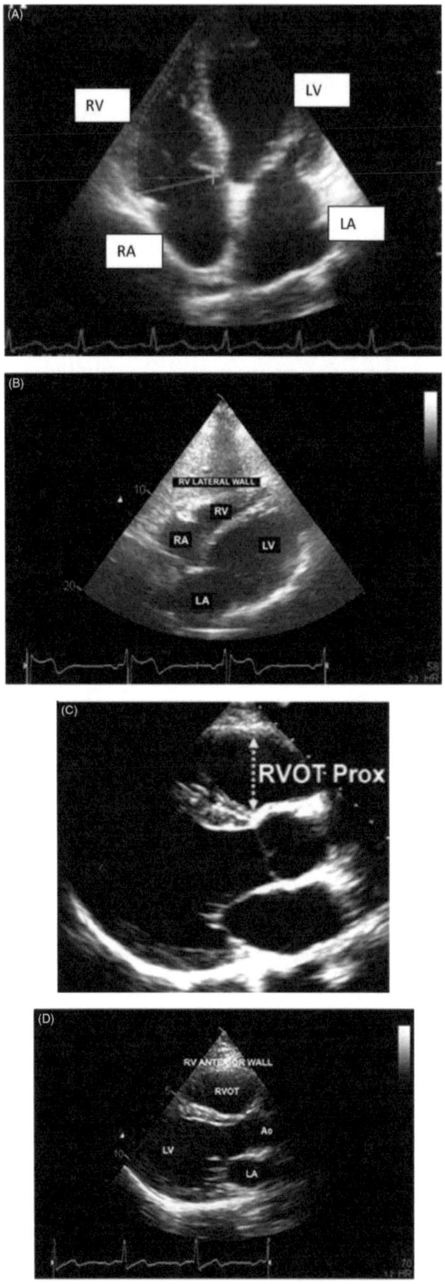

Figure 2. (A) RV basal apical four-chamber view: illustrating the plane of the tricuspid valve and RV endocardial border. **(B) RV wall thickness** (subcostal long axis view): illustrates the LA, left atrium; LV, left ventricle; RA, right atrium; RV, right ventricle; and RV lateral wall. **(C) Proximal RVOT** (parasternal short-axis view PSAX at the great vessels level): illustrates the Ao, aorta; PA, pulmonary artery; LV, left ventricle; RVOT, right ventricular outflow tract; and RV anterior wall. **(D) Distal RVOT** (parasternal long axis view PLAX): illustrates the Ao, aorta; LA, left atrium; LV, left ventricle; RVOT, right ventricular outflow tract, RV anterior wall.

2.5. Right ventricular outflow tract

The RVOT includes the pulmonic valve and subpulmonary infundibulum or conus that extends from the crista supraventricularis to the pulmonary valve [21, 22]. RVOT is usually imaged from the left parasternal short axis view. In patients with congenital heart disease and arrhythmogenic RV dysplasia, parasternal long axis view may be added to assess the proximal and distal diameter of RVOT. There is no standard window for measurement of RVOT size; oblique imaging may interfere in the accurate estimation of its size. The upper reference limit for the PSAX distal RVOT diameter is 27 mm and for PLAX is 33 mm (**Table 5**).

2.6. Interventricular septal morphology

Normally the LV has circular shape throughout the cardiac cycle. During systole, the LV protrudes into the RV. Compliance of one ventricle can modify the other through diastolic ventricular interaction. However, interventricular septum gets flattened and curved into LV cavity secondary to volume and pressure overload of the RV. The LV cavity, therefore, appears D-shaped at end-systole and end-diastole in RV pressure overload and RV volume overload (e.g., tricuspid regurgitation), respectively [17, 19] (**Figure 3**).

2.7. Volumetric assessment of RV

Two-dimensional TTE approximates complex RV geometry and underestimates MRI-derived RV volume. Assessment of RV volume using 3D TTE is superior and more accurate because 3D echo uses disc summation and apical rotational methods for RV volume and EF assessment [20]. However, the accuracy of RV volume assessment is less definite when the RV is dilated.

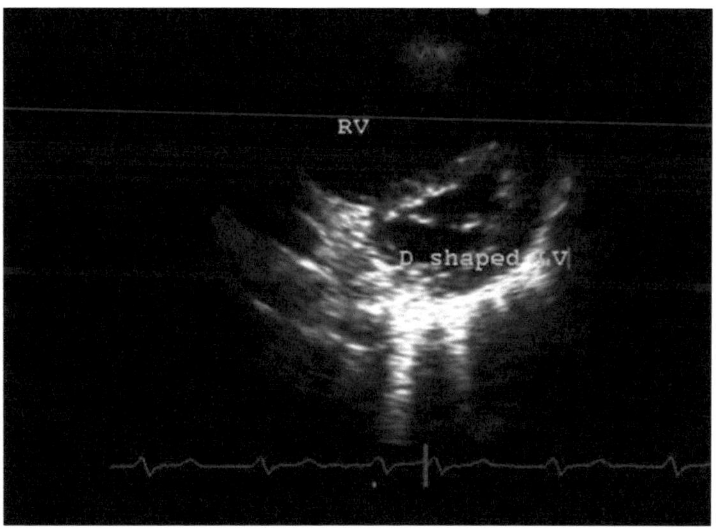

Figure 3. Example of RV with D-shaped LV cavity. RV, right ventricle; LV, left ventricle.

3. Intracardiac pressure measurement

Echocardiography can provide an estimate of right heart hemodynamics.

3.1. Estimated right atrial (RA) pressure

Estimation of right atrial pressure can be derived from the size of the inferior vena cava (IVC) and its response to changes in spontaneous respiration [23, 24]. Using a dilated IVC to assess elevated RA pressures is not accurate in mechanically ventilated patients. However, a small IVC of less than 1.2 cm in mechanically ventilated patient is 100% specific for an RA pressure of less than 10 mm Hg. Normal IVC is <2 cm in diameter, approximately 1 cm from RA-IVC junction and collapses by at least 50% with inspiration or sniff. A flat IVC indicates low RA pressure [0–5 mm Hg]. IVC <2 cm with normal inspiratory collapse indicates RA pressure of 5 mm Hg, and an IVC of >2 cm with normal inspiratory collapse suggests an RA pressure of 10 mm Hg. IVC <2 cm but without inspiratory collapse suggests 15 mm Hg RA pressure; IVC >2 cm but without inspiratory collapse suggests an RA pressure of 20 mm Hg. The normal RA pressure is 0–5 mm Hg.

3.2. Pulmonary artery systolic pressure (PASP)

Pulmonary artery (PA) systolic pressure can be determined from tricuspid regurgitation peak velocity. Provided there is no tricuspid valve obstruction, peak TR velocity depends on the pressure gradient between the right ventricle and right atrium [the difference between peak right ventricular systolic pressure (RVSP) and RA pressure] (**Table 4**). Therefore, estimated RVSP is equal to pressure difference (determined from peak TR velocity using Bernoulli equation) and estimated RA pressure [25]. (**Figure 4**) When there is no obstruction across the pulmonic valve, RVSP will be similar to PASP. PASP = 4 × peak TR velocity^2 + estimated RA pressure. For example, if TR velocity is 2.5 m/sec and IVC is normal in size and collapses with inspiration the estimated PASP would be 33 mm Hg [$4(2.5)^2$ mm Hg = 25 mm Hg + 5 mm Hg (estimated RA pressure)]. If the estimated PASP is >35 to 40 mm Hg, pulmonary HTN is considered to be present.

3.3. Pulmonary artery diastolic pressure (PADP)

Pulmonary regurgitation (PR) represents the pressure difference between pulmonary artery and right ventricle. Hence, the end-diastolic pulmonary regurgitation velocity can be utilized to measure the end-diastolic pressure difference between PA and right ventricle. PA diastolic pressure can be estimated from the spectral Doppler signal of pulmonary regurgitation. The right ventricular end-diastolic pressure is the same as RA pressure; therefore, PADP can be estimated by addition of the estimated RA pressure to the end-diastolic pressure difference between PA and right ventricle. Thus, PADP = 4 × (end-diastolic pulmonary regurgitation velocity)^2 + estimated RA pressure.

http://dx.doi.org/10.5772/64781

Color flow regurgitant jet area of 30% or more of RA area
Annulus dilation (≥4 cm) or inadequate cusp coaptation
Late systolic concave configuration of the continuous-wave signal
Late systolic flow reversals in the hepatic vein
ERO of 0.4 cm^2 or larger
Regurgitant volume of 45 mL or more
Width of vena contracta of 6.5 mm or more

Abbreviations: ERO, effective regurgitant orifice; RA, right atrium.

Table 4. Severe TR is defined by echocardiography on the basis of the following criteria.

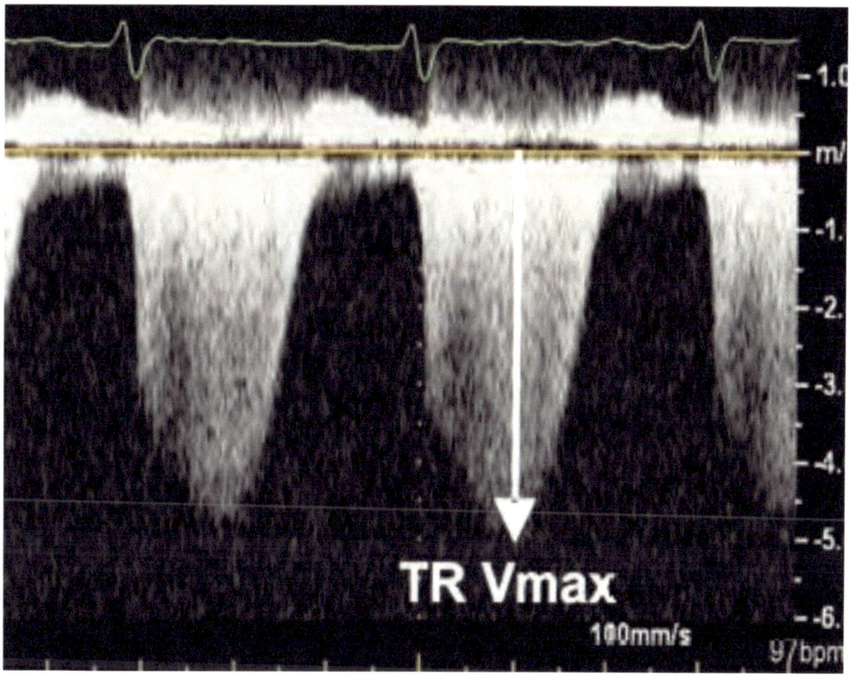

Figure 4. Peak TR velocity. RVSP = $4(V_{max})^2$ + RAP. In the absence of pulmonic stenosis: RVSP = PASP. Peak TR velocity depends on pressure gradient between right ventricle and right atrium [difference between peak RVSP and RA pressure] provided there is no tricuspid valve obstruction. TR, tricuspid regurgitation; RAP, right atrium pressure; RVSP, right ventricle systolic pressure; V_{max}, peak TR velocity.

3.4. Mean pulmonary artery pressure

There are various formulae to estimate mean PA pressure [26–28]. Mean PA pressure = 1/3(PASP) + 2/3 (PADP). Mean PA pressure can be estimated by pulmonary acceleration time

(AT) measured by pulsed Doppler of the pulmonary artery in systole. Mean PA pressure = 79 × (0.45 × AT) or if AT <120 ms, mean PA pressure = 90 – (0.62 × AT). Mean PA pressure = 4 × (early PR velocity)^2 + estimated RA pressure. Mean PA pressure = estimated RA pressure + velocity-time integral of the TR jet to calculate a mean systolic pressure.

3.5. Pulmonary vascular resistance (PVR)

As per the formula $P = QR$, where pressure (P) equals the product of flow (Q) and resistance (R), PASP can be elevated in the setting of increased stroke volume without PVR being elevated. PVR can be calculated by the ratio of peak TR velocity (m/s) to RVOT VTI (velocity time integral) (cm) [29, 30]. PVR = [(TR velocity/RVOT VTI) × 10] + 0.16. PVR value is in Woods units (WU) and correlates well with invasively measured PVR up to approximately 8 WU [30]. However, when PVR is >8 WU by invasive hemodynamic measurement the relationship is not reliable. This method is not validated and should not be used for routine clinical purposes in place of invasive hemodynamic measurements. It can be used when PASP is elevated from increased stroke volume or PASP is low (despite increased PVR) from decreased stroke volume.

4. Assessment of RV function

Most of the RV contraction occurs longitudinally from base to apex (contributing to most of the RV stroke volume), along with radial thickening/inward motion. The following techniques are used to assess RV function [15, 16, 31, 32].

4.1. Tricuspid annular planar systolic excursion (TAPSE)

TAPSE is a diagnostic and prognostic tool of mortality and morbidity in patients with precapillary pulmonary hypertension, RV infarction associated with inferior myocardial infarction, and chronic left-sided heart failure [33, 34]. TAPSE is assessed in an apical four-chamber view by placing the M-mode on the lateral tricuspid annulus; maximum systolic excursion of the lateral annulus along its longitudinal plane toward the apex is recorded [33, 35]. The displacement of the basal segment from the reference point reflects longitudinal contraction of the RV. Normal reference limit is TAPSE of >1.6 cm [36, 37]. This is the most commonly used method as it is a simple, easily obtainable, reproducible with a low interobserver variability. For accurate estimation of TAPSE, one should place M-mode cursor parallel to the plane of longitudinal motion carefully measuring the magnitude of displacement from the M-mode image. The limitations of this method are that TAPSE estimates only the longitudinal contraction within one segment of RV and hypothesizes that the function of a single RV segment reflects the entire RV function which is not true in conditions like RV infarction and pulmonary embolism (**Figure 5**).

http://dx.doi.org/10.5772/64781

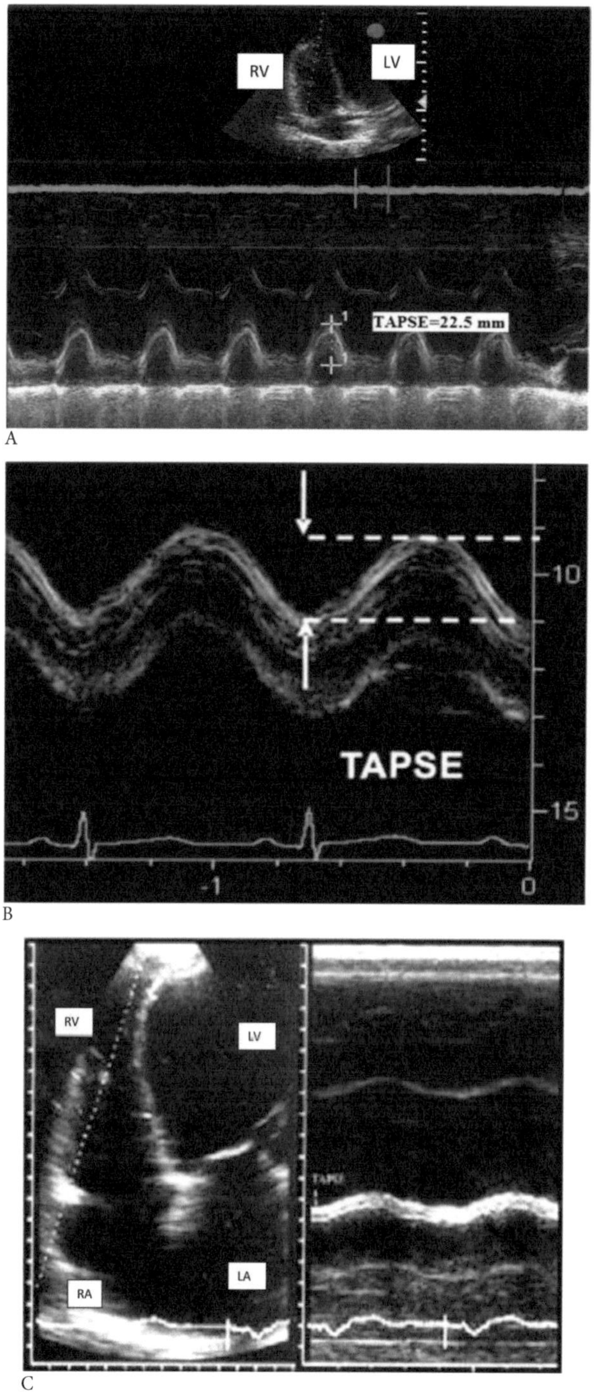

Figure 5. A: Example of a normal TAPSE (tricuspid annular planar systolic excursion) value >1.6 cm; B: normal TAPSE; C: reduced TAPSE.

4.2. Tricuspid annular velocity S'

The tricuspid annular velocity is also known as systolic excursion velocity S'. In an apical four-chamber view, the cursor of pulsed tissue Doppler or color-coded tissue Doppler is placed on the lateral tricuspid annulus to measure the longitudinal velocity of excursion of basal-free wall segment and tricuspid annulus in systole. Normal reference limit (**Table 5**) of S′ is >9.5 cm/s. Color-coded tissue Doppler yields lower velocities and is analyzed off-line on specific platforms. The advantages and disadvantages are similar to TAPSE.

RV systolic dysfunction
TAPSE ≤ 1.6 cm
Pulse Doppler peak annular velocity at tricuspid annulus S′ <9.5 cm/s
2D RV FAC <35%
Tei index/RIMP >0.40 by pulsed Doppler and >0.55 by tissue Doppler
RVEF 3D ≤44%
RV diastolic dysfunction
E/A <0.8 by tissue Doppler
E/A >2.1 by tissue Doppler
Dilated RV chamber
Basal RV diameter >4.2 cm
Mid-level diameter >3.5 cm
Longitudinal dimension >8.6 cm
Abnormal RVOT value
RVOT in PSAX distal diameter >2.7 cm
RVOT in PLAX proximal diameter >3.3 cm
Increased RV subcostal wall thickness >0.5 cm

Abbreviations: 2D, two-dimensional; 3D, three-dimensional ; FAC, fractional area change; MPI, myocardial performance index; PLAX, parasternal long-axis; PSAX, parasternal short-axis; RA, right atrium; RV, right ventricle; RVOT, right ventricular outflow tract; TAPSE, tricuspid annular plane systolic excursion; RIMP, right ventricular index of myocardial performance.

Table 5. Echocardiographic parameters for assessment of right ventricle based on ASE recommendations.

4.3. Myocardial performance index (MPI)

The myocardial performance index is also denoted as the right ventricular index of myocardial performance (RIMP) or right ventricular Tei index. It is an index of global ventricular function and is independent of the geometry of the ventricle [38]. The MPI is calculated by the ratio of isovolumetric time interval over ventricular ejection time as follows: MPI = (isovolumetric

http://dx.doi.org/10.5772/64781

relaxation time + isovolumetric contraction time)/ventricular ejection time = (tricuspid closure to opening time − ejection time)/ejection time. Lower MPI values indicate healthy RV function as less time is utilized in isovolumetric state and more time is consumed in ejecting blood. MPI can be measured through pulsed Doppler or tissue Doppler methods (**Figure 6**).

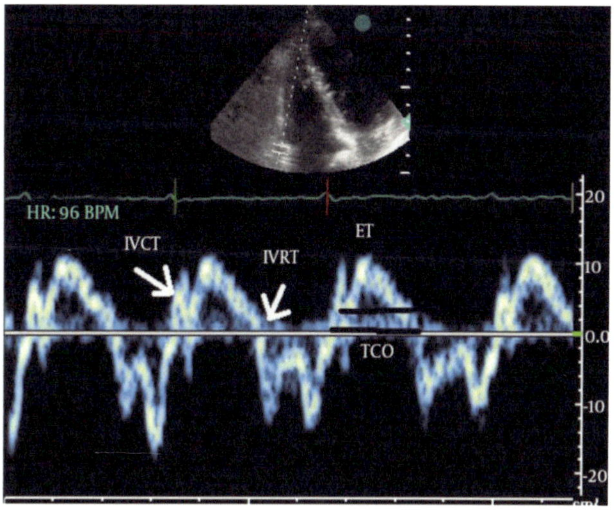

Figure 6. Pulse Doppler MPI. Calculation of RIMP by pulse tissue Doppler imaging RIMP = (TCO - ET)/ET or IVRT + IVCT/ET. RIMP, right ventricular index of myocardial performance; TCO, tricuspid valve closure to opening time; IVCT, isovolumetric contraction time; IVRT, isovolumetric relaxation time; ET, ejection time.

4.3.1. Pulsed Doppler method

In the pulsed Doppler method, pulsed wave Doppler tracing of the distal RVOT is used to obtain ejection time, while the tricuspid-closure-opening time is calculated from the pulsed wave Doppler tracing of the tricuspid inflow (time from end of the A wave to the onset of the following E wave) or the continuous wave Doppler tracing of the tricuspid regurgitation jet. The total isovolumetric time is calculated from the difference between the tricuspid-closure-opening time and the ejection time. The normal reference limit for the pulsed Doppler MPI is <0.40.

4.3.2. Tissue Doppler method

Tissue Doppler method obtains the ejection time, tricuspid-closure-opening time, and total isovolumetric time from the pulsed tissue Doppler tracing of the lateral tricuspid annulus. The normal reference limit for the tissue Doppler MPI is <0.54.

MPI is a sensitive parameter to evaluate subclinical or early RV dysfunction even in poorly visualized RV because it depends on time intervals [39]. However, MPI is observer dependent as delineating time intervals can be challenging [40].

4.4. Fractional area change (FAC)

FAC is the percent change in RV area from diastole to systole.

FAC = [(end-diastolic RV area – end-systolic RV area)/end-diastolic RV area] × 100. FAC is best correlated with MRI-derived RVEF. RV endocardium is traced both in systole and diastole from the annulus, along the free wall to the apex and then back to the annulus, along the interventricular septum. The RV wall should be carefully traced under the trabeculations. FAC has prognostic value and is an independent predictor of all-cause mortality in patients with acute myocardial infarction and low left ventricular ejection fraction. The reference value for normal RV systolic function is >35%.

5. Pulse Doppler MPI

5.1. Three-dimensional echocardiogram

3D echo combined with intravenous contrast agents can improve endocardial border delineation and RV end-diastolic and end-systolic volumes.

$$\begin{aligned}\text{RVEF} = & \left[\text{end}-\text{diastolic RV volume} - \text{end}-\text{systolic RV volume}\right]/ \\ & \text{end}-\text{diastolic RV volume.}\end{aligned} \tag{1}$$

The RV volumes measured by 3D echo use disk summation or surface modeling method. Although 3D echo-derived RVEF correlates well with MRI-derived RVEF, the method is complex, time-consuming, and very much dependent on image quality [20]. The normal reference limit for 3D-derived RVEF is >45%.

5.2. Strain imaging by 2D

The strain is the degree of myocardial deformation, while strain rate represents the rate of myocardial deformation over time [38]. In echocardiography, RV longitudinal strain can be assessed reliably from apical views, whereas the assessment of radial strain is challenging from the parasternal views because of near-field artifacts and extremely small computational distance. The crescent shape of thin-walled RV contributes to inhomogeneous strain rate and values with the highest values in the apical segments and outflow tract. One-dimensional strain is measured using a tissue Doppler (angle-dependent) [18], while 2D strain is measured by speckle tracking (non-angle-dependent). 2D strain imaging estimates global and regional RV function, reflects intrinsic contractility of the RV (with contractility defined as the less stress-strain interplay), and evaluates diastolic properties [39, 41].

Disadvantages are a dearth of normative data, challenges in the adequate image acquisition and analysis requiring high frame rates, high signal-to-noise ratio, minimal image dropout, and most notably the need for experienced observers for reproducible measurements. As it is not highly reproducible, this technique is not recommended for routine use. Given high variability, no reference limits are available [40].

6. Clinical and prognostic significance of assessment of right ventricle

Quantitative assessment of RV size and function has prognostic value regarding exercise tolerance and outcome in various cardiac and pulmonary diseases [3, 36, 42, 43]. RV pump function depends on contractility, afterload, preload, heart rate, rhythm, and valve function. Being a thin-walled chamber, it is not suited to sustain high pressure (**Tables 1** and **2**). RV dysfunction can be acute or chronic, secondary to RV volume overload, pressure overload, or decreased contractility.

6.1. RV overload

RV overload can be related to pressure overload or volume overload. RV overload, in turn, reduces LV diastolic function and causes higher filling pressures.

6.1.1. Volume overload

Volume overload can result from tricuspid regurgitation, pulmonary regurgitation, ASD, and VSD and is assessed through the movement of IVS. Normally during systole, IVS thickens and moves into the left ventricle and during diastole, it moves into the RV cavity. In RV volume overload, RA and RV are enlarged, and IVS is pushed into the LV during end-systole and early diastole as RV pressure exceeds LV pressure. This leads to IVS flattening and a D-shaped LV only during early diastole. At the outset of systole, LV contraction increases LV pressure pushing the IVS in the direction of RV cavity [12].

6.1.2. Pressure overload

Pressure overload can be acute or chronic. Acute pressure overload can be from adult respiratory distress syndrome (ARDS) or massive pulmonary embolism. Echocardiographic findings of RV pressure overload are the same as volume overload. RA and RV are enlarged with no hypertrophy of RV-free wall; there is a flattening of the IVS in diastole. The peak RV systolic pressures rarely exceed 50 mm Hg in acute pressure overload. Chronic pressure overload is secondary to chronic lung diseases, chronic thromboembolism, or chronic pulmonary venous hypertension from left heart pathology. RV is enlarged with thickening of the RV-free wall and increased trabeculation. The RV can generate higher peak systolic pressures, usually exceeding 50 mm Hg. The IVS remains flattened into the LV cavity during the entire cardiac cycle.

6.2. Right ventricular diastolic function

RV diastolic dysfunction has prognostic value and has been associated with both acute and chronic conditions. RV diastolic function is assessed like that of the left ventricle. Techniques used are Doppler velocities of the trans tricuspid flow (E, A, E/A), tissue Doppler velocities of the tricuspid annulus (E', A', and E'/A'), deceleration time, and isovolumetric relaxation time [20, 40]. Estimation of RA pressure by measurement of IVC diameter and collapse with inspiration is to be considered while determining the RV diastolic function.

6.3. Cardiac rhythm and the RV

RV function is dependent on cardiac rhythm. RV function is compromised by atrial fibrillation and ventricular tachycardia originating from the RV examples of which are arrhythmogenic RV dysplasia, RV myocardial infarction, idiopathic ventricular tachycardia, or ventricular tachycardia occurring after surgical repair of congenital heart disease [44].

6.4. Cardiac markers

The elevated B-type natriuretic peptide is associated with RV failure secondary to pulmonary hypertension, congenital heart disease, or pulmonary disease [45–47]. Elevated troponin levels indicate poor prognosis in pulmonary embolism and pulmonary hypertension [48].

6.5. Evaluation of pulmonary arterial hypertension

Pulmonary arterial hypertension is a clinical entity that is seen as a consequence of both left heart disease and pulmonary pathology, as well as occurring without an underlying etiology such as primary pulmonary arterial hypertension. Estimation of pulmonary artery pressure can be performed by TTE in the majority of patients [37, 49].

6.6. Evaluation of patients with pulmonary embolism

Pulmonary embolism is associated with high mortality and morbidity; hence, prompt diagnosis and treatment is imperative. When a patient has had a large pulmonary embolism, this may place acute pressure overload on the right ventricle. The right ventricle handles pressure poorly and may undergo acute dilation with decreased right ventricular systolic function as a result of an acute increase in afterload. Usually, peak systolic pressures in the pulmonary artery do not exceed 50 mm Hg unless there is a baseline chronic RV pressure overload. The size and function of the RV are among the most important factors in determining the initiation of either thrombolysis or referral for surgical embolectomy. A classic pattern of RV systolic dysfunction in acute pulmonary embolism has been described. This is known as McConnell sign and is characterized by akinesis of the free wall of the right ventricle with sparing of the apical segment. This phenomenon has 77% sensitivity and 94% specificity for the diagnosis of acute pulmonary embolism (**Figure 7**).

6.7. Evaluation of RV dyssynchrony

Echocardiographic indices of dyssynchrony are assessed by measuring time delay in mechanical activity between segments. Tissue Doppler imaging is limited to the assessment of the septum-RV free wall.

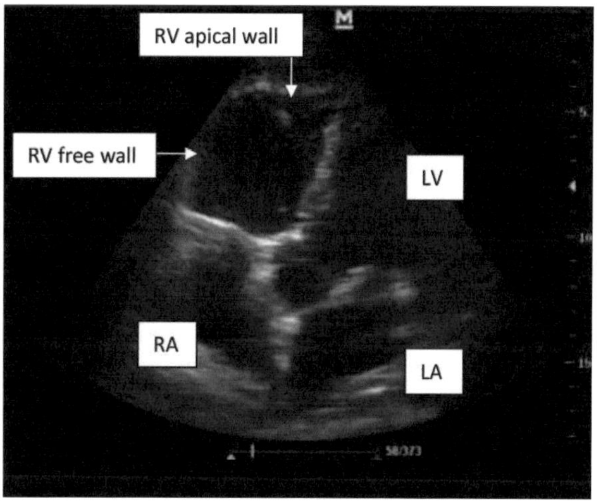

Figure 7. McConnell sign. McConnell sign: akinesis of the free wall of the right ventricle with sparing of the apical segment seen in acute pulmonary embolism causing right ventricle systolic dysfunction.

7. Conclusion

Accurate quantitative assessment of right ventricular size and function remains difficult given its unique shape despite significant advances in echocardiography. RV dysfunction is an important diagnostic and prognostic indicator in many cardiac and pulmonary diseases [42, 43, 50, 51]. Qualitative evaluation of RV systolic function is through visual assessment. For quantitative assessment of RV, FAC, TAPSE, pulsed tissue Doppler S', and MPI are available and at least one of them should be routinely performed and reported as recommended by the ASE. If more than one of these measurements is used in conjunction, RV function can be more reliably and accurately assessed [36, 40, 52].

Author details

Gunjan Choudhary[1*], Arushi A. Malik[2], Dwight Stapleton[1] and Pratap C. Reddy[3]

*Address all correspondence to: dgc678@gmail.com

1 Robert Packer Hospital/Guthrie Clinic, Sayre, USA

2 Dr. S.N. Medical College, Jodhpur, India

3 Louisiana State University Health Science Center, Shreveport, USA

References

[1] Ghio S, Klersy C, Magrini G, et al. Prognostic relevance of the echocardiographic assessment of right ventricular function in patients with idiopathic pulmonary arterial hypertension. Int J Cardiol 2010; 140:272.

[2] Graham T P, Jr, Bernard Y D, Mellen B G, et al. Long-term outcome in congenitally corrected transposition of the great arteries: a multi-institutional study. J Am Coll Cardiol 2000; 36:255–261.

[3] Burgess M I, Mogulkoc N, Bright-Thomas R J, et al. Comparison of echocardiographic markers of right ventricular function in determining prognosis in chronic pulmonary disease. J Am Soc Echocardiogr 2002; 15:633–639.

[4] D'Alonzo G E, Barst R J, Ayres S M, et al. Survival in patients with primary pulmonary hypertension. Results from a national prospective registry. Ann Intern Med 1991; 115:343–349.

[5] Mehta S R, Eikelboom J W, Natarajan M K, et al. Impact of right ventricular involvement on mortality and morbidity in patients with inferior myocardial infarction. J Am Coll Cardiol 2001; 37:37–43.

[6] Zehender M, Kasper W, Kauder E, et al. Eligibility for and benefit of thrombolytic therapy in inferior myocardial infarction: focus on the prognostic importance of right ventricular infarction. J Am Coll Cardiol 1994; 24:362–369.

[7] de Groote P, Millaire A, Foucher-Hossein C, et al. Right ventricular ejection fraction is an independent predictor of survival in patients with moderate heart failure. J Am Coll Cardiol 1998; 32:948–954.

[8] Gavazzi A, Berzuini C, Campana C, et al. Value of right ventricular ejection fraction in predicting short-term prognosis of patients with severe chronic heart failure. J Heart Lung Transplant 1997; 16:774–785.

[9] Afilalo J, Flynn AW, Shimony A, et al. Incremental value of the preoperative echocardiogram to predict mortality and major morbidity in coronary artery bypass surgery. Circulation 2013; 127:356.

[10] Hamon M, Agostini D, Le Page O, et al. Prognostic impact of right ventricular involvement in patients with acute myocardial infarction: meta-analysis. Crit Care Med 2008; 36:2023.

[11] Rudski LG, Lai WW, Afilalo J, et al. Guidelines for the echocardiographic assessment of the right heart in adults: a report from the American Society of Echocardiography endorsed by the European Association of Echocardiography, a registered branch of the European Society of Cardiology, and the Canadian Society of Echocardiography. J Am Soc Echocardiogr 2010; 23:685.

[12] Bleeker G B, Steendijk P, Holman E R, Yu C M, Breithardt O A, Kaandorp T A, et al. Assessing right ventricular function: the role of echocardiography and complementary technologies. Heart 2006; 92:19–26.

[13] Nagel E, Stuber M, Hess O M. Importance of the right ventricle in valvular heart disease. Eur Heart J 1996; 17:829–836.

[14] Ho S Y, Nihoyannopoulos P. Anatomy, echocardiography, and normal right ventricular dimensions. Heart 2006; 92(Suppl 1): i2–i13.

[15] Ostenfeld E, Flachskampf FA. Assessment of right ventricular volumes and ejection fraction by echocardiography: from geometric approximations to realistic shapes. Echo Res Pract 2015; 2(1):R1–R11.

[16] Haddad F, Hunt SA, Rosenthal DN, Murphy DJ. Right ventricular function in cardiovascular disease, part I: anatomy, physiology, aging, and functional assessment of the right ventricle. Circulation 2008; 117:1436.

[17] Kaul S. The interventricular septum in health and disease. Am Heart J 1986; 112:568–581.

[18] Lindqvist P, Morner S, Karp K, Waldenstrom A. New aspects of septal function by using 1-dimensional strain and strain rate imaging. J Am Soc Echocardiogr 2006;19:1345–1349.

[19] Klima U, Guerrero JL, Vlahakes GJ. Contribution of the interventricular septum to maximal right ventricular function. Eur J Cardiothorac Surg 1998; 14:250–255.

[20] Lang RM, Badano LP, Tsang W, et al. EAE/ASE recommendations for image acquisition and display using three-dimensional echocardiography. J Am Soc Echocardiogr 2012; 25:3.

[21] Grant RP, Downey FM, MacMahon H. The architecture of the right ventricular outflow tract in the normal human heart and in the presence of ventricular septal defects. Circulation 1961; 24:223–235.

[22] Foale R, Nihoyannopoulos P, McKenna W, et al. Echocardiographic measurement of the normal adult right ventricle. Br Heart J 1986; 5:633–644.

[23] Brennan JM, Blair JE, Goonewardena S, et al. Reappraisal of the use of inferior vena cava for estimating right atrial pressure. J Am Soc Echocardiogr 2007; 20:857.

[24] Beigel R, Cercek B, Luo H, Siegel RJ. Noninvasive evaluation of right atrial pressure. J Am Soc Echocardiogr 2013; 26:1033.

[25] Yock PG, Popp RL. Noninvasive estimation of right ventricular systolic pressure by Doppler ultrasound in patients with tricuspid regurgitation. Circulation 1984; 70:657.

[26] Abbas AE, Fortuin FD, Schiller NB, et al. Echocardiographic determination of mean pulmonary artery pressure. Am J Cardiol 2003; 92:1373.

[27] Mahan G, Dabestani A, Gardin J, Allfie A, Burn C, Henry W. Estimation of pulmonary artery pressure by pulsed Doppler echocardiography. Circulation 1983;68:367.

[28] Dabestani A, Mahan G, Gardin JM, Takenaka K, Burn C, Allfie A, et al. Evaluation of pulmonary artery pressure and resistance by pulsed Doppler echocardiography. Am J Cardiol 1987; 59:662–668.

[29] Rajagopalan N, Simon MA, Suffoletto MS, et al. Noninvasive estimation of pulmonary vascular resistance in pulmonary hypertension. Echocardiography 2009; 26:489.

[30] Abbas AE, Franey LM, Marwick T, et al. Noninvasive assessment of pulmonary vascular resistance by Doppler echocardiography. J Am Soc Echocardiogr 2013; 26:1170.

[31] Lindqvist P, Calcutteea A, Henein M. Echocardiography in the assessment of right heart function. Eur Heart J 2008; 9(2):225–234.

[32] Kaul S, Tei C, Hopkins JM, Shah PM. Assessment of right ventricular function using two-dimensional echocardiography. Am Heart J 1984; 107:526.

[33] Ghio S, Recusani F, Klersy C, et al. Prognostic usefulness of the tricuspid annular plane systolic excursion in patients with congestive heart failure secondary to idiopathic or ischemic dilated cardiomyopathy. Am J Cardiol 2000; 85:837.

[34] Damy T, Kallvikbacka-Bennett A, Goode K, et al. Prevalence of, associations with, and prognostic value of tricuspid annular plane systolic excursion (TAPSE) among outpatients referred for the evaluation of heart failure. J Card Fail 2012; 18:216.

[35] Alam M, Wardell J, Andersson E, et al. Right ventricular function in patients with first inferior myocardial infarction: assessment by tricuspid annular motion and tricuspid annular velocity. Am Heart J 2000; 139:710.

[36] Miller D, Farah MG, Liner A, et al. The relation between quantitative right ventricular ejection fraction and indices of tricuspid annular motion and myocardial performance. J Am Soc Echocardiogr 2004; 17:443.

[37] Sato T, Tsujino I, Ohira H, et al. Validation study on the accuracy of echocardiographic measurements of right ventricular systolic function in pulmonary hypertension. J Am Soc Echocardiogr 2012; 25:280.

[38] Blanchard DG, Malouf PJ, Gurudevan SV, et al. Utility of right ventricular Tei index in the noninvasive evaluation of chronic thromboembolic pulmonary hypertension before and after pulmonary thromboendarterectomy. JACC Cardiovasc Imaging 2009; 2:143.

[39] López-Candales A, Rajagopalan N, Dohi K, et al. Abnormal right ventricular myocardial strain generation in mild pulmonary hypertension. Echocardiography 2007; 24:615.

[40] Lang RM, Badano LP, Mor-Avi V, et al. Recommendations for cardiac chamber quantification by echocardiography in adults: an update from the American Society of Echocardiography and the European Association of Cardiovascular Imaging. J Am Soc Echocardiogr 2015; 28:1.

[41] D'hooge J, Heimdal A, Jamal F, Kukulski T, Bijnens B, Rademakers F, Hatle L, Suetens P, Sutherland GR. Regional strain and strain rate measurements by cardiac ultrasound: principles, implementation and limitations. Eur J Echocardiogr. 2000; 1:154–170.

[42] Mendes LA, Dec GW, Picard MH, Palacios IF, Newell J, Davidoff R. Right ventricular dysfunction: an independent predictor of adverse outcome in patients with myocarditis. Am Heart J 1994; 128:301–307.

[43] Ghio S, Gavazzi A, Campana C, Inserra C, Klersy C, Sebastiani R, et al. Independent and additive prognostic value of right ventricular systolic function and pulmonary artery pressure in patients with chronic heart failure. J Am Coll Cardiol 2001; 37:183–188.

[44] Hoch DH, Rosenfeld LE. Tachycardias of right ventricular origin. Cardiol Clin 1992; 10:151–164.

[45] Nagaya N, Nishikimi T, Uematsu M, Satoh T, Kyotani S, Sakamaki F, Kakishita M, Fukushima K, Okano Y, Nakanishi N, Miyatake K, Kangawa K. Plasma brain natriuretic peptide as a prognostic indicator in patients with primary pulmonary hypertension. Circulation 2000; 22;102:865–870.

[46] Yap LB, Mukerjee D, Timms PM, Ashrafian H, Coghlan JG. Natriuretic peptides, respiratory disease, and the right heart. Chest 2004; 126:1330–1336.

[47] Oosterhof T, Tulevski II, Vliegen HW, Spijkerboer AM, Mulder BJ. Effects of volume and/or pressure overload secondary to congenital heart disease (tetralogy of Fallot or pulmonary stenosis) on right ventricular function using cardiovascular magnetic resonance and B-type natriuretic peptide levels. Am J Cardiol 2006; 1(97):1051–1055.

[48] Konstantinides S, Geibel A, Olschewski M, Kasper W, Hruska N, Jackle S, Binder L. Importance of cardiac troponins I and T in risk stratification of patients with acute pulmonary embolism. Circulation 2002; 106:1263–1268.

[49] Kittipovanonth M, Bellavia D, Chandrasekaran K, et al. Doppler myocardial imaging for early detection of right ventricular dysfunction in patients with pulmonary hypertension. J Am Soc Echocardiogr 2008; 21:1035.

[50] Kjaergaard J, Akkan D, Iversen KK, et al. Right ventricular dysfunction as an independent predictor of short- and long-term mortality in patients with heart failure. Eur J Heart Fail 2007; 9:610.

[51] Baker BJ, Wilen MM, Boyd CM, Dinh H, Franciosa JA. Relation of right ventricular ejection fraction to exercise capacity in chronic left ventricular failure. Am J Cardiol 1984; 54:596–599.

[52] Tamborini G, Pepi M, Galli CA, Maltagliati A, Celeste F, Muratori M, et al. Feasibility and accuracy of a routine echocardiographic assessment of right ventricular function. Int J Cardiol 2007; 115:86–89.

Chapter 10

Role of Echocardiography in the Critically Ill Patients

Manivannan Veerasamy

Additional information is available at the end of the chapter

http://dx.doi.org/10.5772/65068

Abstract

Since its inception in 1950s, echocardiography has evolved significantly. Its role has expanded beyond cardiology into operating theaters, intensive care units, and emergency departments. It is an easy, inexpensive, noninvasive, and portable technique, which can be rapidly performed at bedside. It is devoid of complications and, for the most part, universally available. This review focuses on growing importance of echocardiography for critically ill patients in the intensive care and high dependency unit settings including indications, modalities, measurements, and therapeutic impact. Literature review of echocardiography use for the cardiovascular assessment of the critically ill patients was done and various indications are discussed including appropriate use scores. Methods being used include transthoracic and transesophageal echo with various modes. This does include assessment of volume status of the hemodynamically unstable patients, myocardial function, global left ventricular systolic function, regional wall motion abnormalities, cardiac output, cardiac tamponade, valvular function, left ventricular outflow obstruction, and right ventricular function. Other diagnostic assessments include aortic dissection, thromboembolisms, pleural effusions, and septal defects. Echocardiography is now considered as an indispensable tool for diagnosis and management including hemodynamic monitoring in critically ill patients. It provides advantages including noninvasiveness and real-time anatomical and functional assessment of the cardiovascular system.

Keywords: echocardiography, critically ill, ventricular function, hemodynamics

1. Introduction

Echocardiography (echo) is one of the most powerful diagnostic and monitoring tools available to the modern emergency/critical care practitioner. The provision of echo is fundamental to the management of patients with acute cardiovascular disease. Since its inception in 1950s, echocardiography has evolved significantly. Its role has expanded beyond cardiology into operating theaters, intensive care units, and emergency departments [1]. It is an easy, inexpensive, noninvasive, and portable technique, which can be rapidly performed at bedside. It is devoid of complications and, for the most part, universally available. This review focuses on growing importance of echocardiography for critically ill patients in the intensive care and high dependency unit settings including indications, modalities, measurements, and therapeutic impact.

Echocardiography has been included in international guidelines regarding the management of cardiac arrest and in the universal definition of acute myocardial infarction (AMI). In the acutely ill and critical care settings, echocardiography can be used to measure/monitor cardiac output (CO) and to determine abnormalities of cardiac physiology and coronary perfusion, as well as providing more standard anatomical information related to diagnosis.

This chapter is not intended to be a comprehensive review of echocardiographic techniques. Instead, it focuses on the indications, therapeutic impact, and some of the most common scenarios (**Table 1**) where dilemmas can be answered using echocardiography in critically ill patients.

Hypovolemia/hypotension
Hemodynamic instability
Ventricular dysfunction
Evaluation of cardiac thrombus or embolus
Pulmonary embolism infective endocarditis
Acute valvular regurgitations
Pericardial effusions/cardiac tamponade
Complications after cardiac procedures/cardiothoracic surgery
Acute aortic syndromes

Table 1. General indications for echocardiographic examination in the intensive care unit.

2. Types of echo

The challenges of imaging in the acute settings are well studied and may influence echocardiographic findings and interpretation in critically ill patients. These include a number of factors such as filling status, metabolic status, patient habitus and positioning, positive pressure ventilation, intubation/mechanical ventilation, different ventilation modalities, weaning inotropic status, lung injury, the presence of lines/dressings and/or drains, and extracorporeal support. The echocardiographic data should be interpreted in the case scenario of the acutely/critically ill patient, particularly when time-specific factors further challenge the echocardiographer (i.e., cardiac arrest).

http://dx.doi.org/10.5772/65068

2.1. Transthoracic echocardiography

Transthoracic echocardiography (TTE) is a widely available, inexpensive tool, which is generally the initial imaging modality in the assessment of acute cardiac conditions (**Table 2**). It is used in the majority of clinical scenarios associated with cardiac emergencies. Findings can be overlooked if the study is restricted to standard imaging only. The study should be comprehensive and undertaken with a fully equipped echocardiographic machine. The easiest and least invasive way to image cardiac structures is echocardiography using the transthoracic approach [2]. This noninvasive imaging modality is of great value in the critical care settings because of its portability, widespread availability, and rapid diagnostic capability.

Indication	AUS
Assessment of volume status in critically ill patient	U
Hypotension/hemodynamic instability of uncertain or suspected cardiac etiology	A
Suspected complication of MI	A
Acute chest pain with suspected MI, inconclusive ECG during pain	A
Respiratory failure/hypoxemia of uncertain etiology	A
Respiratory failure/hypoxemia when noncardiac etiology is already established	U
To guide therapy of known acute PE	A
To establish diagnosis of suspected PE	I
Reevaluation of known PE change RV function and PAP after therapy	A
Routine surveillance of prior PE, with normal RV function and PAP	I
No chest pain but laboratory and/or other features indicative of MI	A
Severe deceleration injury/chest trauma with suspected or possible pericardial effusion, valvular, or cardiac injury	A
Routine evaluation in mild chest trauma without ECG or biomarker changes	I

Note: I: inappropriate test for that indication (not generally acceptable and not a reasonable approach. Score 1–3 out of 9); U: uncertain for specific indication (may be acceptable and may be a reasonable approach. Also implies that further patient information/research needed to classify indication definitively. Score 4–6 out of 9); A: appropriate test for that indication. (Test is generally acceptable and is a reasonable approach for the indication. Score 7–9 out of 9.) MI: myocardial infarction, PE: pulmonary embolism, RV: right ventricle, PAP: pulmonary arterial pressure.

Table 2. Indications for echocardiography in acute care settings, evaluated using appropriate use scores (AUS).

2.2. Transesophageal echocardiography

A nondiagnostic TTE usually requires a transesophageal echocardiography (TEE). TEE allows better imaging of the posterior structures and heart in general, due to the position of the probe and better acoustic transmission. Certain situations that warrant TEE include acute aortic syndromes, unexplained hypotension, trauma, morbid obesity, prosthetic valve dysfunction, valvular regurgitations/vegetation, and mechanical ventilation with high-level positive end-expiratory pressure and source of cardiac emboli. TEE should be done cautiously in patients with coagulopathy, potential trauma to airway or esophagus, and in patients who are unable to protect their own airways or severely hypoxic without mechanical ventilation. During the study, the airway and hemodynamics should be monitored. In the ICU, transthoracic echocardiography (TTE) may, in certain cases, fail to provide adequate image quality because of different factors that can potentially hinder the quality of the ultrasound signal, be it air, bone, calcium, a foreign body, or any other type of interposed structure.

Other imaging modalities include contrast echocardiography, 3D-echo, lung ultrasound examination, focused cardiac ultrasound, and pocket imaging devices.

3. Hemodynamic evaluation

3.1. Ventricular function

3.1.1. Left ventricular systolic function

Patients may present with a spectrum of conditions ranging from cardiogenic shock, acute pulmonary edema, isolated RV dysfunction, or heart failure (HF) complicating an ACS. Since HF is not a diagnosis *per se*, but rather a syndrome, additional investigations are required to determine the underlying cause. Rapid diagnosis of the underlying cause, and distinction between HF due to systolic versus isolated diastolic dysfunction, should be obtained since identification of these features determines immediate treatment in the acute settings.

Assessment of the left ventricular (LV) systolic function is an integral part of the medical management of hemodynamically unstable critically ill patients. Assessment of the global LV function can be quickly obtained by "eyeballing" from the parasternal long- and short-axis, apical two- and four-chamber, and subcostal views and real-time visualization of the kinetics and size of the cardiac cavities, a combination of ejection fraction/fractional shortening, Doppler patterns of ventricular filling and tissue. Doppler imaging supplements to the information from the echocardiogram. Assessment of the chamber size and LV wall thickness is also done. Findings may include increase in the left ventricular end-systolic and diastolic volume, increase in end-systolic and diastolic diameter and abnormal wall motion. Two other modes of imaging that are relatively easy to obtain for the assessment of the LV function are the atrioventricular plane displacement (AVPD) and systolic tissue Doppler velocities (sTD) [3].

TTE was shown to be an excellent diagnostic tool for assessment of the LV function in the ICU, even when positive end expiratory pressure was present [4]. However, if the TTE provides suboptimal imaging for evaluation of ventricular function, TEE can be obtained for better assessment. It is important to remember that significant LV dysfunction is common in critically ill patients and the "normal" values quoted from noncritical care studies may not be valid.

http://dx.doi.org/10.5772/65068

3.1.1.1. Sepsis-related cardiomyopathy

Bedside echocardiography is an important tool for identification of the cause of hemodynamic instability (which may be of cardiogenic, hypovolemic, or distributive origin) and for the further management (i.e., administration of fluid, vasoactive, or inotropic agent infusion). Classically, septic shock has been considered to be a hyperdynamic state characterized by normal or high cardiac output (CO). But echocardiographic studies indicate that ventricular performance is often diminished in those patients. LVEF might not be a reliable index of LV systolic function in patients with early septic shock.

3.1.1.2. Stress-induced cardiomyopathy (Takotsubo syndrome)

Defined as a transient, stress-induced dysfunction of the LV apex, it predominantly affects female patients (90%). Takotsubo cardiomyopathy mimics an ACS, echo findings show a reversible LV dysfunction with regional wall motion abnormalities, but these patients have no angiographic evidence of ACS. Akinesia has also been demonstrated in the LV mid-cavity, LV base, and RV, with or without sparing of the other LV segments (**Figure 1**). Echo is a useful tool for the follow-up as the LV function must completely recover over time to confirm the diagnosis.

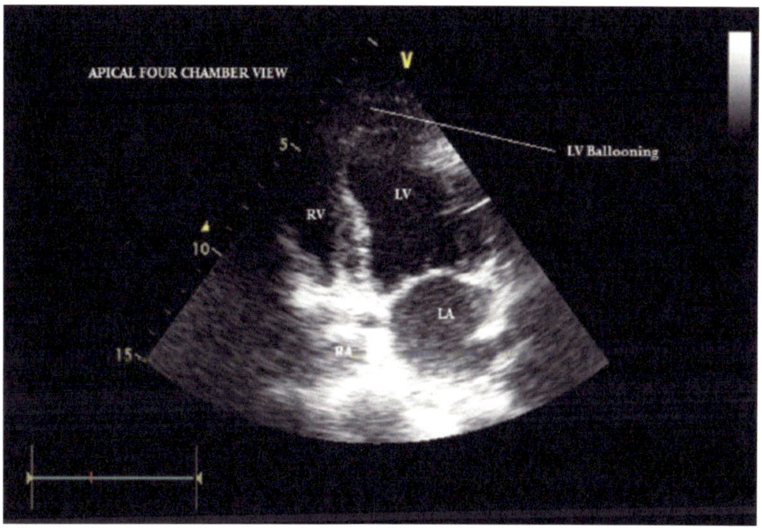

Figure 1. Takotsubo's cardiomyopathy.

LV measurements also provide data on myocardial injury, cardiomyopathies, and fluid status. The left atrial size is evaluated as an enlarged Left atrium (LA) may indicate significant valvular disease, intra-atrial shunting and atrial fibrillation, all of which may in turn cause hemodynamic instability. Finally, the aortic and mitral valves are assessed to complete the examination of left ventricular function. Two-dimensional speckle tracking echocardiography (STE) offers potentially useful information in acute HF patients with underlying cardiomyopathies.

3.1.2. LV diastolic function

In the ICU, when EF is normal or supernormal and ventricular filling pressure (pulmonary artery occlusion pressure) is elevated, diastolic dysfunction should be suspected. The filling patterns related to the diastolic function can be influenced by different factors such as heart rate, ischemia, left atrial pressure, ventricular hypertrophy, and valvular pathologies. In patients with an abnormal relaxation pattern ($E/A < 1$), and peak E velocity <50 cm/s, LV filling pressures are usually normal [5]. With restrictive filling ($E/A \geq 2$, mitral E deceleration time <150 ms), mean LA pressure is often increased. Patients with heart failure with preserved LV ejection fraction (HFpEF) present with signs and/or symptoms of HF and several echocardiographic findings.

In both acute systolic and diastolic HF, interstitial edema may be diagnosed at the bedside by the demonstration of an abnormally high number of bilateral sonographic B-lines (also called ultrasound lung comets). Two-dimensional speckle tracking echocardiography offers diagnostic data in acute heart failure associated with cardiomyopathies, specifically when ejection fraction appears preserved [5].

3.1.3. Cardiac arrest

Echo is a very useful tool in the management of critically ill patients with cardiac arrest. The use of echo in an advanced cardiac life support (ACLS) is supported by international evidence-based recommendations. Peri-resuscitation echocardiography does not impact upon high-quality cardiopulmonary resuscitation (CPR) when appropriately applied and requires special training in advanced cardiac life support (ACLS) compliant manner. Images should be obtained only during the pulse/rhythm check. It can provide data to diagnose or exclude certain potential reversible causes of cardiac arrest (including severe LV/RV dysfunction, myocardial infarction, hypovolemia, pulmonary embolism (PE), tension pneumothorax, or tamponade). Echo is particularly useful in situations of pulseless electrical activity (electromechanical dissociation—EMD) to differentiate between pseudo-EMD and true EMD. Though there is extensive data, we need further recommendations regarding how to use echo during a code situation and specific guidelines for termination of resuscitation.

3.2. Right ventricular function

Right ventricular (RV) function can be altered by massive pulmonary embolism and acute respiratory distress syndrome (ARDS), the two main causes of acute cor pulmonale, in the critical care settings [6]. Other causes of acute RV dysfunction include RV infarction associated with inferior myocardial infarction, myocardial contusion, fat or air embolism, acute sickle-cell crisis, and sepsis. In unstable critically ill patients, specifically those with massive PE and acute respiratory distress syndrome, a diagnosis of RV dysfunction may guide therapy (e.g., use of thrombolytics, vasopressors, volume resuscitation, and catheter-directed interventional therapy). RV size and function are frequently evaluated by visual comparison with the left ventricle. RV kinetics of the cavity and septum, and diastolic dimensions are also measured, using either TTE or TEE. Measuring the ratio between the RV and LV end diastolic areas from apical four-chamber view is one of the best ways to evaluate RV dilation [7]. The diastolic ventricular ratio of 0.6–1.0 is consistent with moderate RV dilation and a ratio of 1 is consistent with severe RV dilation. Tricuspid regurgitation, right atrial dilation, and inferior vena caval dilation are commonly associated with RV diastolic enlargement.

3.2.1. Pulmonary embolism

Though pulmonary angiography remains the gold standard for diagnosis of pulmonary embolism (PE), other available imaging modalities include ventilation-perfusion scanning, spiral computed tomography (CT), and magnetic resonance imaging (MRI) angiography. TTE can help to establish a prompt diagnosis to identify patients with high-risk features, especially if the patient is hemodynamically unstable. Overall, the sensitivity of TTE for the diagnosis of pulmonary embolism is about 50–60% while the specificity is around 80–90%. In some situations, that is, in critically ill patients, TEE may improve the sensitivity.

The main indirect findings for pulmonary embolism (**Table 3**) are the consequences of acutely increased pulmonary artery/right heart pressures [5]. In pulmonary embolism, RV hypokinesia is not necessarily global but can be limited to the mid-RV free wall while the contraction of the RV apex may be normal or hyperdynamic (McConnell sign) (**Figure 2**).

Thrombus into right chambers
RV systolic dysfunction/global RV hypokinesia
Dilatation RA, RV (end-diastolic RV/LV diameter.0.6 or area.1.0)
Mild to severe TR
Pulmonary arterial dilatation
Abnormal septal motion toward LV
McConnell sign—mid-RV wall hypokinesia with apical sparing
Pulmonary hypertension around 40–50 mm Hg (60 mm Hg in the case of pre-existing pulmonary hypertension)
Lack of respiratory variation of the inferior vena cava

Table 3. Echocardiographic finding in pulmonary embolism.

As other clinical conditions can produce acute cor pulmonale in the ICU, better visualization of the pulmonary arteries is needed to achieve high accuracy for the diagnosis of PE. This goal can be achieved by using TEE. TEE helps to achieve a better visualization of the pulmonary arteries and detecting emboli that are lodged in the main and right pulmonary arteries. The diagnosis is made when an embolus is visualized. When the index of suspicion for PE is high and TEE is negative, then pulmonary angiography or helical computed tomography should be considered as the next step. The demonstration of acute cor pulmonale with echocardiography has important prognostic and therapeutic implications. The presence of cor pulmonale with massive PE is associated with increased mortality, whereas the absence of RV dysfunction is associated with a better prognosis.

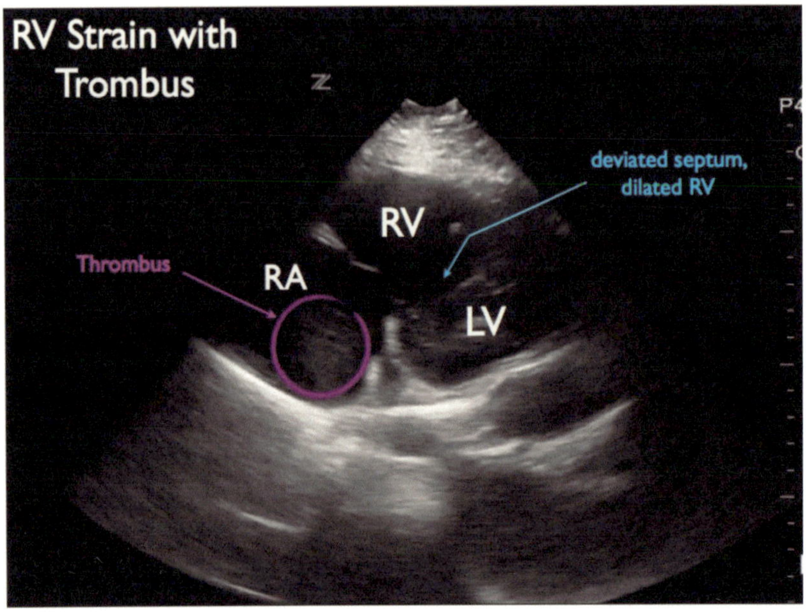

Figure 2. Thrombus in the right ventricle.

3.3. Assessment of cardiac output (CO)

Measurement of CO is an important data in the assessment of critically ill patients with unstable hemodynamics. Cardiac output and stroke volume can be established by combining Doppler data derived from blood flow velocity through a conduit and the cross-sectional area of the conduit. The most common and most reliable technique is using the left ventricular outflow tract and aortic valve. Another method using an esophageal probe inserted in sedated patients, to measure blood flow velocity waveforms in the descending aorta combined with a nomogram, is particularly useful in adult patients to provide continuous monitoring of cardiac function.

3.4. Assessment of filling pressures and volume status

Accurate measurement of volume status and LV preload is important for management of critically ill patients. Besides, invasive pressure measurements to assess LV filling may not correlate well with LV volume. Echo can be very useful in adequately evaluating preload. Measurements from two-dimensional and Doppler echo include LV end-diastolic volume (EDV), LV end-diastolic area (EDA), transmitral diastolic filling pattern, and mitral and pulmonary venous flow.

"Eyeballing" LV end-diastolic (LVED) and end-systolic (LVES) areas provide a quick assessment of intracardiac volume status. Findings in hypovolemic patients include hyperdynamic LV with a reduced end-diastolic volume and "kissing" papillary muscles in systole, suggesting an increased ejection fraction with an empty ventricle at end-systole. Septic patients tend to have a reduced afterload, which is usually demonstrated by a normal LVED area, but a reduced LVES area. Patients with chronic cardiac failure have a dilated LV and may be hypovolemic even with a higher LVED area.

Right atrial pressure measurement is also helpful in the evaluation of the circulating volume status and often measured by the diameter and change in caliber with inspiration of the inferior vena cava. A dilated vena cava (diameter of 20 mm) without a normal inspiratory decrease in caliber (50% with gentle sniffing) usually indicates elevated right atrial pressure. Available data suggest inferior vena cava diameter variation with inspiration can be used a guide to fluid therapy [8]. A small vena cava in mechanically ventilated patient excludes the presence of elevated right atrial pressure, as these patients usually have dilation of the inferior vena cava [9].

3.5. Assessment of pulmonary artery pressure

Pulmonary hypertension is usually diagnosed when systolic pulmonary pressure is ~35 mm Hg, diastolic pulmonary pressure is ~15 mm Hg, and mean pulmonary pressure is ~25 mm Hg. Critically ill patients commonly have pulmonary arterial hypertension, possibly from various cardiac, pulmonary, and systemic processes. Several echocardiographic methods have been validated for noninvasive estimation of pulmonary artery pressure [10], which are useful in critically ill patients. A large number of ICU patients have some degree of tricuspid and pulmonary regurgitation, which are needed to measure pulmonary arterial pressure. The tricuspid and pulmonary regurgitation velocities determine systolic and diastolic pulmonary artery pressures.

3.6. Assessment of valvular function

Significant valvular abnormalities can be present in the critically ill patient without being clinically recognized. In the ICU, TTE can provide valuable information concerning valvular integrity and function [11] but may be suboptimal and TEE may be indicated. Adequate and accurate evaluation of the valvular structures may often be required in the critically ill patients. The most common indications for bedside echocardiography for evaluation of the valvular apparatus in this population are for suspected endocarditis, acute valvular stenosis or regurgitation, critical aortic stenosis, significant mitral stenosis, or prosthetic valve dysfunction including regurgitation and obstruction. Information regarding etiology, pathogenesis, and severity of the valvular lesions, valvular anatomy and function, chamber size, function, and wall thickness of the ventricles can be readily obtained by echo. Abnormalities such as vegetation, thrombus, fibrosis, calcification, immobile, or prolapsing leaflets or prosthetic valve dehiscence can be detected by echo [5].

3.7. Evaluation of the pericardial space

Suspected tamponade is the most common indication for assessment of the pericardium in the critically ill patient. The pericardial space can be filled with a variety of substances including fluid, pus, blood, or air. Presence of fluid in this space is detected as an echo-free space. TTE easily detects pericardial effusion (**Figure 3**), usually in the parasternal long and short-axis and the apical views. But, given higher chances of suboptimal TTE in critically ill patients, TEE may be warranted, particularly in patients with poor acoustic windows or post cardiothoracic surgical patients.

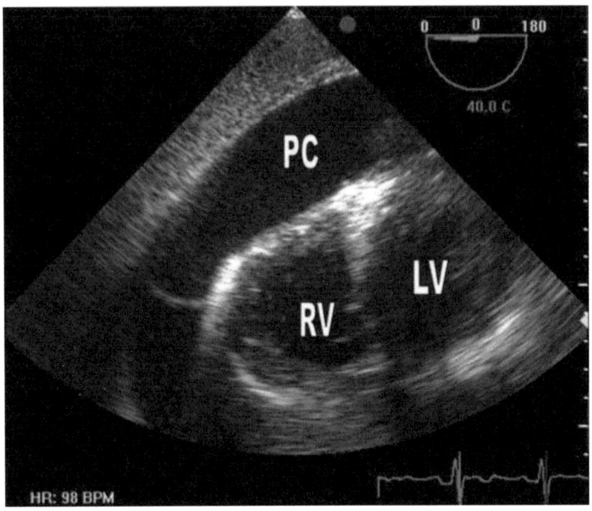

Figure 3. Pericardial effusion.

Echocardiography is also useful in the management of pericardial effusion, as pericardiocentesis can be performed safely under echocardiographic guidance [12]. Echocardiography also can be used to accurately place the needle during the drainage, immediately monitor the results of the pericardiocentesis, and serially monitor to evaluate the reaccumulation of the effusion.

3.7.1. Cardiac tamponade in the ICU

The most common causes of cardiac tamponade in the ICU are listed in **Table 4**.

Complication of myocardial infarction (e.g., ventricular rupture)
Blunt or penetrating chest trauma
Proximal ascending aortic dissection
Myocardial or coronary perforation secondary to catheter-based interventions (i.e., after
intravenous pacemaker lead insertion, central catheter placement, or percutaneous coronary interventions)
Uremic or infectious pericarditis
Compressive hematoma after cardiac surgery
Pericardial involvement by metastatic disease or other systemic processes

Table 4. Common causes of cardiac tamponade in intensive care unit.

There are several 2D-echo findings that suggest a hemodynamically significant pericardial fluid collection (**Table 5**). The rate of accumulation of the pericardial fluid, and collection and size of the collection determine the intrapericardial pressure. Although diastolic RV collapse (inward diastolic motion of the RV free wall) occurs later, it is a more specific sign and is best appreciated from the parasternal or subcostal long-axis views [13] (**Figure 4**).

Usually large pericardial effusion
Swinging heart
RA collapse (rarely LA)
Diastolic collapse of the anterior RV-free wall (rarely LV)
IVC dilatation (no collapse with inspiration)
TV flow increases and MV flow decreases during inspiration (reverse in expiration)
Systolic and diastolic flows are reduced in systemic veins in expiration and reverse flow with atrial contraction is increased

Table 5. Echo findings of hemodynamically significant pericardial effusion.

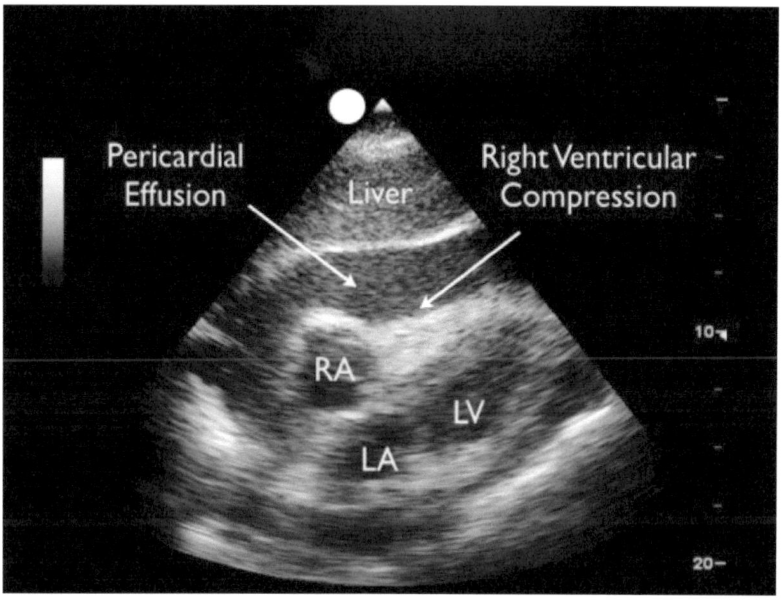

Figure 4. Cardiac tamponade.

If the patient's condition requires urgent pericardiocentesis, the procedure may be echocardiographically guided, as this has been shown to reduce complications. Echocardiography can additionally be used to verify whether the collection has been completely drained. TEE is rarely indicated in this setting.

4. Some other common conditions/scenarios

4.1. LVOT obstruction

In patients who develop dynamic Left Ventricular Outflow Tract (LVOT) obstruction with resultant decrease in cardiac output, particularly the ones who fail to respond to inotropic support, echo is a valuable diagnostic tool. In these patients, right heart catheterization can often be misleading, resulting in inappropriate management.

4.2. Cardiogenic shock

The commonest cause of cardiogenic shock is severe systolic dysfunction from acute myocardial infarction and echo remains an excellent initial diagnostic tool. Shock due to LV dysfunction remains the leading cause of mortality in AMI (50–70%) [14]. Other etiologies include mechanical complications of AMI, myocarditis, cardiomyopathy, valvular heart disease, RV dysfunction, myocardial contusion, and acute aortic dissection. TTE should be obtained first in this set of patients and TEE may be warranted when TTE is suboptimal. Common findings of cardiogenic shock complicating acute myocardial infarction are shown in **Table 6**.

LV dysfunction	Depressed EF, regional wall motion abnormalities, decrease in stroke volume, CO, elevated LV pressures, mitral regurgitation infarction
RV infarction	RV dilatation, dyssynergy, paradoxical septal motion, and McConnell sign, decrease of tricuspid annulus systolic excursion (TAPSE)
Free ventricular wall rupture	Obvious cardiac tamponade or only pericardial collection in subacute free wall rupture (30% of rupture)
Acute mitral regurgitation	Complete or partial rupture of the posterior papillary muscle with partial or complete flail of the mitral valve. Also from acute systolic anterior motion of the mitral valve secondary to dynamic LVOT obstruction

Table 6. Echo findings in cardiogenic shock complicating acute myocardial infarction.

4.3. Complications after cardiac surgery/procedures

In patients with hemodynamic instability after cardiothoracic operations, bedside echocardiography has been shown as a valuable tool in the critical care management [15]. TTE is often suboptimal and TEE is warranted as it obtains information that can help determine the etiology of hypotension in this set of patients. Most frequently encountered echocardiographic findings of LV dysfunction, cardiac tamponade, RV failure, hypovolemia, and valvular dysfunction have been described in earlier sections of this chapter.

Echo is useful in other situations such as evaluation of coronary arteries in suspected coronary disruption, RV dysfunction, and TAPSE (pre-, intra-, and postoperative TAPSE) evaluation, immediately after heart transplant (to rule out early rejection, early RV dysfunction, tamponade, or other causes of instability). Echo is an initial modality of imaging in patients who

http://dx.doi.org/10.5772/65068

underwent catheterization/electrophysiology procedures presenting with potential acute complications include ventricular failure, cardiogenic shock, tamponade, displacement of implanted devices, and occlusion of coronary stents.

4.4. Extracorporeal support

Extracorporeal support is increasingly used to support critically ill patients with severe cardiac and/or respiratory failure. Echocardiography for extracorporeal support is highly specialized. Thus echocardiography has a vital role in excluding any potentially treatable underlying cause for cardiorespiratory failure, essential to determine the requirement for the RV and/or LV support and level of support required, mandatory to exclude cardiovascular contraindications for initiation of the support. Echocardiography subsequently has a vital role in its successful implementation, including confirming/guiding correct cannula placement, ensuring the goals of support are met, detecting complications, and assessing tolerance to assistance. Finally, in patients requiring extracorporeal cardiac support, various echocardiographic parameters have been proposed to be used in conjunction with clinical and hemodynamic assessment in order to attempt to predict those patients who can be successfully weaned.

4.5. Cardiac arrhythmias

In the critically ill patient population, heart rates of 100–120/min may be required to maintain adequate cardiac output.

4.5.1. Atrial arrhythmias

Atrial arrhythmias, common in the acute settings, present challenging conditions for assessing cardiac function and hemodynamics, especially when irregular (as in atrial fibrillation). Use of echo in critically ill patients is done with caution. In atrial fibrillation, measurements are obtained from an average of about 10 consecutive heartbeats, to permit the use of echocardiographic parameters usually used in sinus rhythm, to predict elevated filling pressures. The "index beat" method using the measurement performed on the cardiac cycle following a pair of equal preceding cardiac cycles, is also being used in practice.

4.5.2. Ventricular arrhythmias

Echocardiography is one of the first investigations to be performed as soon as the arrhythmia is successfully terminated. Etiologies include ischemic and nonischemic causes that require echocardiographic evaluation.

4.6. Assessment of the aorta

TTE is a good initial investigation tool for evaluation of the proximal aorta (ascending aorta and arch). Because of the close anatomic relationship between the thoracic aorta and the esophagus, TEE allows optimal visualization of the entire thoracic aorta.

4.6.1. *Aortic dissection and rupture*

Diagnosis and management of aortic dissection is an emergency and these patients are often critically ill. Of the various available imaging modalities, echo, particularly TEE has been recommended for evaluation of suspected aortic dissection (**Figure 5**). TEE has the ability to assess the following, including extension of dissection into the proximal coronary arteries, the point of entry and exit between the true and false lumens, the presence of thrombus in the false lumen, the presence of pericardial or mediastinal hematoma or effusion, severity, and mechanism of associated aortic valve regurgitation, and ventricular function.

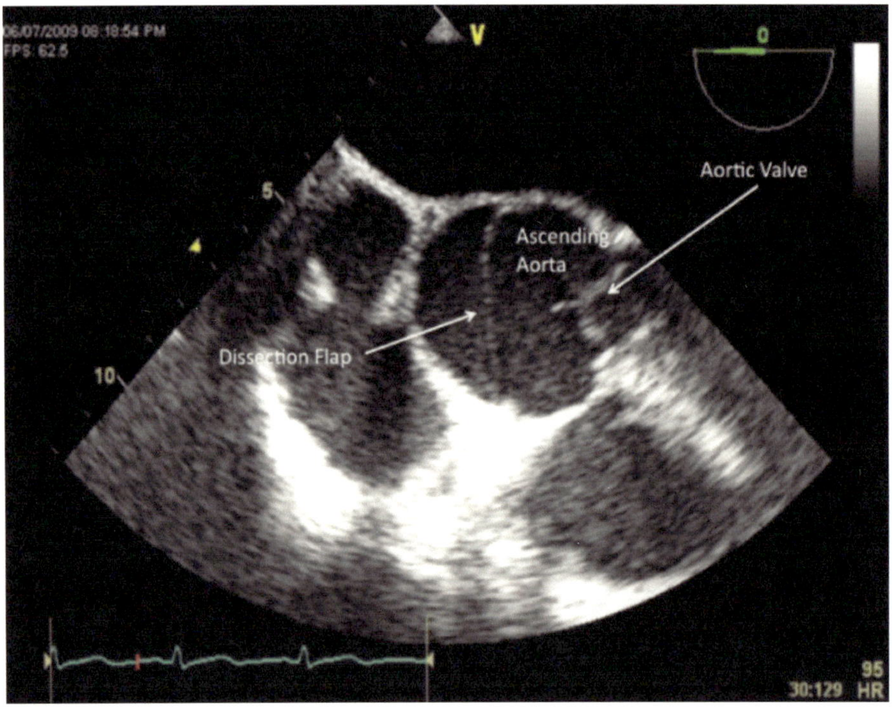

Figure 5. Ascending aortic dissection on TEE.

4.6.2. *Intraaortic balloon pump*

TEE is useful in various phases of management including evaluation of aortic regurgitation as a contraindication prior to insertion, to confirm the position of the catheter, to ensure correct functioning of the balloon, and to rule out complications such as aortic dissection.

4.6.3. *Traumatic injuries of the heart and aorta*

Blunt or penetrating chest trauma may cause severe injury to the heart and great vessels. A rapid, focused assessment with echocardiography can detect pericardial collection, myocardial contusion, mediastinal hematomas, aortic intramural hematomas, aortic dissection or transection, and pleural collections. Both TTE and TEE play an important role in the assessment of patients with chest trauma, and TEE may be indicated in patients with polytrauma and/or on mechanical ventilation or when a traumatic, acute aortic syndrome is suspected. It is important to distinguish aortic from cardiac injuries. Also, traumatic pseudoaneurysms must be differentiated from true aneurysms. Trauma may cause aortic rupture, dissection, or intramural hematoma. Partial disruption of the aortic wall may lead to pseudoaneurysm. Once pericardial tamponade is excluded, a standard echocardiogram is useful in other conditions, like cardiac contusion/dysfunction, myocardial rupture, septal and valvular injury. Acute MI from coronary artery dissection and arrhythmias in acute trauma patients warrant echocardiographic evaluation.

4.7. Infective endocarditis

Febrile illness in critically ill patients warrants evaluation including infective endocarditis. See section on valvular lesions evaluations. Echocardiography is the test of choice for the noninvasive diagnosis of endocarditis. The echocardiographic findings may include new valvular regurgitation, an oscillating intracardiac mass on a valve or supporting structure or in the path of a regurgitant jet or an iatrogenic device, valve abscesses and new partial dehiscence or vegetation of a prosthetic valve. TEE has also been clearly shown to be superior to TTE for diagnosing complications of endocarditis, such as aortic root abscess, fistulas, and ruptured chordae tendineae of the mitral valve.

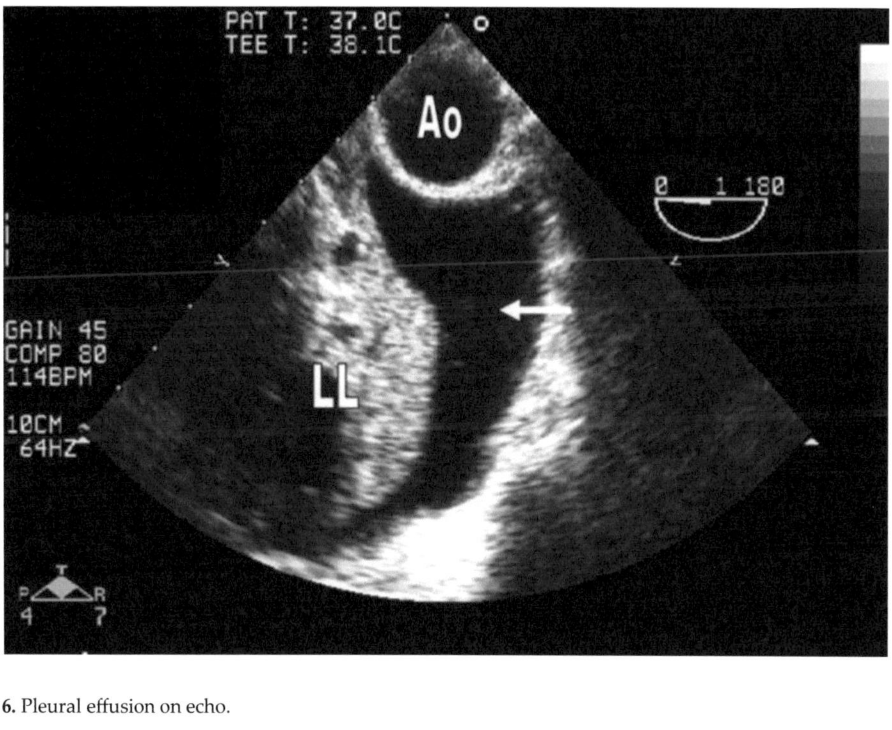

Figure 6. Pleural effusion on echo.

4.8. Pleural effusions

Echocardiogram often finds the presence of pleural effusions (**Figure 6**) and can be used as a diagnostic tool while evaluating the cardiovascular system, especially in patients with acute dyspnea and decompensated heart failure.

4.9. Assessment for intracardiac and intrapulmonary shunts

In critically ill patients with unexplained embolic stroke or refractory hypoxemia, the presence of a right-to-left shunt needs to be excluded. Common positions of right-to-left shunt are atrial septal defect or patent foramen ovale at the cardiac level, arteriovenous fistula at the pulmonary level and pulmonary arteriovenous fistulas. Bubble study, color Doppler studies, and contrast-enhanced studies are done to increase the detection rate of intracardiac shunt.

4.10. Source of embolus

Patients presenting with acute unexplained embolic stroke and arterial occlusions, echocardiography should be obtained to investigate a potential embolic source of cardiac origin. In this situation, TEE is the preferred imaging of choice. Possible cardiac sources of emboli include thrombus in the left atrial or appendage, LV thrombus, valvular vegetation, right-sided clots (right atrium, right ventricle, vena cava) combined with a right-to-left intracardiac shunt (leading to a paradoxical embolus), thoracic atheromatosis, and cardiac tumors. TEE is a valuable tool in evaluating the left atrium and appendage for the presence of thrombus, for patients with atrial fibrillation or flutter in whom cardioversion is considered.

5. Conclusion

Echocardiography is now considered as an indispensable tool and primary imaging modality for diagnosis and management of hemodynamic monitoring in critically ill patients. However, echocardiography is subject to variations in interpretation, which can potentially lead to errors, as with any diagnostic and monitoring tool and caution need to be undertaken during interpretation. Nevertheless, it provides advantages including noninvasiveness and rapid and accurate real-time anatomical and functional assessment of the cardiovascular system under stressful situations and is very useful in assisting therapeutic procedures.

Author details

Manivannan Veerasamy

Address all correspondence to: manivannan22@gmail.com

Spectrum Health, GRMEP/Michigan State University, Grand Rapids, MI, USA

References

[1] Roscoe, A., Strang, T. (2008). Echocardiography in intensive care. *Continuing Education in Anaesthesia, Critical Care & Pain, 8* (2), 46–49. doi: 10.1093/bjaceaccp/mkn002

[2] Poelaert, J., Schmidt, C., Colardyn, F. (1998). Transoesophageal echocardiography in the critically ill. *Anaesthesia, 53*(1), 55–68. doi:10.1111/j.1365-2044.1998.00285

[3] Parker, M.M., Suffredini, A.F., Natansan, C., et al. (1989). Responses of left ventricular function in survivors and nonsurvivors in septic shock. *Journal of Critical Care, 4*, 19–25. doi:10.1016/0883-9441(89)90087-7

[4] Beaulieu, Y. (2007). Bedside echocardiography in the assessment of the critically ill. *Critical Care Medicine, 35*(5 Suppl), S235–S249. doi:10.1097/01.CCM.0000260673.66681.AF

[5] Lancellotti, P., Price, S., Edvardsen, T., Cosyns, B., Neskovic, A.N., Dulgheru, R., et al. (2015). The use of echocardiography in acute cardiovascular care: Recommendations of the European association of cardiovascular imaging and the acute cardiovascular care association. *European Heart Journal Cardiovascular Imaging, 16*(2), 119–146. doi: 10.1093/ehjci/jeu210

[6] Vieillard-Baron, A., Schmitt, J.M., Augarde, R., Fellahi, J.L., Prin, S., Page, B., et al. (2001). Acute cor pulmonale in acute respiratory distress syndrome submitted to protective ventilation: Incidence, clinical implications, and prognosis. *Critical Care Medicine, 29*(8), 1551–1555. doi:10.1007%2Fs00134-013-3045-2

[7] Vieillard-Baron, A., Prin, S., Chergui, K., Dubourg, O., Jardin, F. (2002). Echo-doppler demonstration of acute cor pulmonale at the bedside in the medical intensive care unit. *American Journal of Respiratory and Critical Care Medicine, 166*(10), 1310–1319. doi: 10.1164/rccm.200202-146CC

[8] Feissel, M., Michard, F. et al. (2004). The respiratory variation in inferior vena cava diameter as a guide to fluid therapy. *Intensive Care Medicine, 30* (9), 1834–1837. doi: 10.1007/s00134-004-2233-5

[9] Jardin, F., Vieillard-Baron, A. (2006). Ultrasonographic examination of the venae cavae. *Intensive Care Medicine, 32*(2), 203–206. doi:10.1007/s00134-005-0013-5

[10] Stevenson, J.G. (1989). Comparison of several non-invasive methods for estimation of pulmonary artery pressure. *Journal of American Society Echocardiography, 2*, 157–171. doi: 10.1016/S0894-7317(89)80053-7

[11] Alam, M. (1996). Transesophageal echocardiography in critical care units: Henry ford hospital experience and review of the literature. *Progress in Cardiovascular Diseases, 38*(4), 315–328. doi: S0033-0620(96)80016-8

[12] Callahan, J. A., Seward, J. B. (1997). Pericardiocentesis guided by two-dimensional echocardiography. *Echocardiography (Mount Kisco, N.Y.), 14*(5), 497–504. doi/10.1111/j. 1540-8175. 1997.tb00757

[13] Troianos, C.A., Porembka, D.T. (1996). Assessment of left ventricular function and hemodynamics with transesophageal echocardiography. *Critical Care Clinics, 12*(2), 253–272. doi :10.1016/S0749-0704(05)70248-7

[14] Klein, T., Ramani, G.V. (2012). Assessment and management of cardiogenic shock in the emergency department. *Cardiology Clinics, 30*(4), 651–664. doi:10.1016/j.ccl. 2012.07.004

[15] Wake, P.J., Ali, M., Carroll, J., Siu, S.C., Cheng, D.C. (2001). Clinical and echocardiographic diagnoses disagree in patients with unexplained hemodynamic instability after cardiac surgery. *Canadian Journal of Anaesthesia, 48*(8), 778–783. doi:10.1007/BF03016694